nw
ML
(20)

9406675   MBCS BN

DNA Topoisomerases in Cancer

DNA Topoisomerases in Cancer

Edited by
MILAN POTMESIL, M.D., Ph.D.
KURT W. KOHN, M.D., Ph.D.

and the Editorial Board
LEROY F. LIU, Ph.D.
FRANCO M. MUGGIA, M.D.
WARREN E. ROSS, M.D.
ROBERT SILBER, M.D.

New York   Oxford
OXFORD UNIVERSITY PRESS
1991

Oxford University Press

Oxford   New York   Toronto
Delhi   Bombay   Calcutta   Madras   Karachi
Petaling Jaya   Singapore   Hong Kong   Tokyo
Nairobi   Dar es Salaam   Cape Town
Melbourne   Auckland
and associated companies in
Berlin   Ibadan

Copyright © 1991 by Oxford University Press, Inc.

Published by Oxford University Press, Inc.,
200 Madison Avenue, New York, New York 10016

Oxford is a registered trademark of Oxford University Press

Library of Congress Cataloging-in-Publication Data
DNA topoisomerases in cancer /
edited by Milan Potmesil, Kurt W. Kohn,
and the editorial board, Leroy F. Liu . . . [et. al.].
p. cm.   Includes index.   ISBN 0-19-506106-3
1. DNA topoisomerase I—Inhibitors—Therapeutic use—Testing.
2. DNA topoisomerase II—Inhibitors—Therapeutic use—Testing.
3. Cancer—Chemotherapy.   I. Potmesil, Milan.   II. Kohn, Kurt W.
[DNLM: 1. Antineoplastic Agents—therapeutic use.
2. DNA Untwisting Proteins—therapeutic use.
3. Neoplasms—therapy.
QZ 266 D629] RC271.D54D53 1991 616.99'4061—dc20
DNLM/DLC for Library of Congress   90-7992

1 2 3 4 5 6 7 8 9
Printed in the United States of America
on acid-free paper

Preface

DNA topoisomerases, ubiquitous cellular enzymes, continue to interest scientists and clinicians alike, the former because of intrinsic involvement in biological functions of the cell, and the latter for presenting a target of successful chemotherapy of certain cancers. In this book the reader finds a series of chapters written by researchers actively involved in an emerging and expanding research field. The volume should provide information for those who wish to gain an in-depth understanding of various aspects of topoisomerase biology and biochemistry. The book also offers background information that can serve as a reference guide to investigators and clinicians who would like to obtain better insight into various processes linked to topoisomerase biology and interaction with chemotherapeutic agents.

The editors wish to acknowledge the invaluable help of colleagues who provided critical reviews and constructive comments of contributions in this monograph: William T. Beck, Robert P. Hertzberg, Tao-Shih Hsieh, Kenneth N. Kreuzer, Michael R. Mattern, Neil Osheroff, Yves Pommier, and James C. Wang; and to thank Ms. Gloria Elugardo for her expert editorial and secretarial assistance.

New York, New York   M.P.
Bethesda, Maryland   K.W.K.

Contents

PART I GENETICS AND BIOCHEMISTRY OF DNA TOPOISOMERASES

PART II INHIBITORS OF TOPOISOMERASE I

PART III INHIBITORS OF TOPOISOMERASE II

PART IV DRUG RESISTANCE AND TOPOISOMERASES

PART V DEVELOPMENT AND CLINICAL USE OF TOPOISOMERASE INHIBITORS

Contributors

Toshiwo Andoh
Division of Biochemistry
Aichi Cancer Center Research Institute
Nagoya, Japan

William T. Beck
Department of Biochemical and Clinical
  Pharmacology
St. Jude Children's Research Hospital
Memphis, Tennessee

Terry A. Beerman
Grace Cancer Drug Center
Roswell Park Memorial Institute
Buffalo, New York

Christian Bendixen
Department of Molecular Biology and
  Plant Physiology
University of Aarhus
Aarhus, Denmark

Annette Bodley
Department of Biological Chemistry
Johns Hopkins University School of
  Medicine
Baltimore, Maryland

Bjarne Juul Bonven
Department of Molecular Biology and
  Plant Physiology
University of Aarhus
Aarhus, Denmark

Giovanni Capranico
Laboratory of Molecular Pharmacology
Developmental Therapeutics Program
Division of Cancer Treatment
National Cancer Institute
National Institutes of Health
Bethesda, Maryland

Mary J. Caranfa
Department of Biochemistry
SmithKline Beecham
Philadelphia, Pennsylvania

Pierre Chartrand
Canadian Red Cross Society
Montreal, Quebec, Canada

Kuan-Chih Chow
The James G. Brown Cancer Center
University of Louisville
Louisville, Kentucky

Kent Christiansen
Department of Molecular Biology and
  Plant Physiology
University of Aarhus
Aarhus, Denmark

Thomas D. Y. Chung
Departments of Molecular Pharmacology
  and Biomolecular Discovery
SmithKline Beecham
King of Prussia, Pennsylvania

Joseph M. Covey
Laboratory of Molecular Pharmacology
Division of Cancer Treatment
Developmental Therapeutics Program
National Cancer Institute
National Institutes of Health
Bethesda, Maryland

Stanley T. Crooke
Departments of Molecular Pharmacology
and Biomolecular Discovery
SmithKline Beecham
King of Prussia, Pennsylvania

Mary K. Danks
Department of Biochemical and Clinical
Pharmacology
St. Jude Children's Research Hospital
Memphis, Tennessee

Fred H. Drake
Departments of Molecular Pharmacology
and Biomolecular Discovery
SmithKline Beecham
King of Prussia, Pennsylvania

Paul T. Englund
Department of Biological Chemistry
Johns Hopkins University School of
Medicine
Baltimore, Maryland

Parkash S. Gill
Department of Medicine
Divisions of Hematology and Medical
Oncology
University of Southern California School
of Medicine
Los Angeles, California

Beppino C. Giovanella
Stehlin Foundation for Cancer Research
Houston, Texas

Bonnie S. Glisson
Department of Medical Oncology
The University of Texas
M.D. Anderson Cancer Center
Houston, Texas

Jack D. Griffith
Lineberger Cancer Center
University of North Carolina
Chapel Hill, North Carolina

Sidney M. Hecht
Department of Biochemistry
SmithKline Beecham
Philadelphia, Pennsylvania

Caroline R. Heise
Laboratory of Molecular Pharmacology
Developmental Therapeutics Program
National Cancer Institute
National Institutes of Health
Bethesda, Maryland

Robert P. Hertzberg
Department of Biomolecular Discovery
SmithKline Beecham
King of Prussia, Pennsylvania

Christine Holm
Laboratory of Molecular Pharmacology
Developmental Therapeutics Program
National Cancer Institute
National Institutes of Health
Bethesda, Maryland

Michael Howard
Lineberger Cancer Research Center
University of North Carolina
Chapel Hill, North Carolina

Yaw-Huei Hsiang
Highland Hospital of Rochester
Rochester, New York

Tao-Shih Hsieh
Department of Biochemistry
Duke University Medical Center
Durham, North Carolina

Anne C. Huff
Department of Microbiology and
Immunology
Duke University Medical Center
Durham, North Carolina

Kazuyuki Ishii
Meiji College of Pharmacy
Tokyo, Japan

Mervyn Israel
Departments of Pharmacology and
  Medicinal Chemistry and the
  Cancer Center
University of Tennessee
College of Medicine
Memphis, Tennessee

Christine Jaxel
Laboratoire d'Enzymologie des Acides
  Nucléiques
Université Pierre et Marie Curie
Paris, France

Randall K. Johnson
Departments of Molecular Pharmacology
  and Biomolecular Discovery
SmithKline Beecham
King of Prussia, Pennsylvania

Donna Kerrigan
Laboratory of Molecular Pharmacology
Developmental Therapeutics Program
National Cancer Institute
National Institutes of Health
Bethesda, Maryland

William D. Kingsbury
Department of Biochemistry
SmithKline Beecham
Philadelphia, Pennsylvania

Eigil Kjeldsen
Department of Molecular Biology and
  Plant Physiology
University of Aarhus
Aarhus, Denmark

Viiu A. Klein
Department of Biological Chemistry
Johns Hopkins University School of
  Medicine
Baltimore, Maryland

Kurt W. Kohn
Laboratory of Molecular Pharmacology
Developmental Therapeutics Program
National Cancer Institute

National Institutes of Health
Bethesda, Maryland

Kenneth N. Kreuzer
Department of Microbiology and
  Immunology
Duke University Medical Center
Durham, North Carolina

Paul E. Kroeger
Department of Pharmacology and
  Therapeutics
University of Florida College of Medicine
Gainesville, Florida

Maxwell P. Lee
Department of Biochemistry
Duke University Medical Center
Durham, North Carolina

Erich K. Lehnert
Department of Chemistry
University of Virginia
Charlottesville, Virginia

Leroy F. Liu
Department of Biological Chemistry
Johns Hopkins University School of
  Medicine
Baltimore, Maryland

John T. Loper
Department of Chemistry
University of Virginia
Charlottesville, Virginia

Timothy L. Macdonald
Department of Chemistry
University of Virginia
Charlottesville, Virginia

Michael R. Mattern
Departments of Molecular Pharmacology
  and Biomolecular Discovery
SmithKline Beecham
King of Prussia, Pennsylvania

Mary M. McHugh
Department of Experimental
   Therapeutics
Grace Cancer Drug Center
Roswell Park Memorial Institute
Buffalo, New York

Christopher K. Mirabelli
Departments of Molecular Pharmacology
   and Biomolecular Discovery
Division of Research and Development
SmithKline Beecham
King of Prussia, Pennsylvania

Franco M. Muggia
Division of Oncology
Norris Cancer Center of the University
   of Southern California School of
   Medicine
Los Angeles, California

Ole Frederik Nielsen
Department of Molecular Biology and
   Plant Physiology
University of Aarhus
Aarhus, Denmark

John L. Nitiss
Department of Biochemistry and
   Molecular Biology
Harvard University
Cambridge, Massachusetts

James M. Nolan
Department of Biology
Indiana University
Bloomington, Indiana

Kosuke Okada
Division of Blood Transfusion
Hiroshima University Hospital
Hiroshima, Japan

Neil Osheroff
Department of Biochemistry
Vanderbilt University School of Medicine
Nashville, Tennessee

Steven R. Per
Departments of Molecular Pharmacology
   and Biomolecular Discovery
SmithKline Beecham
King of Prussia, Pennsylvania

Yves Pommier
Laboratory of Molecular Pharmacology
Developmental Therapeutics Program
National Cancer Institute
National Institutes of Health
Bethesda, Maryland

Milan Potmesil
Laboratory of Experimental Therapy
Department of Radiology
New York University School of Medicine
New York, New York

Megan J. Robinson
Department of Biochemistry
Vanderbilt University School of Medicine
Nashville, Tennessee

Warren E. Ross
Department of Medicine
The James G. Brown Cancer Center
University of Louisville
Louisville, Kentucky

Thomas C. Rowe
Department of Pharmacology and
   Therapeutics
University of Florida College of Medicine
Gainesville, Florida

Ramakrishan Seshadri
Departments of Pharmacology and
   Medicinal Chemistry and the
   Cancer Center
University of Tennessee-Memphis
College of Medicine
Memphis, Tennessee

Theresa A. Shapiro
Department of Biological Chemistry and
   Internal Medicine
Division of Clinical Pharmacology

Johns Hopkins University School of
    Medicine
Baltimore, Maryland

Michael J. Siciliano
Department of Biochemical Genetics
University of Texas
M.D. Anderson Cancer Center
Houston, Texas

Robert Silber
Department of Medicine
Division of Hematology
New York University Medical Center
New York, New York

Brian Smith
Department of Biochemistry
SmithKline Beecham
Philadelphia, Pennsylvania

John S. Stehlin
Stehlin Foundation for Cancer Research
Houston, Texas

Kong B. Tan
Departments of Molecular Pharmacology
    and Biomolecular Discovery
SmithKline Beecham
King of Prussia, Pennsylvania

Bo Thomsen
Department of Molecular Biology and
    Plant Physiology
University of Aarhus
Aarhus, Denmark

Monroe E. Wall
Research Triangle Institute
Research Triangle Park, North Carolina

James C. Wang
Department of Biochemistry and
    Molecular Biology
Harvard University
Cambridge, Massachusetts

Mansukh C. Wani
Research Triangle Institute
Research Triangle Park, North Carolina

Karsten Wassermann
Laboratory of Molecular Pharmacology
Developmental Therapeutics Program
National Cancer Institute
National Institutes of Health
Bethesda, Maryland

Ole Westergaard
Departments of Molecular Biology and
    Plant Physiology
University of Aarhus
Aarhus, Denmark

R. D. Woessner
Departments of Molecular Pharmacology
    and Biomolecular Discovery
SmithKline Beecham
King of Prussia, Pennsylvania

Jan M. Woynarowski
Grace Cancer Drug Center
Roswell Park Memorial Institute
Buffalo, New York

Elizabeth Wyckoff
Department of Cellular, Molecular, and
    Viral Biology
University of Utah Medical Center
Salt Lake City, Utah

E. Lynn Zechiedrich
Department of Biochemistry
Vanderbilt University School of Medicine
Nashville, Tennessee

DNA Topoisomerases in Cancer

Chapter 1
Introduction

MILAN POTMESIL
AND KURT W. KOHN

This volume is an extension of international conferences on DNA topoisomerases in cancer chemotherapy, held in 1986 and 1988 in New York City under the auspices of New York University Post-Graduate Medical School and the Rita and Stanley H. Kaplan Cancer Center. The articles are organized in five sections, each containing contributions with related topics. The first section deals with basic aspects of genetics and biochemistry of prokaryotic and eukaryotic topoisomerases. The second and third sections focus on inhibitors of DNA topoisomerase I and II, their chemistry, mechanism of action, and molecular correlates. Drug resistance, as it reflects on DNA topoisomerase I and II, is addressed in the fourth section, and the fifth section reviews preclinical development of two groups of analogs targeted at DNA topoisomerases. This part also discusses the utility of topoisomerase II–directed drugs in clinical hematology.

DNA topoisomerases have emerged as important therapeutic targets of drugs ranging from antimicrobial to antineoplastic compounds. As amply documented by L. F. Liu and J. C. Wang (Chapter 2), all the drugs share the same principal mechanism of action: they interfere with the enzyme-mediated breakage-rejoining of DNA strands by blocking the rejoining step. Different from inhibitors of other enzymes, topoisomerase-targeting therapeutics kill cells by a mechanism unrelated to the inhibition of enzyme catalytic activity. Instead, the drugs convert an essential cellular topoisomerase into DNA breaking poison, thus starting a series of events that lead to cell death. For the convenience of the reader, brief overviews of individual contributions follow.

GENETICS AND BIOCHEMISTRY OF DNA TOPOISOMERASE (CHAPTERS 2–7)

In the general introduction to the book, L. F. Liu and J. C. Wang (Chapter 2) review some of the most recent developments in topoisomerase biochemistry and the studies of drug–topoisomerase interaction. Although only topoisomerases I and II are reviewed here, the same basic principles may apply to other, less extensively studied topoisomerase enzymes.

3

A comparison of sequence homology among DNA topoisomerase II of various species indicates that the structure of the enzymes is conserved during the course of evolution (J. M. Nolan et al., Chapter 3). The Drosophila *TOP2* gene, encoding DNA topoisomerase II, was analyzed by locating the gene in both the cytogenetic and molecular maps. The mapping experiments, which use the available deficiency chromosomes, indicate that the *TOP2* is located in a cytogenetic region between 37D2 and 37D5–6 in the left arm of chromosome 2. Expression of both *TOP2* mRNA and protein is elevated during developmental periods characterized by active DNA synthesis. The majority of topoisomerase II is located in the cytoplasm in early embryos and moves into the nuclei as development progresses.

M. H. Howard and J. Griffith (Chapter 4) studied the complex relation between topoisomerase II binding sites on DNA, the position of weak and strong cleavage sites, and the way in which topoisomerase II arranges DNA into loops. DNA is now known to contain many different variations in structure that differ from the classic B form owing to unique sequence arrangements. How these unusual structures influence the way in which topoisomerase II moves along DNA, loops DNA, and where drug-induced cleavages occur, is not yet fully understood. It seems likely, however, that novel DNA structures will be found to play an important role.

Topoisomerase I and II cleavage sites were mapped *in vivo* on the Hsp70 heat-shock genes of *Drosophila melanogaster* cells using the drugs camptothecin and VM-26 (P. E. Kroeger and T. C. Rowe, Chapter 5). The authors found that topoisomerase I and II may play different roles in the transcription of these genes. Topoisomerase I cleavage, confined within the transcribed region of the Hsp70 gene, only occurred when the Hsp70 gene was transcriptionally active. In contrast, topoisomerase II cleavage was present near the ends of the Hsp70 gene, and it occurred in the presence or absence of Hsp70 transcription. Prior to activation of Hsp70 transcription, topoisomerase II cleavage was primarily localized at the 5' end of the gene. However, following heat-induced activation of Hsp70 transcription, cleavage in this region disappeared with a concomitant increase in cleavage at the 3' end of the gene. During the recovery from heat-shock, there was a gradual repression of Hsp70 RNA synthesis with a corresponding return of topoisomerase II cleavage to the 5' end of the gene. This suggests that enzyme binding in this region may be involved in suppressing Hsp70 transcription.

The effects of inhibitors on DNA topoisomerase II in mitochondria are reviewed by T. A. Shapiro and P. T. Englund (Chapter 6). Treatment of intact *Trypanosoma equiperdum* with compounds known to be active against mammalian type II topoisomerases results in DNA cleavage. Since minicircle DNA is present in the cleaved complex, DNA topoisomerase II that has been trapped must be mitochondrial in origin. As is characteristic of topoisomerase II–DNA complexes, the enzyme from *T. equiperdum* mitochondria binds to both 5' ends of the substrate DNA. Furthermore, VP-16 inhibits the catalytic activity of the enzyme, resulting in an accumulation of multimeric replicating minicircle forms. Inhibitors of DNA gyrase (bacterial DNA topoisomerase II), even at concentrations 25 times greater than those effective against *E. coli,* do not promote minicircle linearization or give evidence of topoisomerase II inhibition. In terms of inhibitor susceptibility, the mitochondrial topoisomerase II of *T. equiperdum* closely resembles topoisomerase II present in the nuclei of higher eukaryotes, rather than DNA gyrase. The inhibitors of DNA topoisomerase II will undoubtedly prove important in understanding the role of topoisomerases in trypanosomes, and may also provide much needed new approaches to anti-trypanosomal chemotherapy.

J. L. Nitiss and J. C. Wang (Chapter 7) discuss the use of yeast permeability mutants as a genetic system that facilitates the study of antitumor drugs targeted at DNA topoisomerases. Purified yeast DNA topoisomerases I and II are similar to their mammalian counterparts in the interactions with the antitumor drug camptothecin, which acts on the former, and amsacrines, etoposide and teniposide, which act on the latter enzyme. Sensitivity of yeast cells to the drugs is strongly dependent on mutations affecting drug uptake, as well as on mutations that affect the *RAD52* DNA repair pathway. The latter is implicated in the chain of events that lead to cell killing by antitopoisomerase drugs. In contrast to the hypersensitivity of the *rad52* mutants, mutations in *RAD2* and *RAD6* have little effect on drug sensitivity. When *RAD52*+ cells, permeable to both camptothecin and *m*-AMSA, are treated with a combination of the two drugs over a long period relative to the generation time, cell killing is significantly greater than that achieved with either drug alone.

INHIBITORS OF TOPOISOMERASE I (CHAPTERS 8–15)

Topoisomerase I was brought dramatically to the forefront of the field of anti-cancer drug development by the discovery by Y. H. Hsiang, R. Hertzberg, S. Hecht, and L. F. Liu (J. Biol. Chem. **260:** 14873, 1985) of the specific action exerted by a previously abandoned natural product, camptothecin. This finding is striking because the mechanism by which camptothecin blocks topoisomerase I through the formation of covalent DNA cleavage complexes is analogous to the manner in which topoisomerase II had previously been found to be blocked by several notable anticancer drugs. Investigations of drug actions against the two types of topoisomerases have been progressing largely in parallel directions, and many similarities, as well as some differences, have emerged. The papers in this section review several of the major new findings on inhibitors of topoisomerase I and also include comparative results on inhibitors of topoisomerase II.

There is renewed interest in the chemistry of camptothecin: the synthesis of new derivatives, structure–activity relationships, and chemical mechanisms. A better understanding of these matters could resolve the problems that had been encountered in the clinical testing of camptothecin: insolubility, high plasma protein binding, and toxicity to the urinary tract. The solubility problem might be alleviated by the development of active derivatives that have greater water solubility or more potent compounds that would require lower drug concentrations. The plasma protein binding and urinary tract toxicity problems might also be resolved by applying chemical knowledge that is available. M. E.

Wall and M. C. Wani (Chapter 8) review the relationships between chemical structure and the preclinical antitumor activities of camptothecin derivatives, and show the features of the molecule that must be increased by certain substitutions, and suggest that active water-soluble compounds could be obtained by hydrophilic substitution at specific positions. Y. Pommier et al. (Chapter 10) examine the relationship between structure and action on topoisomerase I, and find agreement with the antitumor data, independent of whether the assay is inhibition of topoisomerization activity or stabilization of cleavage complexes. The findings give strong support to the notion that topoisomerase I is the effective target in the antitumor activity of camptothecins. R. P. Hertzberg et al. (Chapter 9) add further important chemical information, especially regarding the possible key role of the camptothecin lactone ring and the importance of pH, and also present evidence that camptothecin binds to topoisomerase I–DNA complexes.

In analogy with topoisomerase II inhibitors, camptothecin may cause potentially lethal lesions in cells in the form of drug-stabilized covalent DNA cleavage complexes, in this case involving topoisomerase I. The magnitude of the lethal effect can, according to the current evidence, be viewed as depending upon (1) the amount of topoisomerase I present, (2) the extent to which the forms of the enzyme present in a cell are susceptible to drug-stabilization of complexes, and (3) the activity of processes in the cell that interact with complexes so as to produce a lethal catastrophe. C. K. Mirabelli et al. (Chapter 11) discuss regulatory mechanisms that may alter the phosphorylation state of topoisomerase I and thereby alter its ability to form camptothecin-stabilized complexes. C. Holm et al. (Chapter 13) present evidence that DNA replication may be the major process that interacts with the complexes to kill cells. These and other reports elsewhere in this volume are beginning to clarify the complex metabolic factors that influence drug–topoisomerase interaction and have lethal consequences.

E. Kjeldsen et al. (Chapter 12) and C. Jaxel et al. (Chapter 15) address the question of factors which determine where in a DNA sequence is the location of various topoisomerase I cleavage sites in the presence or absence of camptothecin. Kjeldsen et al. identified a 16 base pair element at strong cleavage sites in nucleosome-free regions of Tetrahymena ribosomal genes. Since the cleavages occurred at the same position in chromatin as in DNA purified from the chromatin, chromatinic structure did not seem to influence the sites. The sites were only slightly stimulated by camptothecin, and were quite different in sequence from the sites that were strongly stimulated. The sequenced sites compiled in the two articles show some features that may be required for strong cleavage. Most of the available sites are of the camptothecin-stimulated type, and little can be said with certainty about the few prominent cleavage sites in the absence of the drug. The data agree in the identity of three positions occurring in sequences where cleavage was strongly stimulated by camptothecin: G at -3, T at -1, and G at $+1$ relative to the cleavage site. Of these three features, only the T at -1 was present in the strong sites identified in the absence of drug. These features appear to be necessary but not sufficient for strong camptothecin-stimulated cleavage. There must be other requirements that do not reveal a simple sequence dependency. It is increasingly suspected that these may have something to do with the conformation, bending, or flexibility of the DNA over a region flanking the binding site.

The effects of topoisomerase inhibitors can be modified by the presence of other DNA binders such as polyamines or DNA minor-groove binders. Since the sites required for topoisomerase interaction could be blocked or conformationally perturbed, it comes as no surprise that high concentrations of DNA binders inhibit topoisomerase actions. It is all the more notable that T. A. Beerman et al. (Chapter 14), in their exploration of the effects of minor-groove binders on both types of topoisomerases, find a modest concentration of distamycin enhancing topoisomerase II actions. This finding suggests that topoisomerase activities can, in some cases, be enhanced by conformational alterations caused by DNA binders.

INHIBITORS OF TOPOISOMERASE II (CHAPTERS 16–19)

More knowledge is becoming available concerning the mechanism by which topoisomerase II–active agents interact with DNA and produce species termed "cleavable complexes." T. L. Macdonald et al. (Chapter 16) have identified a composite pharmacophore for five classes of agents that induce the formation of cleavable complexes. The existence of such pharmacophore for topoisomerase II–active agents implies a common drug target site in the cleavable complex. The authors postulate that this site resides on DNA and that the drug–DNA interaction, the initial event in the formation of a cleavable complex, causes a specific distortion of the DNA duplex. This distortion, induced in DNA upon drug association, may present an altered DNA structure, an intermediate in the cleavage–resealing sequence of the enzyme. At some point in the catalytic cycle, the drug–DNA complex forms so-called transition state analog of DNA.

Bacteriophage T4 represents a uniquely informative system suitable for studies of the mechanism of antitumor drug action. The experimental advantages of this prokaryotic system have permitted A. C. Huff and K. N. Kreuzer (Chapter 17) to demonstrate conclusively that viral-encoded DNA topoisomerase is the intracellular target of antitumor agent 4′(9-acridinylamino)methanesulfon-m-anisidide (m-AMSA) in T4-infected *Escherichia coli*. In addition, the coincidence of a frameshift mutation hotspot and a strong T4 topoisomerase cleavage site directly implicates the topoisomerase itself in the generation of frameshift mutations. Finally, the mutation alters enzyme sensitivity to m-AMSA, to several other antitumor agents, and to a DNA–gyrase inhibitor. One of the most provocative findings of this contribution is the evidence that m-AMSA–resistance mutations alter the drug-independent DNA cleavage site specificity of T4 topoisomerase. This and other results stress the importance of DNA site recognition by a topoisomerase and support the proposal that drug action is mediated through a ternary complex consisting of DNA, a topoisomerase, and a drug.

The ability to induce and relegate double-stranded breaks in DNA is central to the physiological functions of DNA topoisomerase II. This activity serves as the primary target reaction for a number of antineoplastic agents, and their chemotherapeutic activities correlate well with drug potency to stabilize covalent enzyme–DNA cleavage complexes. Despite the importance of the topoisomerase II–mediated DNA cleavage–religation cycle to the survival of the eukaryotic cell and to the treatment of human cancers, little is known concerning its detailed mechanism. N. Osheroff et al. (Chapter 18) have employed a novel DNA religation assay and characterized both the kinetic pathway of the reaction and the mechanism by which two potent antineoplastic drugs (*m*-AMSA and etoposide) affect the DNA cleavage–religation equilibrium. Results indicate that the enzyme mediates DNA cleavage–religation by making two sequential single-stranded breaks. The antineoplastic agents stabilize the covalent topoisomerase II–DNA cleavage complex, at least in part, by inhibiting the rate of religation of both cleaved DNA strands.

DRUG RESISTANCE AND TOPOISOMERASES (CHAPTERS 20–22)

Acquired and *de novo* resistance to chemotherapy represent a serious problem in the management of patients with many types of cancer or leukemia. Although the multidrug resistance phenotype seems to be the most damaging, other types of resistance also present a serious problem. These types include, among others, the resistance operating against topoisomerase I– and topoisomerase II–directed drugs.

T. Andoh et al. (Chapter 20) purified DNA topoisomerase I from a "wild" line of human lymphoblastic leukemia cells and from a line resistant to camptothecin. The resistance appears to be directly associated with the enzyme. Using several criteria, e.g., efficacy of the cleavage and salt sensitivity of the cleavable complex, the cleavable complex formed by topoisomerase I isolated from resistant cells was compared to that of the wild-type. The "resistant" enzyme formed the cleavable complex in the absence of divalent cations that were required for the complex formation by the wild-type enzyme. The results indicate that DNA topoisomerase I is the cellular target of camptothecin, and a change in its properties may be a factor in drug resistance.

The objective of a paper by W. T. Beck and M. K. Danks (Chapter 21) was to summarize current knowledge concerning the biochemistry of multidrug resistance (MDR) associated with alterations in topoisomerase II activity (at-MDR). The results were primarily obtained from studies of a human leukemic lymphoblastic cell line selected for its resistance to teniposide (VM-26). It was shown that at-MDR is a different entity from the well-characterized form of MDR associated with overexpression of the integral membrane P-glycoprotein. This is despite the fact that cells with at-MDR phenotypes can express resistance and cross-resistance to several classes of anticancer drugs, including the epipodophyllotoxins, aminoacridines, and anthracyclines. Nuclear extracts from cell lines with the at-MDR phenotype are altered in both cleavage and catalytic activities. Specifically, they are relatively resistant to drug inhibition of strand-passing activity, drug stimulation of topoisomerase II–mediated DNA breaks, and drug stabilization of enzyme–DNA ("cleavable") complexes. It also appears that topoisomerase II activities from human leukemic at-MDR cell lines, compared to drug-sensitive cells, are altered in ATP requirements. The authors discuss possible mechanisms of at-MDR.

Previous studies of a mutant CHO cell line by B. S. Glisson et al. (Chapter 22) suggest that the resistance to epipodophyllotoxins and intercalating agents may be mediated through a qualitative change in topoisomerase II. This change may confer resistance to drug-stimulated DNA cleavage activity. In order to define the genetic basis for the resistance, the authors have analyzed human lymphocyte somatic cell hybrid lines for reconstitution of drug sensitivity. Partial loss of resistance to etoposide, mitoxantrone, adriamycin, and 5-iminodaunorubicin was identified in 3/16 hybrid lines, all of which retained complete resistance to m-AMSA. Their data suggest that loss of drug resistance in a hybrid line is relatively specific for each drug, and it involves both increased cleavable complex formation as well as altered postcleavable complex processing.

DEVELOPMENT AND CLINICAL USE OF TOPOISOMERASE INHIBITORS (CHAPTERS 23–25)

In addition to the clinically useful topoisomerase-targeted drugs doxorubicin, VP-16, and VM-26, there are several inhibitors of topoisomerase I or II in various stages of preclinical or early clinical studies. Four groups of doxorubicin and daunorubicin analogs, differing by their substituents on the chromophore and sugar moieties, were used in studies by A. Bodley et al. (Chapter 23). It is shown that DNA intercalation, be it of high or low strength, is required but not sufficient for the activity by topoisomerase II–targeted anthracyclines. In addition to the planar chromophore that is involved in intercalation, two other domains of the anthracycline molecule are important for the interaction with the enzyme: (1) substitution on the C14 position totally inhibits drug activity in the purified system but enhances cytotoxicity by aiding drug uptake and presumably acting on other cellular targets; (2) substitutions on the 3'-N position of the sugar ring can, depending on the nature of the substituent, inhibit intercalation and/or topoisomerase II–targeting activity. These findings may provide guidance for anthracycline taxonomy and for the synthesis and development of new active analogs.

Drug development is needed to improve chemotherapy of patients with locally advanced or metastatic colon cancer, who otherwise have unfavorable prognosis. Two camptothecin analogs, 9-amino-20(RS) and 10,11-methylene-dioxy-20(RS), were selected by tests with the purified topoisomerase I and tissue-culture screens. Unlike other anticancer drugs or parent camptothecin, both analogs induced long-term disease-free remissions, which resulted from single-agent treatment of human colon cancer lines carried by immunodeficient mice (M. Potmesil et al., Chapter 24). Drug toxicity was low and allowed for repeated courses of therapy. The compounds effectively reduced the size of bulky tumors and decreased the incidence of liver metastases. The experiments have also demonstrated that camptothecin and 9-amino-20(RS) bypass the MDR1–related cell resistance in cancer, and overcome a less-defined resistance to alkylating agents. Further studies of camptothecin analogs are necessary to evaluate their clinical usefulness. The drugs can be a much needed addition to cancer chemotherapy, and also a tool that allows detail studies of the molecular pathology of cancer.

In a review of clinical data, F. M. Muggia and P. S. Gill (Chapter 25) show that the majority of known DNA topoisomerase II–inhibiting drugs are most active against tumors with high growth fraction, such as large cell lymphoma, acute nonlymphocytic leukemia, and the blast crisis of chronic myelogenic leukemia. Traditionally, these drugs have played a lesser role in neoplasms with low growth fraction. The authors review the current regimens and discuss the contributions of topoisomerase II–drug interaction to the success or failure of treatments. New concepts that may influence future treatment strategies are outlined.

PART I

GENETICS AND BIOCHEMISTRY OF DNA TOPOISOMERASES

Chapter 2
Biochemistry of DNA Topoisomerases and Their Poisons

LEROY F. LIU
AND JAMES C. WANG

ENZYME MECHANISMS

DNA topoisomerases were originally discovered as activities that change the superhelical structure of closed circular DNAs (1–4). Studies using purified DNA topoisomerases have demonstrated additional DNA topoisomerization reactions such as knotting/unknotting and catenation/decatenation of DNA rings (5–9). Based on the fundamental differences in their mechanisms of action, DNA topoisomerases have been classified into two types (6,10). During their catalytic cycles, type I DNA topoisomerases introduce transient single-strand DNA breaks, while type II topoisomerases break both DNA strands to allow another duplex DNA segment to pass through. A hallmark of type II DNA topoisomerases is that they change the linking number of a circular DNA in steps of two, which is a consequence of the strand-passing mechanism (6,10). Some of the enzymatic properties of topoisomerases are listed in Table 2.1.

One of the major catalytic functions of topoisomerases is the relaxation of DNA supercoils (or supercoiling in the case of bacterial DNA gyrase or topoisomerase II), which are generated during various DNA transactions (see the section on Biological Functions). In addition to the fundamental differences in their mechanism of action, DNA topoisomerases are also different in their specificity for DNA conformation. While bacterial DNA topoisomerase I and II are specific for negatively and positively supercoiled DNAs, respectively, eukaryotic DNA topoisomerases are equally active on either form of super-coiled DNA (reviewed in 18). The DNA conformation specificity of bacterial DNA topoisomerase I is most likely due to its mode of DNA binding, which appears to be rate limiting in the topoisomerization reactions (19). Partial unwinding of the duplex DNA in the enzyme–DNA complex has been proposed (19). Since unwinding of duplex DNA is favored on a negatively supercoiled DNA, bacterial DNA topoisomerase I relaxes negative supercoils preferentially (1). Binding of bacterial DNA topoisomerase II to DNA involves the formation of a complex in which the DNA duplex is wrapped around the enzyme

Table 2.1. Enzymatic Properties of Prokaryotic and Eukaryotic DNA Topoisomerase I and II[a]

| | Bacterial | | Eukaryotic | |
	Type I	Type II	Type I	Type II
Relaxes positive supercoils	no[b]	yes	yes	yes
Relaxes negative supercoils	yes	no[c]	yes	yes
Introduces negative supercoils	no	yes	no	no
Catenation/decatenation of DNA	no[d]	yes	no[d]	yes
Requires ATP hydrolysis	no	yes[e]	no	yes
Requires divalent ions (e.g., Mg)	yes	yes	no[f]	yes
DNA end covalently linked to tyrosine	5'-P	5'-P	3'-P	5'-P
Subunit structure[g]	M	A_2B_2	M	D

[a]Topoisomerase III, which is a type I DNA topoisomerase, is not included (11,12).
[b]Bacterial DNA topoisomerase I relaxes positive supercoils only when an unpaired region (e.g., a heteroduplex region) is present (13).
[c]Bacterial DNA topoisomerase II (DNA gyrase) relaxes negative supercoils only in the absence of ATP (14).
[d]Both eukaryotic and prokaryotic DNA topoisomerase I can catenate and decatenate DNA provided that at least one of the duplex circle contains a nick or a gap (15,16).
[e]Negative supercoils are slowly relaxed in the absence of ATP (14).
[f]Stimulated by Mg(II) (17).
[g]M, monomer; A and B, different subunits; D, homodimer.

surface in a right-handed manner (20). The formation of this complex is presumably responsible for the unidirectional decrease of the DNA linking number during ATP-dependent topoisomerization reaction (21). Purified eukaryotic DNA topoisomerases do not show DNA conformation specificity (2,22). Either eukaryotic DNA topoisomerase I or II relaxes positive and negative supercoils with roughly equal rates (2,22). This absence of detectable winding or unwinding of DNA upon enzyme binding explains the lack of DNA conformation specificity of eukaryotic DNA topoisomerases (reviewed in 18).

A number of prokaryotic and eukaryotic DNA topoisomerase genes have been cloned and sequenced (reviewed in 23, 24–26). No sequence homology is found between prokaryotic and eukaryotic DNA topoisomerase I (23). The lack of homology explains the significant difference in their enzymatic reactions (see Table 2.1). On the other hand, prokaryotic and eukaryotic DNA topoisomerase II share significant sequence homology (23); eukaryotic topoisomerase II has apparently evolved from bacterial DNA topoisomerase II by fusion of the *GyrA* and *GyrB* subunits into a single polypeptide. It is not readily explainable, however, why eukaryotic DNA topoisomerase II has lost the ability to negatively supercoil DNA and yet retain its DNA-dependent ATPase function. The possibility that eukaryotic DNA topoisomerase II may exhibit supercoiling activity at certain DNA sequences, cellular locations, or in the presence of additional factors cannot be ruled out. Recently, a new DNA topoisomerase, DNA topoisomerase III, has been identified in *Saccharomyces cerevisiae* and has been shown to share sequence identity with bacterial DNA topoisomerases I and III (12). However, both yeast and bacterial DNA topoisomerase III appear to play a minor role in maintaining DNA conformation *in vivo*.

BIOLOGICAL FUNCTIONS

DNA topoisomerases are involved in many aspects of DNA functions. One of their most important roles is in DNA replication. The intertwined parental DNA strands have to be completely resolved before the segregation of the two daughter DNA molecules. For a closed circular DNA molecule, the linking number of the parental strands decreases continuously during DNA replication and is reduced to zero when the two daughter molecules are completely segregated. The reduction of the linking number of the parental DNA strands during the elongation phase of DNA replication can be achieved by either of the two DNA topoisomerases (28,29). Segregation of the daughter DNA molecules, however, often involves the separation of two multiply intertwined intact duplex DNA molecules and is specifically carried out by DNA topoisomerase II (28,29).

Studies in yeast have also suggested that topoisomerase II is involved in mitosis (30). Topoisomerase II activity coupled with spindle pulling is presumably required for the complete separation of the two multiply intertwined daughter chromosomes. In the absence of topoisomerase II, pulling of the two multiply intertwined daughter chromosomes results in chromosome loss, DNA breakage, and cell death (30,31). The formation of double minute chromosomes in certain mammalian cells undergoing gene amplification may be due to incomplete segregation of multiply linked daughter minichromosomes. In this case, the lack of centromeres on the double minutes, and thus the absence of spindle, is presumably responsible for the failure in separating the pairs.

The role of topoisomerases in transcription is less clear. According to the twin-supercoiled-domain model of RNA transcription, topoisomerase activities may be required to avoid excessive supercoiling of the DNA template by transcription (32). However, the role of topoisomerases in transcription and local DNA supercoiling can be quite complex. It seems likely that transcription may affect other DNA functions (e.g., DNA replication and recombination) indirectly through its effect on DNA conformation (33,34). The interplay among topoisomerases, transcription, DNA conformation, and possibly histone–DNA interactions needs further clarification.

DNA TOPOISOMERASE POISONS

The importance of topoisomerases as therapeutic targets has become increasingly evident (see reviews 35,36). Various inhibitors of topoisomerases have been shown to have antibacterial, antiparasitic, antifungal, antiviral, and antitumor activities. Interestingly, all these therapeutic drugs act by a similar mechanism: they interfere with the breakage–reunion reaction of topoisomerases by stabilizing the cleaved state. The trapped intermediate, which is an enzyme–DNA–drug ternary complex, termed the "cleavable complex," apparently mediates drug action, while inhibition of the catalytic activity of topoisomerases by drug is unrelated to drug action. It is almost certain that this unique mechanism of action of topoisomerase poisons is responsible for their rapid action and broad spectrum of activities.

DNA Topoisomerase II Poisons

The first characterized topoisomerase poison was nalidixic acid, a bacterial DNA topoisomerase II inhibitor (37,38). The target of nalidixic acid is the *GyrA* subunit of DNA gyrase (DNA topoisomerase II). Using the purified enzyme, nalidixic acid has been shown to induce gyrase-mediated DNA cleavage. The cleavage reaction requires SDS treatment, and the majority of cleavages produce double-strand DNA breaks. Like all other topoisomerase poison–mediated DNA breakage, one end of the broken DNA strand is covalently linked to the enzyme. In this case, *GyrA* subunit is covalently linked to the 5′ phosphoryl end of each broken DNA strand. Studies of the bactericidal action of nalidixic acid has suggested that the enzyme–DNA–drug ternary complex is essential for the strong bactericidal action of the drug.

Studies in cultured mammalian cells and using purified mammalian DNA topoisomerase II have established that a number of antitumor drugs interfere with the breakage–reunion reaction of mammalian DNA topoisomerase II by a mechanism analogous to that of nalidixic acid (reviewed in 36; see Table 2.2). They interfere with the breakage–reunion reaction of DNA topoisomerase II by trapping a ternary topoisomerase–drug–DNA complex, the cleavable complex, which upon exposure to a strong protein denaturant such as SDS or alkali results in single- and double-strand DNA breaks and the covalent linking of a topoisomerase II polypeptide ($M_r = 170$ kDa) to the 5′ phosphoryl end of the broken DNA strand (reviewed in 36).

How topoisomerase II poisons interfere with the breakage–reunion reaction is still not known. A working model has been proposed (39) in which the intercalative mode of drug binding to DNA is assumed to be essential for trapping topoisomerase II cleavable complexes (40). The intercalation of a topoisomerase II poison in the vicinity of the breakage–reunion site on DNA may misalign the two transiently broken DNA ends by about 10–30 degrees (depending on the unwinding angle of the intercalator); this misaligned state of the

Table 2.2. Some Known Mammalian DNA Topoisomerase II Poisons

Drug	Examples
Acridines	*m*-AMSA
Actinomycins	Actinomycin D
Anthracenediones	Mitoxantrone
Anthracyclines	Adriamycin
Benzisoquinolinediones	Amonafide
Ellipticines	Ellipticine
Epipodophyllotoxins	VP-16 (etoposide)
	VM-26 (teniposide)
Isoflavonoids	Genistein

enzyme–drug–DNA complex may in turn prolong the disjoined state of the DNA strands. This model does not explain the action of nonintercalative epipodophyllotoxins, which are also an important class of topoisomerase II poisons. Some recent results, however, suggest that epipodophyllotoxins may also bind DNA (41). It remains to be determined whether epipodophyllotoxins also weakly intercalate DNA.

Drug intercalation into duplex DNA appears to be the common determinant for many topoisomerase II poisons. It is interesting to note that topoisomerase II enzymes isolated from different organisms are sensitive to different DNA intercalators. For example, topoisomerase II enzymes isolated from human and bacteriophage T4 infected *E. coli* cells are sensitive to *m*-AMSA, but topoisomerase II isolated from *E. coli* and Drosophila are not (42). Ethidium bromide, a trypanocidal drug, which does not poison human DNA topoisomerase II, poisons trypanosomal topoisomerase II (43).

Topoisomerase I Poisons

Camptothecin and its derivatives such as 9-amino camptothecin are the only well-characterized DNA topoisomerase I poison (reviewed in 35). Camptothecin was initially identified as an antitumor plant alkaloid from the tree *Camptotheca accuminata* (44). Earlier brief clinical phase I and II trials of the drug yielded discouraging results because of its excessive toxicity (reviewed in 45). Renewed interest in camptothecin as a potential antineoplastic compound was initially due to the identification of its molecular target, DNA topoisomerase I (46), and more recently by the demonstration of unprecedented activity of 9-amino-camptothecin against some of the most refractory human solid tumors transplanted into nude mice (45).

Similar to topoisomerase II poisons, camptothecin inhibits DNA topoisomerase I by trapping a reversible topoisomerase I–drug–DNA ternary complex, the cleavable complex (46). Exposure of the cleavable complex to a strong protein denaturant such as SDS or alkali results in topoisomerase I–linked single-strand breaks. The ternary cleavable complex is highly reversible; removal of the drug (by dilution), challenge with excess DNA, or a brief heating to 65°C leads to a rapid reduction of detectable cleavable complexes (47). The reversibility of the ternary cleavable complex has also been demonstrated in cultured cells treated with camptothecin (47).

MECHANISM OF CELL KILLING BY TOPOISOMERASE POISONS

The reversibility of ternary cleavable complexes in cultured mammalian cells has raised the possibility that cell killing by topoisomerase poisons may be triggered by interaction of the reversible cleavable complexes with other cellular processes (48). Recent studies in cultured cells and in a cell-free SV40 DNA replication system have pointed to the possibility that DNA replication is the key cellular process that converts the reversible topoisomerase I cleavable complexes into lethal DNA lesions (see Fig. 2.1 for a model) (49). The strong S-phase specificity of camptothecin is consistent with this model (50).

The mechanism of cell killing by topoisomerase II poisons is much less clear. Studies of *m*-AMSA have suggested that both DNA and RNA synthesis are involved in drug cytotoxicity (P. D'Arpa and L. F. Liu, unpublished results). At lower concentrations of *m*-AMSA, active DNA replication appears to be a major cellular process that is crucial for *m*-AMSA cytotoxicity. However, at higher *m*-AMSA concentrations, additional cellular processes, including RNA synthesis, may be involved in cell killing. The drug concentration effect cannot be easily explained. However, earlier cell cycle studies have shown that *m*-AMSA specifically kills S-phase cells only at lower concentrations (51). At higher *m*-AMSA concentrations, S-phase specific cytotoxicity appears minimal; cells are killed effectively at all phases of the cell cycle (51). It seems likely that topoisomerase II poisons may have multiple cell killing mechanisms. The drug concentration effect remains to be explained.

Recently, the lower eukaryote, *Saccharomyces cerevisiae,* has been used for studies of topoisomerase poisons (52). Strains that are more permeable and sensitive to topoisomerase poisons have been constructed (52,53). It was shown that mutations in *RAD52,* a gene required for double-strand break repair, dramatically sensitizes yeast strains to topoisomerase poisons. It is now firmly established that topoisomerase I is the sole cytotoxic target of camptothecin in yeast (52,53). Cell cycle studies showed that DNA replication was crucial for both camptothecin and *m*-AMSA cytotoxicity in *RAD52* mutant strain. The polymerase inhibitor, aphidicolin, abolished camptothecin and *m*-AMSA–mediated cytotoxicity in mating factor arrested yeast cells (see Nitiss and Wang, this volume). These results are in general agreement with the results obtained from studies in mammalian cells and suggest that lethal double-strand DNA breaks may be generated in cells treated with topoisomerase II poisons. However, the non–S-phase cytotoxicity of topoisomerase II poisons was not demonstrated in yeast. It seems plausible that double-strand DNA breaks may be responsible for only one pathway of cell killing by topoisomerase poisons, which is accentuated in *RAD52* mutant yeast. The possible existence of other cytotoxic pathway(s) remains to be determined. The major action of topoisomerase poisons through DNA damage is also evidenced by the induction of a DNA-damage-inducible gene, *DIN3* (52). It appears that yeast can be a powerful genetic system for studies of topoisomerase poisons.

Like topoisomerase II poisons, topoisomerase I poison camptothecin also exhibits antiviral activity (29,54). Since both topoisomerase I and II can also act on viral DNA, the destruction of viral DNA template by topoisomerase poisons is expected. However, topoisomerase poisons are probably inactive against RNA viruses.

Future Studies

The importance of topoisomerase poisons in chemotherapy is well established. Biochemical studies of topoisomerases and topoisomerase poisons have provided a satisfactory explanation of the initial steps in drug action. However,

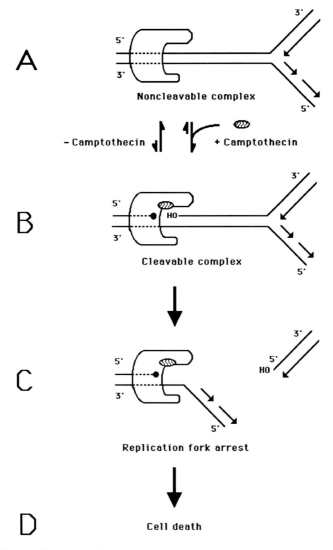

Figure 2.1. Processing of topoisomerase I-camptothecin-DNA cleavable complexes by replication forks. In this model, topoisomerase I is trapped by camptothecin on a replicating DNA molecule. The horseshoe shape of topoisomerase I is to emphasize the asymmetry of topoisomerase I relative to the cleavage site. In the camptothecin–topoisomerase I–DNA ternary complex, topoisomerase I is presumably covalently linked to the 3′ phosphoryl end of the broken DNA strand through a tyrosine residue (#723 on the human enzyme) (55). The 5′ hydroxyl end is minimally protected by the enzyme as compared to the enzyme-linked 3′ phosphoryl end. The strand containing the 5′ hydroxyl end is primarily held in place through its base-pairing with the complementary strand. The advancing fork may separate the two complementary strands (e.g., through its associated helicase action), resulting in the production of a double-strand break at the interface of the ternary complex and the fork.

little is known about the subsequent events from the cleavable complexes to cell death. Other cellular responses such as elevated levels of sister chromatid exchange, chromosomal aberration, G2 delay/arrest, and stimulation of differentiation of some cell lines may be tightly linked to the cell killing mechanism of topoisomerase poisons. Studies of the cell killing mechanisms and the complex cellular responses to topoisomerase poisons are likely to expand our understanding of DNA damage response in general and drug resistance to topoisomerase poisons in particular. The cloning of human topoisomerase genes and their overexpression will undoubtedly lead to more detailed understanding of the chemistry of drug–enzyme–DNA interactions. Furthermore, expression of foreign (e.g., human or parasite) DNA topoisomerases in microorganisms (e.g., yeast or *E. coli*) may make possible inexpensive screening of topoisomerase poisons against various diseases. The future of topoisomerase research in clinical pharmacology requires a multidisciplinary approach.

REFERENCES

1. Wang, J. C. Interaction between DNA and an *Escherichia coli* protein ω. J. Mol. Biol. 43: 263–272, 1969.
2. Champoux, J. J. and Dulbecco, R. An activity from mammalian cells that untwists superhelical DNA—A possible swivel for DNA replication. Proc. Natl. Acad. Sci. USA. 69: 143–146, 1972.
3. Gellert, M., Mizuuchi, K., O'Dea, M. H., and Nash, H. A. An enzyme that introduces superhelical turns into DNA. Proc. Natl. Acad. Sci. USA. 73: 3872–3876, 1976.
4. Liu, L. F., Liu, C. C., and Alberts, B. M. T4 DNA topoisomerase. A new ATP-dependent enzyme essential for the initiation of T4 bacteriophage DNA replication. Nature. 281: 456–461, 1979.
5. Liu, L. F., Depew, R. E., and Wang, J. C. Knotted single-stranded DNA rings: *A novel topological isomer of single-stranded circular DNA formed by E. coli omega protein treatment.* J. Mol. Biol. 106: 439–452, 1976.
6. Liu, L. F., Liu, C. C., and Alberts, B. M. Type II DNA topoisomerases. Enzymes that can unknot a topologically knotted DNA molecule via a reversible double-strand break. Cell. 19: 697–707, 1980.
7. Hsieh, T. S. and Brutlag, D. ATP dependent DNA topoisomerase from *D. melanogaster* reversibly catenates duplex DNA rings. Cell. 21: 115–125, 1980.
8. Kreuzer, K. N. and Cozzarelli, N. R. Formation and resolution of catenanes by DNA gyrase. Cell. 20: 245–254, 1980.
9. Marini, J. C., Miller, K. G., and Englund, P. T. Decatenation of kinetoplast DNA by topoisomerases. J. Biol. Chem. 255: 4976–4979, 1980.
10. Cozzarelli, N. R. DNA topoisomerases. Cell. 22: 327–328, 1980.
11. Dean, F., Krasnow, M. A., Otter, R., Matzuk, M. M., Spengler, S. J., and Cozzarelli, N. R. Escherichia coli type I DNA topoisomerases: Identification, mechanism, and roles in recombination. Cold Spring Harbor Symp. Quant. Biol. 47: 769–777, 1982.
12. Wallis, J. W., Chrebet, G., Brodsky, G., Rolfe, M., and Rothstein, R. A hyper-recombination mutation in *S. cerevisiae* identifies a novel eukaryotic DNA topoisomerase. Cell. 58: 409–419, 1989.
13. Kirkegaard, K. and Wang, J. C. Bacterial DNA topoisomerase I can relax positively supercoiled DNA containing a single-stranded loop. J. Mol. Biol. 185: 625–637, 1985.
14. Brown, P. O. and Cozzarelli, N. R. A sign inversion mechanism for enzymatic supercoiling of DNA. Science 206: 1081–1083, 1979.
15. McCoubrey, W. K., Jr. and Champoux, J. J. The role of single-strand breaks in the catenation reaction catalyzed by the rat type I topoisomerase. J. Biol. Chem. 261: 5130–5137, 1986.
16. Tse, Y. C. and Wang, J. C. *E. coli* and *M. luteus* DNA topoisomerase I can catalyze catenation or decatenation of double-stranded DNA rings. Cell. 22: 269–276, 1980.
17. Liu, L. F. and Miller, K. G. Eukaryotic DNA topoisomerases. Two forms of type I DNA topoisomerases from HeLa cell

nuclei. Proc. Natl. Acad. Sci. USA. **78:** 3487–3491, 1981.

18. Wang, J. C. DNA topoisomerases. Annu. Rev. Biochem. **54:** 665–697, 1985.

19. Wang, J. C. and Liu, L. F. DNA topoisomerases. Enzymes that catalyze the concerted breaking and rejoining of DNA bonds. In H. Taylor, ed. *Molecular Genetics*. New York: Academic Press, 1979, pp. 65–88.

20. Liu, L. F. and Wang, J. C. DNA-DNA gyrase complex. The wrapping of the DNA duplex outside the enzyme. Cell. **15:** 979–984, 1978.

21. Liu, L. F. and Wang, J. C. *Micrococcus luteus* gyrase: Active components and a model for its supercoiling of DNA. Proc. Natl. Acad. Sci. USA. **75:** 2098–2102, 1978.

22. Miller, K. G., Liu, L. F., and Englund, P. T. A homogeneous type II DNA topoisomerase from HeLa cell nuclei. J. Biol. Chem. **256:** 9334–9339, 1981.

23. Wang, J. C. Recent studies of DNA topoisomerases. Biochim. Biophys. Acta. **909:** 1–9, 1987.

24. Pflugfelder, M. T., Liu, L. F., Liu, A. A., Tewey, K. M., Whang-Peng, J., Knutsen, T., Huebner, K., Croce, C. M., and Wang, J. C. Cloning and sequencing of cDNA encoding human DNA topoisomerase II and localization of the gene to chromosome 17q21-22. Proc. Natl. Acad. Sci. USA. **85:** 7177–7181, 1988.

25. D'Arpa, P., Machlin, P. S., Ratrie, H., III., Rothfield, N. F., Cleveland, D. W., and Earnshaw, W. C. cDNA cloning of human DNA topoisomerase I: Catalytic activity of a 67.7-kDa carboxyl-terminal fragment. Proc. Natl. Acad. Sci. USA. **85:** 2543–2547, 1988.

26. Juan, C.-C., Hwang, J., Liu, A. A., Whang-Peng, J., Knutsen, T., Huebner, K., Croce, C. M., Zhang, H., Wang, J. C., and Liu, L. F. Human DNA topoisomerase I is encoded by a single-copy gene that maps to chromosome region 20q12-13.2. Proc. Natl. Acad. Sci. USA. **85:** 8910–8913, 1988.

27. Sundin, O. and Varshavsky, A. Terminal stages of SV40 DNA replication proceed via multiply intertwined catenated dimers. Cell. **21:** 103–114, 1980.

28. DiNardo, S., Voelkel, K., and Sternglanz, R. DNA topoisomerase II mutant of *Saccharomyces cerevisiae:* Topoisomerase II is required for segregation of daughter molecules at the termination of DNA replication. Proc. Natl. Acad. Sci., USA. **81:** 2616–2620, 1984.

29. Yang, L., Liu, L. F., Li, J. J., Wold, M. S., and Kelly, T. J. The roles of DNA topoisomerase in SV40 DNA replication. UCLA Symposia Mol. Cell. Biol. **47:** 315–326, 1986.

30. Uemura, T., Ohkura, H., Adachi, Y., Morino, K., Schiozaki, K., and Yanagida, M. DNA topoisomerase II is required for condensation and separation of mitotic chromosomes in *S. pombe.* Cell. **50:** 917–925, 1987.

31. Holm, C., Stearns, T., and Botstein, D. DNA topoisomerase II must act at mitosis to prevent nondisjunction and chromosome breakage. Mol. Cell Biol. **9:** 159168, 1989.

32. Liu, L. F. and Wang, J. C. Supercoiling of the DNA template during transcription. Proc. Natl. Acad. Sci. USA. **84:** 7024–7027, 1987.

33. Kim, R. A. and Wang, J. C. A subthreshold level of DNA topoisomerases leads to the excision of yeast rDNA as extrachromosomal rings. Cell. **57:** 975–985, 1989.

34. Christman, M. F., Dietrich, F. S., and Fink, G. R. Mitotic recombination in the rDNA of *S. cerevisiae* is suppressed by the combined action of DNA topoisomerase I and II. Cell. **55:** 413425, 1988.

35. Potmesil, M. and Ross, W. E., eds. Proceedings of the First Conference on DNA Topoisomerases in Cancer Chemotherapy. NCI Monographs. **4:** 1–133, 1987.

36. Liu, L. F. DNA topoisomerase poisons as antitumor drugs. Annu. Rev. Biochem. **58:** 351–375, 1989.

37. Sugino, A., Peebles, C. L., Kruezer, K. N., and Cozzarelli, N. R. Mechanism of action of nalidixic acid: Purification of *E. coli nal A* gene product and its relationship to DNA gyrase and a novel nicking-closing enzyme. Proc. Natl. Acad. Sci. USA. **74:** 4767–4771, 1977.

38. Gellert, M., Mizuuchi, K., O'Dea, M. H., Itoh, T., and Tomizawa, J. Nalidixic acid resistance: A second genetic character involved in DNA gyrase activity. Proc. Natl. Acad. Sci. USA. **74:** 4772–4776, 1977.

39. D'Arpa, P. and Liu, L. F. Topoisomerase-targeting antitumor drugs. Biochim. Biophys. Acta. **989:** 163–177, 1989.

40. Bodley, A. L., Liu, L. F., Israel, M., Giuliani, F. C., Silber, R., Kirschenbaum, S., and Potmesil, M. DNA topoisomerase II–mediated interaction of doxorubicin and daunomycin congeners with DNA. Cancer Res. **49:** 5969–5978, 1989.

41. Chow, K.-C., MacDonald, T. L., and Ross, W. E. DNA binding by epipodophyllotoxins and N-acyl anthracyclines: Implications for mechanism of topoisomerase II inhibition. Mol. Pharmacol. **34:** 467–473, 1988.

42. Rowe, T. C., Tewey, K. M., and Liu, L. F. Identification of the breakage and reunion subunit of T4 DNA topoisomerase. J. Biol. Chem. **259:** 9177–9181, 1984.

43. Shapiro, T. A. and Englund, P. T. Selective cleavage of kinetoplast DNA minicircles promoted by antitrypanosomal drugs. Proc. Natl. Acad. Sci. USA. **87:** 950–954, 1990.

44. Wall, M. E., Wani, M. C., Cooke, C. E., Palmer, K. H., McPhail, A. T. and Slim, G. A. S. Plant antitumor agents. I. The isolation and structure of camptothecin, a novel alkaloidal leukemia and tumor inhibitor from *Camptotheca acuminata*. J. Am. Chem. Soc. **88:** 3888–3890, 1966.

45. Giovanella, B. C., Stehlin, J. S., Wall, W. E., Wani, M. C., Nicholas, A. W. L., Liu, L. F., Silber, R., and Potmesil, M. DNA topoisomerase I targeted chemotherapy of human colon cancer in xenografts. Science. **246:** 1046–1048, 1989.

46. Hsiang, Y.-H., Hertzberg, R., Hecht, S., and Liu, L. F. Camptothecin induces protein-linked DNA breaks via mammalian DNA topoisomerase I. J. Biol. Chem. **260:** 14873–14878, 1985.

47. Hsiang, Y.-H. and Liu, L. F. Identification of mammalian DNA topoisomerase I as an intracellular target of the anticancer drug camptothecin. Cancer Res. **48:** 1722–1726, 1988.

48. Nelson, E. M., Tewey, K. M., and Liu, L. F. Mechanism of antitumor drugs. Poisoning of mammalian DNA topoisomerase II on DNA by an antitumor drug *m*-AMSA. Proc. Natl. Acad. Sci. USA. **81:** 1361–1365, 1984.

49. Hsiang, Y.-H., Lihou, M. G., and Liu, L. F. Mechanism of cell killing by camptothecin: Arrest of replication forks by drug-stabilized topoisomerase 1-DNA cleavable complexes. Cancer Res. **49:** 50775082, 1989.

50. Li, L. H., Fraser, T. J., Olin, E. J., and Bhuyan, B. K. Action of camptothecin on mammalian cells in culture. Cancer Res. **32:** 2643–2650, 1972.

51. Wilson, W. R. and Whitmore, G. F. Cell-cycle-stage specificity of 4'-(9-acridinylamino) methanesulfon-*m*-anisidide (*m*-AMSA) and interaction with ionizing radiation in mammalian cell cultures. Radiat. Res. **87:** 121136, 1981.

52. Nitiss, J. and Wang, J. C. DNA topoisomerase-targeting antitumor drugs can be studied in yeast. Proc. Natl. Acad. Sci. USA. **85:** 7501–7505, 1988.

53. Eng, W.-K., Faucette, L., Johnson, R. K., and Sternglanz, R. Evidence that DNA topoisomerase I is necessary for the cytotoxic effects of camptothecin. Mol. Pharmacol. **34:** 755–760, 1989.

54. Horwitz, S. B., Chang, C.-K., and Grollman, A. P. Antiviral action of camptothecin. Antimicrob. Agents Chemother. **2:** 395401, 1972.

Chapter 3
Analyses of the *Top2* Gene from *Drosophila melanogaster:* Structure, Mapping, and Expression

JAMES M. NOLAN, ELIZABETH WYCKOFF,
MAXWELL P. LEE, AND TAO-SHIH HSIEH

Type II DNA topoisomerases modulate the topology of DNA molecules by breaking a DNA duplex, passing another segment of DNA through this transient break, then religating it. This reaction is utilized by eukaryotic and the bacteriophage T4 topoisomerase II to relax supercoiled DNA, to knot or unknot circular DNAs, and to perform catenation and decatenation reactions between DNA circles. In addition to these activities, the bacterial type II topoisomerase, DNA gyrase, can introduce negative supercoils into circular DNA (for reviews of topoisomerases see ref. 1–4). Type II DNA topoisomerases are involved in many aspects of cellular DNA metabolism, most likely through their activity in modulating DNA and chromosome structures. In yeasts, topoisomerase II has been shown to be encoded by an essential gene, *TOP2*, in *Saccharomyces cerevisiae* (5,6) and *Schizosaccharomyces pombe* (7). Temperature-sensitive top2 mutants are defective in chromosome condensation and segregation during mitosis at the restrictive temperature; chromosomes apparently are sheared when cells attempt cytokinesis in the absence of topoisomerase activity (8–10). While DNA topoisomerase I is not an essential enzyme in yeast, strains with both topoisomerases inactivated genetically are immediately disrupted in DNA replication and RNA transcription (7, 11–13). Apparently, either topoisomerase I or II can relieve the superhelical tension generated during the processes of replication and transcription. Recent experiments also demonstrated that the expression of either type I or II topoisomerase can modulate the frequency of recombination in yeast cells (14–16).

The level of expression of DNA topoisomerase II appears to depend critically on the proliferative state of cells. In developing chick erythroid cells, topoisomerase II has been shown to be abundant in cells that are proliferating but undetectable in differentiated and nonproliferating cells (17). Both topoisomerases I and II are present in mammalian cells during all phases of the cell cycle; however, topoisomerase II is depleted in the cells that exit from the cell cycle and are arrested in G_o (18,19).

To establish a genetic system for analyzing the functions of DNA topo-isomerase II during the growth and development of *Drosophila melanogaster* we have cloned and characterized the gene for this enzyme, *Top2*, from Dro-sophila (20). In this paper, we summarize our results on the structural analysis of *Top2* and present its protein sequence homology to several other type II DNA topoisomerases. The Drosophila *Top2* gene has been mapped cytologi-cally to region 37D on the left arm of chromosome 2 (20). Several well-studied genes map near this region including *Dopa decarboxylase (Ddc)* at 37C (21), *Segregation distorter (Sd)* at 37D (22), and refractaire *(2)P (ref(2)P*, resistance to sigma virus) at 37E (23–25). As a result of these studies, there is a wealth of preexisting deficiency and lethal point mutations that map near *Top2*. Here we present a further refinement of the *Top2* map by localizing the *Top2* gene cy-tologically and physically with respect to deficiency mutations that map to this region. In addition we have analyzed the *in vivo* function of topoisomerase II in Drosophila by examining the temporal regulation of *Top2* gene expression throughout development. We present here an investigation of the level of *Top2* expression at both the mRNA and protein levels. These experiments demon-strate that the expression of Drosophila *Top2* is developmentally regulated and appears to correlate with cell division activity during the growth of this organ-ism.

MATERIALS AND METHODS

Fly Strains

All *VA* series deficiencies (T.R.F. Wright, personal communication) were from T.R.F. Wright (University of Virginia, Charlottesville). *Df(2L)TW2* and *Df(2L)TW158* (21), *Df(2L)pr26*, and *Df(2L)Sd57* (22) were from B. Ganetzky (University of Wisconsin, Madison).

Physical Mapping

DNA from various mutants was prepared from adult flies. Five hundred to 1000 frozen adults were lysed by Dounce homogenization in 20 ml 0.2 M sucrose, 50 mM Tris-HC1 (pH 7.9), 50 mM EDTA, 0.1% Triton X-100, filtered through Miracloth, and centrifuged 8 min at 8000 rpm in the HB-4 rotor (DuPont-Sor-vall). Pelleted nuclei were washed in 10 ml homogenization buffer and repel-leted. Nuclei were resuspended in 3 ml homogenization buffer and sarkosyl was added to 0.28%; samples were mixed gently, incubated 10 min on ice, then an equal weight of CsCl was added, followed by 0.03 volumes of 10 mg/ml ethid-ium bromide. Samples were centrifuged 36 h at 35,000 rpm in the AH-650 rotor (DuPont-Sorvall). Fluorescent bands were collected by syringe with a 16-gauge needle and extracted with butanol to remove ethidium. DNA was dialyzed 2 times each against TE + 1 M NaCl and TE (TE = 10 mM Tris-HC1, pH 7.9, 0.1 mM EDTA). Concentrations were measured by UV absorbance. Samples were digested with various restriction enzymes, electrophoresed on agarose gels, and blotted to nylon membrane. The membrane was baked 2 h at 80°C

under vacuum and prehybridized overnight at 42°C in a solution containing 5×
SSCP (1× SSCP = 0.15 M NaCl, 15 mM Na citrate, 10 mM Na phosphate,
pH 7.0), 50% formamide, 10× Denhardt's (1× Denhardt's = 0.02% each bovine serum albumin, Ficoll, and polyvinyl pyrollidone), and 0.5 mg/ml sonicated salmon sperm DNA. Hybridizations were carried out overnight at 42°C
in a mixture containing 10^6 cpm/ml probe DNA, 4× SSCP, 2× Denhardt's, 40%
formamide, 100 μg/ml sonicated salmon sperm DNA, 0.2% SDS, and 10% dex-
tran sulfate. Probes were labeled with [^{32}P] by DNA polymerase I nick-trans-
lation to a specific activity of 10^8 cpm/μg (26). Blots were washed at 55°C 2
times in 1× SSCP, 0.2% SDS for 15 min each, 2 times in 0.1× SSCP, 0.2%
SDS for 15 min each, dried briefly, and autoradiographed with Kodak XAR
film.

For analysis of proximal deficiency breakpoints using pulsed field gel electrophoresis (27), agarose DNA plugs were prepared from 0–24 h embryos. The
dechorionated embryos were homogenized by Dounce at a concentration of
0.25 g/ml in PBS (0.137 M NaCl, 2.68 mM KCl, 8.1 mM Na_2HPO_4 and 1.47 mM
KH_2PO_4, pH 7.0). An equal volume of 1% low gelling temperature agarose
(Sea-Plaque, FMC Bioproducts, Rockland, ME) was added and the agarose
solution was cast in a plastic mold. After gelling, the plugs were incubated in
0.4 M EDTA, 1% sarkosyl, 1 mg/ml proteinase K overnight at 50°C, and were
washed in TE as described (28). The high molecular weight DNA in the agarose
insert was digested with restriction enzymes and the digested DNA was fractionated on a CHEF gel (29) at 240 V with a switching time of 10 sec for 36 h.
DNA was blotted to nitrocellulose membrane and detected as described above.

Isolation of Staged Materials

All studies were performed on wild-type Oregon-R (P2) flies raised at 25°C.
Embryos were collected on yeasted corn syrup–agar plates, incubated on the
plate for the appropriate period of time, dechorionated in 50% chlorox, and
rinsed with 0.01% Triton X-100 and 0.7% NaCl. First and second instar larvae
were collected from plates of 0–24 h embryos incubated for an additional 1 or
2 days, respectively. For third instar larvae, pupae, and adults, 0–24 h embryos
were used to inoculate standard cornmeal media or Instant Drosophila Media
(Carolina Biological Co., Burlington, NC) supplemented with brewer's yeast.
Third instar larvae were collected after 4–5 days; pupae were collected 6–10
days after larval hatching. Adults were collected 0–2 days after eclosion. All
stages were frozen in liquid N_2 or a dry ice–ethanol bath and stored at −70°C.
Samples were ground under liquid N_2 with a mortar and pestle before lysis.

mRNA Isolation and Analysis

Total RNA was isolated from pulverized frozen material by a modification of
the method of Chirgwin et al. (30), substituting 10 mM vanadyl ribonucleoside
complexes (31) for EDTA. RNA was resuspended in water and polyA+ RNA
selected by 2 successive oligo dT cellulose column steps. Eluted mRNA was
quantitated by UV absorbance at 260 nm and was made 0.3 M in Na acetate,
then 2 volumes of ethanol were added and samples stored at −70°C. Five μg

samples from each stage were precipitated, resuspended in formaldehyde gel sample buffer (50% formamide, 2.2 M formaldehyde, 0.2 M MOPS, pH 7.0, 10 mM Na acetate, 2 mM EDTA), and denatured at 55°C for 15 min. RNA samples were analyzed by gel electrophoresis in 1% agarose containing 2.2 M formaldehyde (32). One-third of each sample was loaded onto a 1% agarose, 2.2 M formaldehyde gel run in 0.2 M MOPS, 10 mM Na acetate, 2 mM EDTA (pH 7.0) for ethidium staining; the remaining two-thirds were run on a second gel and blotted to Zeta-Probe membrane (Bio-Rad Laboratories, Richmond, CA) without staining. The blot was processed as described for physical mapping, using pGFc1, a full-length cDNA clone of Drosophila *Top2* as probe. Washes were as described in physical mapping, except that the wash temperature was 60°C. Autoradiograms were scanned on a Zieneth desitometer.

Topoisomerase II Protein Expression Analysis

Frozen, pulverized samples (0.5 g) were disrupted by Dounce homogenization on ice in Western lysis buffer (50 mM Tris-HC1, pH 7.9, 50 mM NaCl, 1 mM EDTA, 1 mM PMSF, 0.1 mM DTT, 0.05% Triton X-100) (fraction F1); an aliquot was mixed with an equal volume of SDS sample buffer (2% SDS, 100 mM DTT, 50 mM Tris-HC1, pH 6.8, 10% glycerol, 0.1% bromophenol blue) and frozen immediately. Protein concentration of F1 was assayed by Bradford method (33). One hundred μg and 50 μg samples of total protein from each stage were run on 6% polyacrylamide–SDS gels for blotting onto nitrocellulose (34). Topoisomerase II polypeptide was visualized by using monospecific antibody and autoradiography as described previously (35). For quantitation, the resulting autoradiograms were scanned as for the mRNA analysis. Then 50 μg samples from each stage were run on an identical gel and stained with Coomassie blue.

For nuclear and cytoplasmic fractionation of protein, a 200 μl aliquot of fraction F1 was centrifuged for 1 min in an Eppendorf microcentrifuge to pellet nuclei. The supernatant (F1S) was removed and an aliquot frozen in SDS sample buffer as before. The pellet was resuspended in 200 μl of Western lysis buffer (F1P), aliquotted, and frozen. Samples were then analyzed by immunoblot as above. For a given developmental stage, equal volumes of F1S and F1P were loaded on the gel. The volume for each stage was equivalent to the volume of F1 which contained 50 μg of total cell protein. Thus, for each developmental stage, equivalent weights of total cell protein were loaded; the bulk of the protein was in the cytoplasmic fraction. An identical gel was run and stained with Coomassie blue.

RESULTS

Structural Homology Among Type II DNA Topoisomerases

The similarity in the physical and biochemical properties of DNA topoisomerases II suggests that these enzymes are both functionally and structurally related. The protein sequences deduced from the sequence analysis of cloned

Top2 genes support this notion. Figure 3.1 summarizes the sequence homology observed by comparing the Drosophila enzyme (36) with *Bacillus subtilis* DNA gyrase (37), and topoisomerase II from bacteriophage T4 (38,39), *S. cerevisiae* (40), *S. pombe* (41), and human (42). Based upon the sequence–homology comparison, the eukaryotic enzymes can be divided into three domains: (1) an amino-terminal domain which is homologous to the B (ATPase) subunit of bacterial DNA gyrase; (2) a central region homologous to the A (DNA breakage and reunion) subunit of gyrase; and (3) a hydrophilic carboxyl-terminal region with alternating stretches of both the positively and negatively charged amino acids. The bacterial DNA gyrase sequence used in Figure 3.1 is from *B. subtilis*. We have also used the DNA gyrase sequence from *Escherichia coli* (43,44) and obtained very similar results. The bacteriophage T4 topoisomerase is encoded by 3 genes, *39, 52,* and *60* (45,46). The gene *39* protein shows homology to the bacterial *gyr*B protein and to the amino-terminal portion of eukaryotic topoisomerase (38). The gene *52* protein, which carries out the DNA breakage-reunion function (47), has homology to bacterial *gyr*A protein and to the central part of the eukaryotic enzyme (39). The sequences from gene *60* protein (48) are not included in the analysis shown in Figure 3.1. However, it contains some limited, but significant, homology to the central portion of eukaryotic enzyme at a region corresponding to the carboxyl terminal of *Gyr*B protein.

Among the eukaryotic type II DNA topoisomerases, there are approxi-

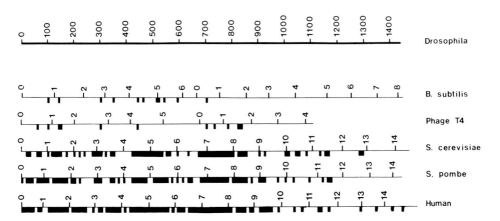

Figure 3.1. Sequence homology comparison among type II DNA topoisomerases. This figure is modified from Figure 5 in ref. 36. Each topoisomerase II was aligned with the Drosophila enzyme by a computer program from Wilbur and Lipman (61). The aligned sequences were divided into segments of 10 amino acids each, and for each segment with 5 or more identical aligned amino acids the line is broadened at a position directly below the homologous region in Drosophila enzyme. To maintain optimal homology, gaps are introduced into the alignment, so that the lengths along the lines are not always proportional to the lengths of amino acid residues. For indicating the locations of the homologies, the lengths along the sequences are marked in hundreds of amino acids. For *B. subtilis* gyrase the amino acid sequence of the B subunit is followed by the A subunit and for phage T4 enzyme, the gene *39* protein is followed by the gene *52* protein. The limited homology between phage T4 gene *60* protein and the regions corresponding to the C-terminal of gyrase B subunit is not shown here.

mately 40–50% of identity in their amino acid sequences. This level of structural homology is also reflected in the functional expression of these enzymes in heterologous hosts. The *Top2* genes from *S. cerevisiae* and *S. pombe* can complement temperature-sensitive mutations in the heterologous yeast (41). The Drosophila *Top2* gene can be functionally expressed in yeast and complements both the temperature-sensitive and disruption mutations in yeast *Top2* gene (49). The yeast system is also used as an efficient expression system for analyzing the structural-functional relationships of the Drosophila enzyme (D. Crenshaw, unpublished results).

Cytogenetic Mapping of *Top2*

Top2 has been mapped to chromosome 2L in a cytological region 37D (20). Cytogenetic localization was further refined by hybridizing *Top2* cDNA probe to salivary gland chromosomes of deficiency mutants whose deletions map to 37D. A summary of hybridizations to various deletions in the 37D region is shown in Figure 3.2; the genetic and cytological map data are summarized from ref. 22 and personal communications from T.R.F. Wright and P. Gay (see also ref. 50). The top line shows the map of the wild-type chromosome with the location of known lethal complementation groups indicated. Bracketed segments denote regions of the chromosome where the exact order of the lethal mutations is not known. Regions deleted from the deficiency chromosomes are

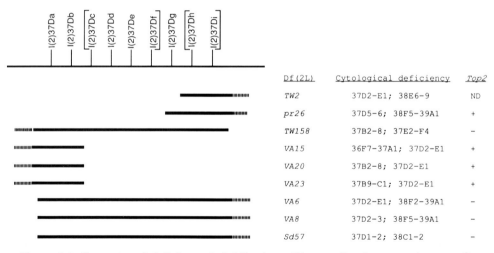

Figure 3.2. Summary of deficiency hybridizations. The top line is a genetic map of lethal point mutations of 37D. Brackets indicate that the exact gene order is not known for these segments. Deficiency chromosomes are listed below with the regions *deleted* by these deficiencies indicated by black bars. Deficiencies extend further in the directions indicated by the broken bars. The chromosomal segments deleted in these deficiencies (50) are shown in the column "cytological deficiency." In the "*Top2* column, "+" denotes deficiency chromosomes that hybridize to *Top2* DNA probes, deficiency chromosomes that do not are designated "−". ND stands for "not determined."

indicated by the horizontal bars; deleted regions continue in the direction of the broken bar. Deficiency chromosomes that hybridize to the *Top2* probe DNA are indicated by a plus sign in the *"Top 2"* column, those which do not are indicated by a minus sign. *Top2* is not deleted by the *Df(2L)VA15,VA20* and *VA23* deficiencies, which have their proximal breakpoints at 37D2-E1, nor by *Df(2L)pr26*, which has a distal breakpoint at 37D5-6. *Top2* is deleted by *Df(2L)VA6,VA8*, and *Sd57* whose distal breakpoints map to the left side of this region at 37D2-E1, 37D2-3, and 37D1-2, respectively. *Top2*, then, is flanked by deficiencies *VA15*, *VA20*, and *VA23* to the left and *pr26* to the right. Another deficiency, *Df(2L)TW2*, which has its distal breakpoint mapped at 37D2-E1, was not tested with *in situ* hybridization by *Top2* probe. However, the data presented in the following section on the physical mapping of this deficiency suggest that *TW2*, similar to *pr26*, does not remove *Top2*. These data, when taken together, indicate that *Top2* maps to a cytogenic region in 37D, most likely between 37D2 to 37D5–6. This region is also characterized by at least 4 existing complementation groups, *l(2)37Dc to l(2)37Df*.

Molecular Mapping

DNA from deficiency mutants was mapped by Southern blotting analysis (51) to define the breakpoints of deficiencies that might map near *Top2*. Figure 3.3 shows a map summarizing these results and also shows the probes used in this analysis. Map coordinate 0 is defined as the start site of *Top2* transcription, approximately 100 bp upstream of the *MluI* site (36); note that *Top2* is transcribed from right to left in this figure, since the map is oriented with the telomeric end of chromosome arm 2L to the left by convention.

DNA from deficiency heterozygotes whose deletions flank the 3' end of *Top2* were digested with *BamHI* or *BamHI* and *NotI* restriction endonucleases. *Df(2L)VA8/CyO* DNA was used as a control since the deficiency homolog does not hybridize to the DNA probes used, thus only sequences from the *CyO* balancer should be detected. One microgram of each of the digested DNAs was electrophoresed, blotted to nylon membrane, and probed with p102-5.3 (probe A in Fig. 3.3), which lies 3' to the *Top2* gene. The results are shown in Figure 3.4A. A single 13.2 kb band corresponding to the wild-type *BamHI* fragment is seen in the *VA8* control as well as the *pr26* and *TW2* proximal flanking deficiencies. The distal flanking deficiencies *VA20* and *VA23* also display this band, in addition, an 11.5 kb band for *VA20* and a 14.5 kb band for *VA23* (marked by arrows in Fig. 3.4A). These additional bands apparently result from loss of the wild-type chromosome segment near the *BamHI* site at map coordinate +22.5 due to the deletion mutation. In the *BamHI/NotI* double digest, the 13.2 kb band is digested to 10.2 kb in all strains, but the 11.5 kb and 14.5 kb bands remain. This indicates that both deletions include the *NotI* site at map coordinate +19.4. Since the physical mapping data show that the *VA20* and *VA23* breakpoints lie at the 3' end of the *Top2* gene and the cytogenetic data indicate that these breakpoints are distal to *Top2* on the left arm of chromosome 2, the *Top2* gene must then be transcribed in the centromere-to-telomere direction.

The deletion endpoints of *VA20* and *VA23* were mapped with a number of

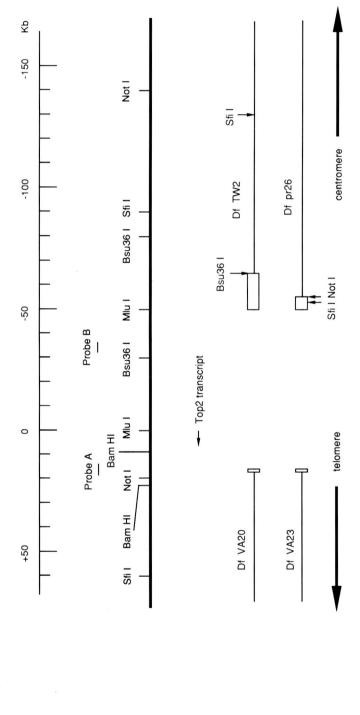

Figure 3.3. Molecular map of *Top2* locus. Map coordinates are given above the map, and they are defined by their distance, in kb, to the start of *Top2* transcription. DNA segments 3′ or 5′ to the *Top2* transcript are marked by positive or negative distance, respectively. A partial restriction map for the wild-type chromosome (thick line) is shown with the relevant restriction cleavage sites indicated above the map. Segments deleted by deficiencies are shown as thin lines below the wild-type map; open boxes designate regions of uncertainty for the breakpoints of the deficiencies. The novel sites in the deficiency segments are indicated by downward arrows in *TW2* and upward arrows in *pr26*. The *Top2* transcript is shown transcribed from right to left. Orientation with respect to the telomere and centromere are indicated by arrows. The DNA probes used in Figure 3.4 are also shown here to indicate their locations in this molecular map.

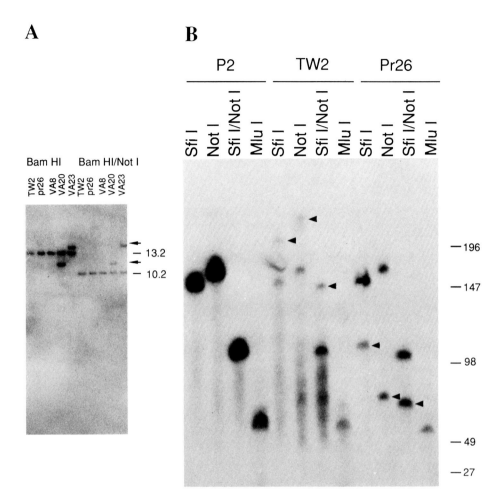

Figure 3.4. Southern blot analysis of deficiencies. **A.** Mapping the deletion endpoints of *Df*(2L)*VA20* and *VA23*. *Bam*HI or *Bam*HI/*Not*I digests of genomic DNA from the indicated deficiencies were resolved on an agarose gel, blotted, probed with p102-5.3 (probe A), and autoradiographed. Molecular weights inferred for labeled wild-type bands are indicated. Arrows denote junction fragments generated by deficiency chromosomes. **B.** Mapping the deletion endpoints of *Df(2L)TW2* and *pr26*. Genomic DNA prepared from wild-type (Oregon R, P2) and deficiencies were digested with *Sfi*I, *Not*I, *Sfi*I/*Not*I, and *Mlu*I. The DNA fragments were resolved by pulsed field gel electrophoresis, blotted, probed with p135A (probe B) and radioautographed. Molecular weights of the DNA size markers are shown, and the arrowheads indicate the novel junction fragments in the deficiency chromosome.

restriction enzymes and hybridization probes. For instance, a similar analysis using either *Bgl*II digests or *Xba*I digests indicated that both breakpoints mapped between the *Xba*I site at + 16.2 and the *Bgl*II site at coordinate + 17.0 (data not shown). Thus, both breakpoints map within 0.8 kb of each other, between + 16.2 and + 17.0 on the physical map. These deletions obviously represent independent events, however, since they have different restriction maps. In addition, their distal breakpoints map to different cytological locations; the distal breakpoint of *VA20* is 37B2-8 and that of *VA23* is 37B9-C1 (T.R.F. Wright, personal communication).

Since we have not cloned the DNA segment that would straddle the distal breakpoints of deficient chromosomes *Df(2)TW2* and *Df(2)pr26*, we used the pulsed field gel electrophoresis to analyze the long restriction DNA fragment generated from this region and deduced the deletion endpoints from these data. Embryonic DNAs from the laboratory Drosophila strain of Oregon R (P2), the heterozygote deficiencies *Df(2)TW2/Cy0* and *Df(2)pr26/Cy0* were isolated *in situ* in the agarose blocks. They were treated with restriction enzymes *Sfi*I, *Not*I, *Mlu*I, and *Sfi*I/*Not*I double digest and analyzed by pulsed field gel electrophoresis to resolve DNA fragments ranging between 20 to 200 kb (Fig. 4B). The gell was then blotted and probed with p135A (probe B in Fig. 3.3), which is located around 32 kb 5' to the *Top2* gene. The Southern blot analysis shows that while *Mlu*I digests yield a DNA band about 50 kb in all 3 samples, there are novel DNA fragments, in comparison with the wild-type chromosome, produced in the DNA digests of *Sfi*I or *Not*I and in the double digest of *Sfi*I/*Not*I. These results suggest that the deletion boundaries map between *Mlu*I (at map coordinate − 50) and *Sfi*I (at − 90) or *Not*I (at − 140). Similar experiments with restriction digest of *Bsu*36I locate the deletion ends to a region between − 50 (*Mlu*I site) and − 80 (*Bsu*36I site). The introduction of new restriction sites in the deficient chromosomes, like *Bsu*36I (at − 65) and *Sfi*I (at − 130) in *TW2* as well as *Sfi*I and *Not*I (at about − 55) in *pr26*, has further allowed us to deduce that the breakpoint of *TW2* maps in a region of 15kb segment between − 50 and − 65 and the breakpoint of *pr26* maps to a 5 kb region between − 50 and − 55 (Fig. 3.3). An assumption essential in interpreting these mapping data is that the alterations in restriction sites are due to the sequence change from the chromosome rearrangement in these deficiency strains, rather than from another mechanism such as restriction site polymorphism. While we cannot rule out the latter possibility, a similar analysis using the DNA from *Sc0/Cy0* heterozygotes gave the same restriction pattern as the P2 Oregon R (data not shown). Neither the *Sc0* nor *Cy0* chromosomes involves any sequence rearrangement in the *Top2* locus based upon the cytogenetic data (52). Another assumption invoked here is the alteration of restriction sites being limited to those located at 5' to *Top2*, rather than the 3' side. It is apparent from Figure 3.4A that the *Not*I at 3' side of *Top2* located at + 19.4 is not changed in *TW2* and *pr26*. We do not have any data directly bearing on the mapping of *Sfi*I site (at + 60) in *TW2* and *pr26;* however, the available restriction digestion data are all consistent with the map shown in Figure 3.3. It is also interesting to note that the breakpoints mapped physically for *VA20*, *VA23*, *TW2*, and *pr26* are also consistent with the cytogenetic map data (see Fig. 3.2).

Developmental Regulation of *Top2* Expression

The temporal regulation of *Top2* gene expression during Drosophila development was investigated by blot analysis of mRNA and protein fractions of Drosophila individuals collected at various time points during development. For
mRNA analysis, polyA$^+$ RNA was prepared and 5 µg samples from each stage
were fractionated on a denaturing formaldehyde agarose gel, blotted to nylon
membrane and probed with labeled *Top2* full-length cDNA. A 5.1 kb band was
seen for all stages (data not shown). For protein analysis, equal amounts of
protein from crude homogenates of various stages were fractionated on SDS–
polyacrylamide gels, blotted to nitrocellulose, and topoisomerase II protein detected with polyclonal rabbit antitopoisomerase antibodies and ^{125}I-protein A;
a 170 kd band was detected for all developmental stages (data not shown).
Figure 3.5 is a graphic comparison of the relative expression levels of *Top2*
message and protein obtained by densitometric scanning of the mRNA and
protein blot autoradiograms.

Topoisomerase II protein levels increase throughout embryogenesis, peak-
ing at 6–12 h, while mRNA levels are highest in early embryos and decrease

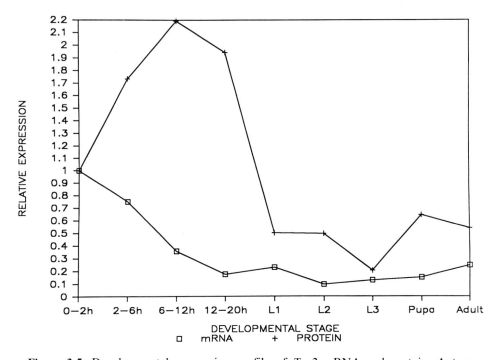

Figure 3.5. Developmental expression profile of *Top2* mRNA and protein. Autoradiograms of mRNA and protein blots were densitometrically scanned to quantitate
relative levels of protein and message expression. For both protein and mRNA, densitometric signals for each time point were normalized to that for the earliest time point,
0–2 h embroys. 0–2h, 2–6h, 6–12h, 12–20h indicate the age in hours of embryo samples;
L1, L2, and L3 indicate 1st, 2nd, and 3rd larval instars, respectively. Pupal and adult
time points are also indicated.

throughout embryogenesis. Both protein and message levels decrease throughout larval stages and rise again in the pupal sample, which includes both prepupae and pupae. These results are similar to those seen previously (53) and indicate that *Top2* expression levels parallel the level of DNA synthesis during development (54,55). *Top2* protein expression more closely parallels the level of DNA synthesis than does *Top2* mRNA expression. DNA synthesis peaks at 6 h after egg deposition (55) and again in prepupae (54). Topoisomerase II protein levels also peak at 6–12 h during embryogenesis and again in prepupae and pupae. This fluctuation in mRNA and protein levels is specific for *Top2*, since the levels of message for a constitutively expressed gene, Dmras 64B (56), are similar among all RNA samples (data not shown). In addition, a Coomassie stained gel of protein samples shows no generalized proteolysis of other proteins during periods of low topoisomerase expression, such as the larval stages (data not shown). Furthermore, only very limited amount of proteolytic fragments of topoisomerase II are detected for all developmental stages, indicating that there is no significant proteolysis of topoisomerase II in samples from various developmental stages.

Localization of Topoisomerase II Protein

Top2 protein expression was further characterized by centrifugation of crude homogenates to separate nuclei and cytoplasm. Nuclear and cytoplasmic fractions from various developmental stages were analyzed by immunoblot; the autoradiogram and densitometric analysis are shown in Figure 3.6A and 3.6B, respectively. The bulk of topoisomerase II is localized in the cytoplasm during early embryogenesis, but shifts to the nucleus as embryogenesis and cell proliferation progress. Topoisomerase II is localized almost exclusively in the nucleus during late embryonic, larval, and pupal stages. Some cytoplasmic distribution is seen again in adults. These results suggest that excess topoisomerase II is stored in the egg cytoplasm, perhaps maternally; as development progresses, stored and newly synthesized topoisomerase II are titrated out of the cytoplasm by increasing amounts of nuclei produced during cell division. This dramatic alteration in the distribution of the bulk topoisomerase II during embryogenesis can also be demonstrated by *in situ* immunostaining of fixed, permeabilized Drosophila embryos (data not shown).

Figure 3.6. Cytological distribution of topoisomerase II during development. **A.** 50 μg of total cell protein from each developmental stage were separated into nuclear and cytoplasmic fractions, then electrophoresed, blotted, and detected with antitopoisomerase antibodies and labeled protein A. CYT, cytoplasmic fraction; NUC, nuclear fraction for the indicated developmental stage. "TOPO II MARKER" lane carries 45 ng of topoisomerase II protein. **B.** The above autoradiogram was scanned and the topoisomerase II marker was used as a standard for topoisomerase protein concentration. This value was used to calculate the percentage of total cell protein for each sample. Developmental time points are as indicated in Figure 3.5.

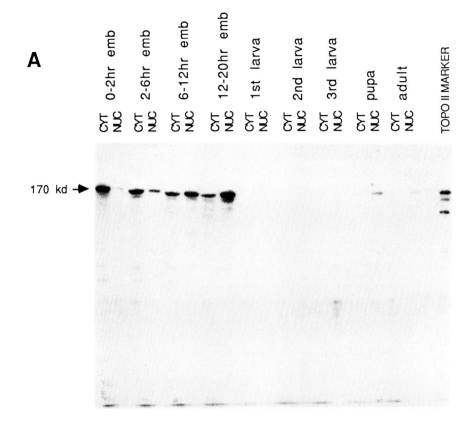

A

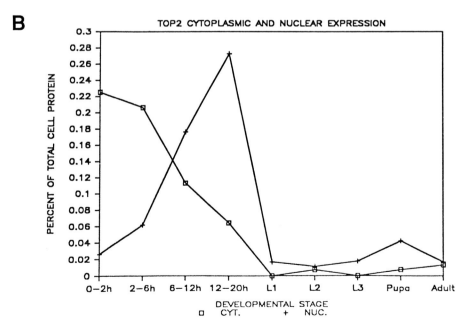

B

DISCUSSION

From the available amino acid sequences of several type II DNA topoisomerases, it is already apparent that these enzymes are fairly conserved during the course of evolution. Therefore, an interesting question is to ask if they share the same spectra of biological functions. The development of heterologous expression systems should facilitate addressing this type of question. A useful application of an efficient expression system is to investigate the structural and functional relationship of these enzymes. An obvious target for the structure–function analysis is the hydrophilic carboxyl-terminal portion of the eukaryotic topoisomerase II. While this general structure is shared by all the eukaryotic enzymes, there is no strong homology at the amino acid sequence level. This is in contrast with the other two domains, namely, the *gyr*B- and *gyr*A- homologous domains, which are highly conserved at the sequence level. It will therefore be interesting to probe the possible biological functions of this C-terminal domain.

In an effort to develop Drosophila as a genetic system to analyze the functions of DNA topoisomerase II, we have further refined the mapping of this gene at both the cytogenetic and molecular levels. From the *in situ* hybridization, *Top2* is located at map position between 37D2 and 37D5–6 on the left arm of chromosome 2. *Top2* is not deleted by the distal deficiencies *VA15, VA20,* and *VA23* nor the proximal deficiency *pr26* which map in the 37D region. It is therefore now possible to screen lethal mutations that map to this region but are not deleted by these deficiencies as putative *Top2* mutations. Four known complementation groups, *1(2)37Dc–1(2)37Df,* map between these deficiencies. These lethal mutants can be studied to determine which, if any, of them, are *Top2* mutations. In addition to these lethal mutations, the meiotic drive mutant, *Segregation distorter (Sd),* maps to this region; segregation distortion involves a number of loci (reviewed in 57). Males carrying *Sd* that are heterozygous for a sensitive responder locus near the centromere of chromosome 2 produce no sperm that carries the sensitive 2nd chromosome, and instead produce almost exclusively sperm with the *Sd*-bearing homolog of chromosome 2. One would expect *Top2* mutations to have some effect on meiosis, given the mitotic phenotype of *TOP2* in yeast. To date, however, there are no data supporting the hypothesis that the *Sd* phenotype is related to any alterations of *Top2* expression.

The breakpoints of *Df(2L)VA20* and *VA23* were mapped physically with respect to the *Top2* gene. Both map 3' to *Top2,* between 16.2 and 17.0 kb downstream of the *Top2* transcription initiation site. These breakpoints map very close to each other physically and may then represent a hot spot for deletion mutations in this region. The breakpoints of *Df(2L)TW2* and *pr26* were also deduced from the restriction digestion data using the pulsed field gel electrophoresis to resolve long DNA fragments ranging up to 200 kb in length. These physical mapping data, when considered in toto, suggest that the cytogenetic region of 37D2–6 likely corresponds to a segment of DNA with the length between 65 to 80 kb. The physical mapping of these breakpoints indicate that *Top2* is transcribed in the centromere-to-telomere direction.

The studies of the developmental expression of *Top2* presented here show a strong correlation between expression of the Drosophila *Top2* gene and periods of increased DNA synthesis, specifically, the embryonic and prepupal stages of development. Both *Top2* mRNA and protein levels are elevated at these developmental stages. DNA polymerase α activity has been shown to increase at these times of development as well (58). Peaks in topoisomerase II protein levels correlate particularly well with peak periods of DNA synthesis; both peak at approximately 6 h during embryogenesis and in prepupae. The high levels of *Top2* mRNA in 0–2 h embryos suggest that this message is transcribed maternally and stored in the egg, since there is little transcription in embryos in the 2 h after egg deposition (55). It is also interesting to note the difference in kinetics of *Top2* protein and mRNA expression. *Top2* message levels are highest in early embryos and decrease throughout embryogenesis; *Top2* protein levels, however, peak 6–12 h into embryogenesis. Since these are steady-state levels, it is not clear if the accumulation of protein is due to altered stability of the enzyme or increased translational efficiency of the message in 6–12 h embryos.

High levels of cytoplasmic topoisomerase II protein are characteristic of early embryonic stages; later in embryogenesis, topoisomerase II is located primarily in the nucleus. The cytoplasmic topoisomerase II may represent stored protein that is taken up by nuclei as they proliferate during development. We do not have any data addressing the quantitative extent of maternal contribution versus zygotic synthesis in the fertilized eggs. Some cytoplasmic topoisomerase II is seen again in pupae and adults. Both male and female adults have cytoplasmic topoisomerase II; however, the proportion of topoisomerase II in the same amount of total cell proteins is 50% higher in females than in males (data not shown).

The larval instars are periods of relatively high levels of transcription but low levels of DNA replication. *Top2* protein and message levels are at a minimum during these periods. This suggests that large amounts of topoisomerase II are not required for transcription. The available data suggest that Drosophila DNA topoisomerase I is specifically associated with transcribed regions of chromatin (59,60). Therefore, our results show a strong correlation between high levels of *Top2* expression and periods of increased DNA replication and cell proliferation; no association is seen between *Top2* expression and periods of transcriptional activation. Developmental studies are limited to such correlations. We are at present attempting to determine whether or not any of the existing mutants that map near *Top2* are *Top2* mutations. Phenotypic characterization of *Top2* mutants from Drosophila will provide a more definitive description of the role of topoisomerase II in the living cell.

Acknowledgments

We are extremely grateful to Drs. Ted Wright, Barry Ganetzky, and Pierre Gay for their generous gift of fly strains and for communicating their unpublished results. We thank Mike Murphy for his dedicated technical assistance in perfecting the *in situ* hybridization techniques, and Gerda Vegara for help in preparing the figures. We also acknowledge the chromosome-walking effort of H. C. Chi from the Molecular Biology Institute, Academia Sinica, Taipei, Taiwan, and his generous supply of plasmid p135A. This work is supported by a grant from NIH (GM29006).

REFERENCES

1. Cozzarelli, N. R. DNA topoisomerases. Science. **207**: 953–960, 1980.
2. Gellert, M. DNA topoisomerases. Annu. Rev. Biochem. **50**: 879–910, 1981.
3. Liu, L. F. DNA topoisomerases-enzymes that catalyze the breaking and rejoining of DNA. CRC Crit. Rev. Biochem. **15**: 1–24, 1983.
4. Wang, J. C. DNA topoisomerase. Annu. Rev. Biochem. **54**: 665–697, 1985.
5. Goto, T. and Wang, J. C. Yeast DNA topoisomerase II is encoded by a single-copy essential gene. Cell. **36**: 1073–1080, 1984.
6. DiNardo, S., Voelkel, K., and Sternglanz, R. DNA topoisomerase II mutant of *Saccharomyces cervisiae:* Topoisomerase II is required for segregation of daughter molecules at the termination of DNA replication. Proc. Natl. Acad. Sci. USA. **81**: 2616–2620, 1984.
7. Uemura, T. and Yanagida, M. Isolation of type I and II DNA topoisomerase mutants from fission yeast: Single and double mutants show different phenotypes in cell growth and chromatin organization. EMBO J. **3**: 1737–1744, 1984.
8. Holm, C., Goto, T. Wang, J. C., and Botstein, D. DNA topoisomerase II is required at the time of mitosis in yeast. Cell. **41**: 553–563, 1985.
9. Uemura, T. and Yanagida, M. Mitotic spindle pulls but fails to separate chromosomes in type II DNA topoisomerase mutants: Uncoordinated mitosis. EMBO J. **5**: 1003–1010, 1986.
10. Uemura, T., Ohkura, H., Adachi, Y., Morino, K.,Shiozaki, K., and Yanagida, M. DNA topoisomerase II is required for condensation and separation of mitotic chromosomes in *S. pombe*. Cell. **50**: 917–925, 1987.
11. Goto, T. and Wang, J. C. Cloning of yeast TOP1 the gene encoding DNA topoisomerase I and the construction of mutants defective in both DNA topoisomerase I and topoisomerase II. Proc. Natl. Acad. Sci. USA **82**: 7178–7182, 1985.
12. Brill, S., DiNardo, S., Voelkel-Meiman, K., and Sternglanz, R. Need for DNA topoisomerase activity as a swivel for DNA replication and for transcription of ribosomal RNA. Nature. **326**: 414–416, 1987.
13. Kim, R. A. and Wang, J. C. Function of DNA topoisomerases as replication swivels in *Saccharomyces cerevisiae*. J. Mol. Biol. **208**: 257–267, 1989.
14. Christman, M. F., Dietrich, F. S., and Fink, G. R. Mitotic recombination in the rDNA of *S. cerevisiae* is suppressed by the combined action of DNA topoisomerases I and II. Cell. **55**: 413–425, 1988.
15. Kim, R. A. and Wang, J. C. A subthreshold level of DNA topoisomerases leads to the excision of yeast and DNA as extrachromosomal rings. Cell. **57**: 975–985, 1989.
16. Wallis, J. W., Chrebet, G., Brodsky, G., Rolfe, M., and Rothstein, R. A hyperrecombination mutation in *S. cerevisiae* identifies a novel eucaryotic topoisomerase. Cell. **58**: 409–419, 1989.
17. Heck, M. M. S. and Earnshaw, W. C. Topoisomerase II: A specific marker for cell proliferation. J. Cell Biol. **103**: 2569–2581, 1986.
18. Hsiang, Y.-H., Wu, H.-Y., and Liu, L. F. Proliferation-dependent regulation of DNA topoisomerase II in cultured human cells. Cancer Res. **48**: 3230–3235, 1988.
19. Heck, M. M. S., Hittelman, W. N., and Earnshaw, W. C. Differential expression of DNA topoisomerases I and II during the eucaryotic cell cycle. Proc. Natl. Acad. Sci. USA. **85**: 1086–1090, 1988.
20. Nolan, J. M., Lee, M. P. Wyckoff, E., and Hsieh, T. Isolation and characterization of the gene encoding Drosophila DNA topoisomerase II. Proc. Natl. Acad. Sci. USA. **83**: 3664–3668, 1986.
21. Wright, T. R. F., Hodgetts, R. B., and Sherald, A. F. The genetics of dopa decarboxylase in *Drosophila melanogaster*. I. Isolation and characterization of deficiencies that delete the dopa decarboxylase dosage sensitive region and the α methyl dopa hypersensitive locus. Genetics. **84**: 267–285, 1976.
22. Brittnacher, J. G. and Ganetzky, B. On the components of Segregation distortion in *Drosophila melanogaster*. II. Deletion mapping and dosage analysis of the Sd locus. Genetics. **103**: 659–674, 1983.
23. Gay, P. Les genes de la Drosophile qui interviennent dans la multiplication du vi-

rus sigma. Mol. Gen. Genet. 159: 269–283, 1978.

24. Nakamura, N. Influence du dosage de l'allele non permissif du gene ref(2)P de la Drosophile sur les souches sensibles du virus sigma. Mol. Gen. Genet. **159**: 285–292, 1978.

25. Nakamura, N., Gay, P., and Contamine, D. Etude du locus ref(2)P de *Drosophila melanogaster*. I. Localisation cytogenetique de ref(2)P. Biol. Cell. **56**: 227–237, 1986.

26. Rigby, P. W. J., Dieckmann, M., Rhodes, C., and Berg, P. Labelling deoxyribonucleic acid to high specific activity in vitro by nick translation with DNA polymerase I. J. Mol. Biol. **113**: 237–251, 1977.

27. Schwartz, D. C. and Cantor, C. R. Separation of yeast chromosome-sized DNAs by pulsed field gradient gel electrophoresis. Cell. **37**: 67–75, 1984.

28. Smith, C. L., Warburton, P. E., Gaal, A., and Cantor, C. R. Analysis of genome organization and rearrangement by pulsed field gradient gel electrophoresis. In J. K. Setlow and A. Hollaender, eds. *Genetic Engineering,* Vol 8 1986, pp. 45–70.

29. Chu, G., Vollrath, D., and Davis, R. W. Separation of large DNA molecules by contour-clamped homogeneous electric fields. Science. **234**: 1582–1585, 1986.

30. Chirgwin, J. M., Przybyla, A. E., MacDonald, R. J., and Rutter, W. J. Isolation of biologically active ribonucleic acid from sources enriched in ribonuclease. Biochemistry. **18**: 5294–5299, 1979.

31. Berger, S. L. and Birkenmeier, C. S. Inhibition of intractable nucleases with ribonucleoside-vanadyl complexes: Isolation of messenger ribonucleic acid from resting lymphocytes. Biochemistry. **18**: 5143–5149, 1979.

32. Lehrach, H., Diamond, D., Wozney, J. M., and Boedtker, H. RNA molecular weight determinations by gel electrophoresis under denaturing conditions: A critical review. Biochemistry. **16**: 4743–4751, 1977.

33. Bradford, M. M. A rapid and sensitive method for the quantitation of microgram quantities of protein utilizing the principle of protein-dye binding. Anal. Biochem. **72**: 248–254, 1976.

34. Towbin, H., Staehelin, T., and Gordon, J. Electrophoretic transfer of proteins to nitrocellulose sheets: Procedure and some applications. Proc. Natl. Acad. Sci. USA. **76**: 4350–4354, 1979.

35. Sander, M. and Hsieh, T. Double-strand cleavage by type II DNA topoisomerase from *Drosophila melanogaster*. J. Biol. Chem. **258**: 8421–8428, 1983.

36. Wyckoff, E., Natalie, D., Nolan, J. M., Lee, M., and Hsieh, T. Structure of the Drosophila DNA topoisomerase II gene: Nucleotide sequence and homology among topoisomerases II. J. Mol. Biol. **205**: 1–13, 1989.

37. Moriya, S., Ogasawara, N., and Yoshikawa, H. Structure and function of the region of the replication origin of the Bacillus subtilis chromosome. III. Nucleotide sequence of some 10,000 base pairs in the origin region. Nucleic Acids Res. **13**: 2251–2265, 1985.

38. Huang, W. M. Nucleotide sequence of a type II DNA topoisomerase gene. Bacteriophage T4 gene 39. Nucleic Acids Res. **14**: 7751–7765, 1986.

39. Huang, W. M. Nucleotide sequence of a type II DNA topoisomerase gene. Bacteriophage T5 gene 52. Nucleic Acids Res. **14**: 7379–7390, 1986.

40. Lynn, R., Giaever, G., Swanberg, S. L., and Wang, J. C. Tandem regions of yeast DNA topoisomerase II share homology with different subunits of bacterial gyrase. *Science* 233: 647–649, 1986.

41. Uemura, T., Morikawa, K., and Yanagida, M. The nucleotide sequence of the fission yeast DNA topoisomerase II gene: Structural and functional relationships to other DNA topoisomerases. EMBO J. **5**: 2355–2361, 1986.

42. Tsai-Pflugfelder, M., Liu, L. F., Liu, A. A., Tewey, K. M., Whang-Peng, J., Knutsen, T., Huebner, K., Croce, C. N., and Wang, J. C. Cloning and sequencing of cDNA encoding human DNA topoisomerase II and localization of the gene to chromosome region 17q21-22. Proc. Natl. Acad. Sci. USA. **85**: 7177–7181, 1986.

43. Adachi, T., Mizuuchi, M., Robinson, E. A., Appella, E., O'Dea, M. H., Gellert, M., and Mizuuchi, K. DNA sequence of the *E. coli gyrB* gene: Application of a new sequencing strategy. Nucleic Acids Res. **15**: 771–783, 1987.

44. Swanberg, S. and Wang, J. C. Cloning and sequencing of *Escherichia coli gyrA* gene coding for the A subunit of DNA gyrase. J. Mol. Biol. **197**: 729–736, 1987.

45. Liu, L. F., Liu, C. C., and Alberts, B. M. T4 DNA topoisomerase: A new ATP-dependent enzyme essential for initiation of T4 bacteriophage DNA replication. Nature. **281**: 456–461, 1979.

46. Stetler, G. L., King, G. J., and Huang, W. M. T4 DNA-delay proteins required for specific DNA replication form a complex that has ATP-dependent DNA topoisomerase activity. Proc. Natl. Acad. Sci. USA. **76**: 3737–3741, 1979.

47. Rowe, T. C., Tewey, K. M., and Liu, L. F. Identification of the breakage-reunion subunit of T4 DNA topoisomerase. J. Biol. Chem. **259**: 9177–9181, 1984.

48. Huang, W. M., Ao, S-H., Casjens, S., Or-

landi, R., Zeikus, R., Weiss, R., Winge, D., and Fang, M. A persistent untranslated sequence within bacteriophage T4 DNA topoisomerase gene 60. Science. **239:** 1005–1012, 1988.

49. Wyckoff, E. and Hsieh, T. Functional expression of a Drosophila gene in yeast: Genetic complementation by DNA topoisomerase II. Proc. Natl. Acad. Sci. USA. **85:** 6272–6276, 1988.

50. Lindsley, D. and G. Zimm. The genome of *Drosophila melanogaster,* Part 2. Drosophila Information Service. **64:** 1–158, 1986.

51. Southern, E. M. Detection of specific sequences among DNA fragments separated by agarose gel electrophoresis. J. Mol. Biol. **98:** 503–517, 1975.

52. Lindsley, D. and Grell, E. H. Genetics variations of *Drosophila melanogaster.* Carnegie Institution of Washington Publication 627, 1968.

53. Fairman, R. and Brutlag, D. L. Expression of the Drosophila type II topoisomerase is developmentally regulated. Biochemistry. **27:** 560–565, 1988.

54. Church, R. B. and Robertson, F. W. A biochemical study of the growth of *Drosophila melanogaster.* J. Exp. Zool. **162:** 337–352, 1967.

55. Anderson, K. V. and Lengyel, J. A. Changing rates of DNA and RNA synthesis in Drosophila embryos. Dev. Biol. **82:** 127–138, 1981.

56. Mozer, B., Marlor, R., Parkhurst, S., and Corces, V. Characterization and developmental expression of a Drosophila ras oncogene. Mol. Cell. Biol. **5:** 885–889, 1985.

57. Sandler, L. and Golic, K. Segregation distortion in Drosophila. Trends in Genetics. **1:** 181–185, 1985.

58. Dusenbery, R. L. and Smith, P. D. DNA polymerase activity in developmental stages of *Drosophila melanogaster.* Dev. Genet. **3:** 309–327, 1983.

59. Fleischman, G., Pflugfelder, G., Steiner, E. K., Javacherian, K., Howard, G. C., Wang, J. C., and Elgin, S. C. R. Drosophila DNA topoisomerase I is associated with transcriptionally active regions of the genome. Proc. Natl. Acad. Sci. USA. **81:** 6958–6962, 1984.

60. Gilmour, D. S., Pflugfelder, G., Wang, J. C., and Lis, J. T. Topoisomerase I interacts with transcribed regions in Drosophila cells. Cell. **44:** 401–407, 1986.

61. Wilbur, W. J. and Lipman, D. J. Rapid similarity searches of nucleic acid and protein data banks. Proc. Natl. Acad. Sci. USA. **80:** 726–730, 1983.

Chapter 4

Possible Roles of DNA Topology in DNA–Topoisomerase II Interactions

MICHAEL HOWARD
AND JACK GRIFFITH

The central role of topoisomerase II in DNA metabolism has been clearly documented by the work of many laboratories, and these contributions are illustrated by the spectrum of studies in this volume. Topoisomerase II is required for the separation of daughter molecules following DNA replication in yeast (1,2) and the replication of closed circular DNAs such as SV40 (3). Topoisomerase I and II play a central role in controlling the superhelical torsion of circular or circularly constrained DNAs, and alterations in the superhelical density have been shown to have profound effects on the transcriptional template capacity of DNAs (reviewed in 4,5). In addition, transcription of DNA in the presence of topoisomerases appears to be a major factor in establishing the superhelical density of DNA in the cell (6). The discovery that the sites on eukaryotic DNA to which it attaches to the nuclear scaffold (SAR or MAR elements) usually contain sites for topoisomerase II cleavage is not surprising if these enzymes regulate the torsional stress of eukaryotic DNA (7,8).

In *Escherichia coli* the circular chromosome is subdivided into roughly 50 independent domains of supertwisting (9,10). Studies of the binding of DNA gyrase to the *E. coli* chromosome have revealed about the same number of cleavage sites for DNA gyrase, suggesting that there may be one gyrase binding site for each looped domain (11). If so, then there would be a close parallel between the SAR or MAR sites in eukaryotes and the DNA anchorage sites in *E. coli.*

Studies of the interaction of topoisomerase II with DNA have been facilitated by the discovery that the cleavage and religation events catalyzed by topoisomerase II can be abrogated at the cleavage step by drugs. The elegant work of Liu, Ross, and their colleagues has shown that a variety of drugs known for their antitumor activity will block topoisomerase II at the stage of DNA cleavage, producing a complex, termed "cleavable complex," in which the enzyme is tightly bound to DNA. The addition of protein denaturants leads to the nonreversible scission of the double-stranded DNA with topoisomerase subunits bound to the ends of the DNA at the cleavage site (for review see 12,13).

The location of topoisomerase II cleavage sites has been mapped on numerous DNAs. In general, a spectrum of specific sites are found, ranging from relatively weak to very strong, with much of the DNA apparently spared. When antitumor drugs such as acridine derivatives, anthracyclines, ellipticines, and epipodophyllotoxins are used to induce DNA cleavage, the pattern of cutting sites is found to be dependent upon the drug used (14). The cleavage pattern produced by the eukaryotic enzymes is similar between species. DNA gyrase of *E. coli* is insensitive to *m*-AMSA, which is a potent inhibitor of the bacteriophage T4 enzyme (15). Thus it would appear that among the factors that determine the nature of a cleavage site, both the drug used and the source of the enzyme contribute.

The DNA sequence is also important in determining whether a site will be cleaved by topoisomerase II. The sequence of 16 strong and 47 weak cutting sites on a DNA plasmid containing the Drosophila transposable P element by Drosophila type II topoisomerase was examined and a consensus derived that was 5' GTN-(A or T)-AY-ATTNATNNG 3' (where Y is a pyrimidine, N is no preferred nucleotide, and / is the position of cleavage) (16). However, among the 63 sites examined, most differed from this consensus, and some strong sites differed considerably. Spitzner and Muller (17) examined the sequence of cleavage sites produced by the chicken erythrocyte type II topoisomerase and derived a consensus sequence that was 5'(A or G)-N-(T or C)-NNCNNG-(T or C)-/NG-(G or T)-TN-(T or C)-N-(T or C) 3'. Yet comparison of the cleavage patterns obtained for the two enzymes and the same DNA reveal many of the strongest cleavage sites to be the same. Studies on the sequence of DNA gyrase cleavage sites show sequence preferences, but the specific determinants of a strong cleavage site are not immediately apparent (18,19).

In vivo, topoisomerase II can be induced to form cleavable complexes by treating cells with drugs such as *m*-AMSA. Here the coverage of the DNA by histones may mask sites that would otherwise by cleaved. For example, Yang et al. (20) found that when protein-free SV40 DNA was cleaved by calf thymus topoisomerase II in the presence of *m*-AMSA, numerous cleavage sites were observed, but when the SV40 DNA was in the form of SV40 minichromosomes, one major site late in the infection cycle, near the origin of replication, became the only predominant strong cleavage site *in vivo*. Similarly, when cells have been treated with antitumor drugs and the cleavage sites near known genetic loci studied, it was found that cleavage was common in upstream control regions of several oncogenes, but not in the protein coding sequences themselves (21,22).

These observations raise a central question as to what factors define the nature of the drug- and detergent-induced cleavage sites. Although the presence of a sequence of bases approximating the consensus sequence may be essential, its presence alone appears insufficient to explain the complex patterns of cleavage. First, there are normally many more sequences present that conform to the consensus than there are cleavage sites, in particular strong sites. Second, it is not always the case that the degree to which a sequence resembles the consensus reflects the strength of cleavage. If the sequence within $+/-$ 20 base pairs of the cleavage site is not sufficient to dictate the degree of DNA–topoisomerase II interaction, then what other features of DNA structure might play a role?

MODELS OF DNA–TOPOISOMERASE II INTERACTION

Several models of how topoisomerase II might interact with DNA are worth considering. In a *tracking model*, the enzyme would bind to the DNA at some point and then move along the DNA for a considerable distance before falling off. In this model, any aberration in DNA structure that would inhibit or slow the movement of the enzyme along the DNA would effectively magnify the exposure of those regions to the enzyme. Clearly a combination of sequence determinants that slow the enzyme tracking and also confer a consensus sequence could generate a strong cleavage site. The nature of sequences that might slow enzyme tracking is discussed later.

In a *wrapping model,* DNA would wrap about the exterior of the topoisomerase molecule just as DNA wraps about the histone core in a nucleosome. Direct evidence for the formation of gyrasomes has been provided by Klevan and Wang (23) studying *E. coli* DNA gyrase. Recent work from this laboratory has shown that certain unusual DNA sequences, termed "bent DNA," preferentially localize nucleosomes by facilitating the energetically difficult task of wrapping DNA in a tight coil around the histone core (24). Were this a common feature of all topoisomerase II enzymes, then one could imagine that a strong cleavage site might involve the conjunction of a consensus sequence and a bent sequence, and that certain potential cleavage sites might be excluded if they were present in segments of DNA that were unusually stiff and unable to form "gyrasomes."

In a *looping model,* when topoisomerase II binds DNA it would form a loop, which, in this model, would be necessary to bring two segments of DNA together for the subsequent cleavage, strand passage, and rejoining steps. Indeed, both DNA gyrase and the T4 phage topoisomerase II have been observed by electron microscopy (EM) to form loops in DNA (25). If DNA is looped by the eukaryotic topoisomerase II molecules, then certain sequence-dependent features of DNA, for example, the presence of bent segments, could affect looping and thus might lead to a nonuniform selection of sites for binding and cleavage. Recent discoveries about unusual sequence-dependent structures have provided new information about DNA that is to be examined in the context of these models.

UNUSUAL SEQUENCE-DEPENDENT STRUCTURES IN DNA

When B form DNA is crystallized, the extreme forces of crystal formation and dehydration force the DNA into a very regular structure with 10.0 bp per turn and thus 3.4 Å per base pair. It has become increasingly clear that in solution the local pitch and rise of DNA may differ significantly from these values, depending on the sequence. For example, poly(dA)·poly(dT) DNA shows a solution structure that is close to the crystal values (26), while most other natural sequences have helical parameters closer to 10.6 bp per turn and 3.0 Å per bp (27–29). Additional evidence that the poly(dA)·poly(dT) duplex is unusual is seen in the fact that it will not form nucleosomes (30). At the other end of the spectrum is the A form of DNA with a 2.55 Å rise and 11.0 bp per turn. Studies by Klug et al. (31) on the internal control region of the Xenopus 5S RNA gene have indicated that a region that binds transcription factor IIIA and is G-C rich may assume a structure that is closer to A form than B form DNA.

Left-handed segments in DNA represent a severe change in structure that is conferred by base sequence and torsional strain. Whether segments of duplex DNA adopt the left-handed form *in vivo* is not well established. Wells and colleagues have demonstrated that in an artificial construct, a plasmid containing a long repeating dGdC segment could be observed in a non-B form in *E. coli* (32). However, long runs of alternating G-C are extremely uncommon in natural DNAs. Alternating G-T segments are more common, but greater superhelical strain is required to induce this DNA to adopt a left-handed form than G-C segments.

Palindromic sequences are a common feature of natural DNAs, particularly in regions that serve as control elements. When present in supertwisted DNA, these segments can adopt a cruciform structure. Another unusual sequence-dependent DNA structure that is driven by superhelical strain consists of segments that have all purines on one strand and all pyrimidines on the other and are also arranged as an inverted repeat. *In vitro* at lowered pH, such segments can rearrange into a triple-stranded structure in which three of the strands pair via Watson-Crick and Hoogstein base pairing, with the fourth strand apparently displaced (33). Such structures would presumably appear as a hairpin along an otherwise linear duplex DNA.

Recently it has been shown that the sequence of bases along a DNA may cause it to have a complex curvature in three dimensions. This sequence-dependent bending or curvature of DNA will have a profound influence on its interaction with proteins. The first evidence that short DNA segments could be curved in space was presented by Wells and colleagues (34,35), who found a change in the helix direction at the junction between B-form and A-form DNA. The first naturally occurring curved DNA segments were found in trypanosome kinetoplast DNA by Englund and colleagues (36,37), who found that certain restriction fragments migrated slower than expected when electrophoresed on 14% acrylamide gels but ran normally on 4% gels. Wu and Crothers (38) proposed that this finding was due to a planar curve that inhibited the DNA from migrating through highly crosslinked gels. DNA sequence analysis revealed a repeating pattern of 4 to 6 As repeated every 10 bp (38). Models for DNA curvature involve junctions between two different helical forms (39,40), wedges in the helix introduced by AA dinucleotides (41,42) and changes due to anisotropic flexibility and altered propeller twist (43). The important experimental finds are (1) these curvatures can be extreme, a segment at the terminus of SV40 DNA replication changes direction by over 180° in 150 bp (24) and a

200 bp segment from the kinetoplast DNA of *Crithidia fasciculata* forms a nearly perfect circle (55); and (2) curved helix segments have been found in many of the control regions of viral and plasmid DNAs—the origins of replication of lambda phage (45,46), SV40 DNA (47), pSC101 (48), in yeast ARS segments (49), at the terminus of SV40 replication (24), and in pBR322 and adenovirus DNAs (50).

Curved DNA segments preferentially localize to the ends of supertwisted DNA domains (51), thus uniquely orienting a population of supertwisted DNA circles, and highly curved DNA strongly positions nucleosomes (38). This is not surprising, since DNA is severely strained as it wraps about the nucleosome or when it is at the end of a supertwisted DNA rod, and any relief of this strain would be preferred.

HOW MIGHT SEQUENCE-DEPENDENT DNA STRUCTURES AFFECT TOPOISOMERASE II–DNA INTERACTIONS?

Topoisomerase Tracking

If topoisomerase II tracks along DNA, then any of the sequence-dependent alterations in DNA structure could change its rate of movement along DNA. Clearly the more severe sequence-dependent variations such as highly bent segments, polypurine–polypyrimidine tracts, and palindromes would have the greatest effects on altering the tracking rate. However, the most important effects might be due to subtle local changes in the helical parameters of the DNA helix due to sequence. This might be the case if the enzyme has a duplex DNA binding groove that senses the "usual" solution structure of DNA. Local deviations from this structure, for example, regions having a more A-like conformation, might either slow the enzyme movement on DNA or cause the enzyme to be released. If tracking was slowed, then the nearby segments would effectively "see" the enzyme at a higher frequency than other regions, and any consensus sequence within this region would appear as a strong cleavage site. On the other hand, local perturbations in the helix that would cause the enzyme to be released would have the opposite effect, reducing the local exposure of the DNA to the enzyme and creating weak cleavage sites. Clearly in such a model, sequences that slow enzyme tracking or induce enzyme release could occur hundreds of nucleotides from the consensus sequence and still have a pronounced effect.

Topoisomerase Wrapping

Klevan and Wang (23) observed that *E. coli* DNA gyrase forms a gyrasome in which DNA is wrapped once about the enzyme. Gyrasomes could be isolated following digestion of the enzyme–DNA complexes with micrococcal nuclease, and it was found that a 145 bp fragment was protected from digestion. As measured by EM, when a DNA segment was bound by gyrase, its total length was shortened by an amount equivalent to 115 bp (52). We demonstrated that highly bent DNA segments will preferentially assemble into nucleosomes (24). By analogy, then, it would be expected that highly bent segments would strongly bind DNA gyrase. This hypothesis has not been tested. There is question, however, as to whether this analogy can be extended to the eukaryotic type II topoisomerases. Nuclease protection studies with the eukaryotic topoisomerase IIs have provided no evidence for the protection of DNA segments as large as 145 bp, in fact the Drosophila enzyme protects only about 30 bp (53). An example of a Drosophila topoisomerase II molecule bound to a short DNA fragment is in Figure 4.1. Measurement of these complexes indicated that the DNA was shortened by only about 20 bp. These observations suggest that DNA may not wrap about the eukaryotic type II enzymes.

From the studies to date, it seems possible that DNA gyrase and the eukaryotic type II enzymes may differ in how they bind DNA. This may relate to the apparently unique ability of DNA gyrase to add supercoils to circular DNAs in addition to being able to remove supertwists as do the other enzymes. If so, then the wrapping model may be highly relevant to DNA gyrase, but not to the eukaryotic topoisomerase IIs.

Topoisomerase Looping

Evidence for the formation of large loops in DNA by DNA gyrase was presented by Moore et al. (25), and similar loops were observed in parallel experiments carried out with the T4 topoisomerase II (54). In recent studies carried out in collaboration with T. Hsieh and M. Lee (Duke University), we have observed that the Drosophila topoisomerase II also has a strong propensity to arrange DNA into looped structures when incubated with linear DNA under ionic conditions typical for relaxation of supercoiled DNA (Fig. 4.2A,B). The size of the loops ranged from a few hundred base pairs to several thousand. Few other DNA binding proteins have been observed to loop DNA except when two binding sites were present on the DNA and when the proteins were known to interact with each other, as, for example, when lambda repressor is bound to its operator sites (44). Proteins such as DNA polymerase I, the histones, RNA polymerase of *E. coli,* RecA and UvsX proteins, when bound to DNA and prepared for EM by the methods used in the topoiosomerase II studies, do not form loops, arguing that the loops are not a simple artifact of the EM preparative conditions. Assuming that the loops observed in the complexes of topoisomerase II and DNA are a necessary feature of topoisomerase II– DNA binding, how might their formation be influenced by local perturbations in DNA structure, and how might this produce a distribution of cleavage sites that would vary in their frequency of cutting (weak to strong cleavage sites)?

To address that question, one must know how the loops are formed. Three possible models need to be considered. In the first, single enzyme molecules bind to DNA and create a tiny loop, which would then grow in size as the DNA is threaded through forming a larger and larger loop. In a second model, the loops form in a manner analogous to the lambda repressor paradigm in which two separate topoisomerase II molecules bind to two different sites on the DNA and then interact with each other to form a loop. Finally, in a third model,

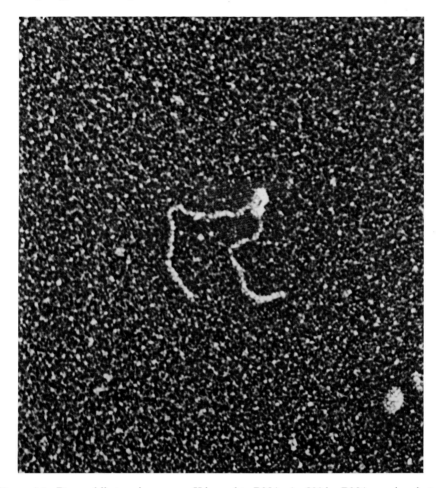

Figure 4.1. Drosophila topoisomerase II bound to DNA. An 890 bp DNA was incubated with Drosphila topoisomerase II under standard relaxation conditions: 10 mM Tris-HCl, pH 7.9, 0.1 mM EDTA, 50 mM KCl, 10 mM MgCl$_2$, 1.25 mM ATP, 0.1 μg DNA, 0.2 μg topoisomerase II in a 20 μl for 5 min at 30°C. Following incubation the samples were fixed in 0.8% glutaraldehyde for 5 min at 30°C, and chromatographed over Sepharose 4B. The protein–DNA complexes were then adsorbed onto freshly glow-charged grids in the presence of a spermidine containing buffer and quick frozen in liquid ethane. Under high vacuum the samples were freeze dried and rotary shadowcast with tungsten. (Bar = 0.05 μm.)

a single molecule of topoisomerase II would bind to the DNA (perhaps while also tracking along the DNA) and then capture a second duplex strand through a "random" collision event.

Data from the literature and recent observations suggest that the third model may best describe the looping process. First, if loops are created by a facilitated threading process (as in the first model), then it is difficult to explain how these enzymes decatenate interlocked DNA circles, and the size of the

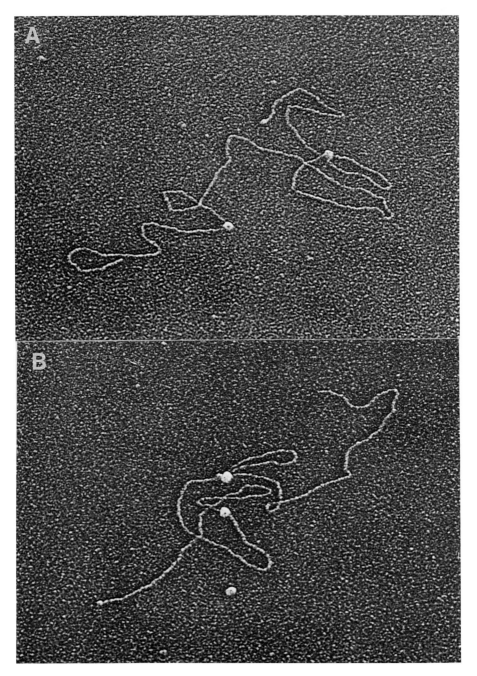

Figure 4.2. A, B. A 7435 bp DNA was incubated with topoisomerase II as described in Figure 4.1. Preparation for electron microscopy was the same as Figure 4.1 except following adsorption to the carbon supports, samples were washed in H_2O and EtOH, air dried, and rotary shadowcast with tungsten. (Bar = 0.1 µm.)

loops would be expected to grow in size with continued incubation in the presence of ATP, an observation that has not been made (unpublished data). If loops were formed by two separate topoisomerase II molecules binding first to DNA and then to each other, it would be expected that the size of the protein complexes observed at a loop would be larger than the complexes at nonlooped sites. In work to be described elsewhere (M. Howard et al., unpublished results) it appears that the size of the Drosophila topoisomerase II molecules seen by EM is the same whether they are at the base of the loops or isolated on linear DNA and these molecules are of a size expected for a single homodimer of the 170 kD peptide. Direct evidence in support of the third model comes from an analysis of the size of the loops formed by the Drosophila topoisomerase II in which it was found that the loop size approximated the Shore and Baldwin distribution (56), which in a simple way describes the probability of forming loops in DNA through a random collision process.

The presence of topoisomerase II molecules bound at the base of loops and bound separately of loops supports the third model of loop formation but makes it even more difficult to consider the relation of topoisomerase II binding to strong and weak cleavage sites since it is not clear whether both forms of the bound enzyme are equally active in forming cleavable complexes in the presence of drugs (e.g., are only those molecules bound at loops active in forming cleavable complexes?). In considering how unusual DNA structures could influence the pattern of topoisomerase binding and loop formation, clearly highly bent sequences would facilitate the formation of loops by topoisomerase. Similarly, unusually stiff DNA segments would inhibit loop formation. If the enzyme tracks along DNA and then forms a loop, then all of the comments on Topoisomerase Tracking would apply to the localization of the first DNA strand bound in the looped complex.

CONCLUSION

The relation between topoisomerase II binding sites on DNA, the position of weak and strong cleavage sites, and the way in which topoisomerase II arranges DNA into loops is complex. DNA is now known to contain many variations in structure that differ from the classic B form owing to unique sequence arrangements. How these unusual structures influence the way in which topoisomerase II moves along DNA, loops DNA, and where drug-induced cleavages occur is not yet understood, but it is likely that these novel DNA structures will be found to play an important role.

Acknowledgments

These studies were supported by grants from the National Institutes of Health (GM31819) and the American Chemical Society (NP-583).

REFERENCES

1. DiNardo, S., Voelkel, K., and Sternglanz, R. DNA topoisomerase II mutant of Saccharomyces cerevisiae: Topoisomerase II is required for segregation of daughter molecules at the termination of DNA replication. Proc. Natl. Acad. Sci. USA. **81:** 2616–2620, 1984.

2. Uemura, T., Ohkura, H., Adachi, Y., Morino, K., Shiozaki, K., and Yanagida, M. DNA topisomerase II is required for condensation and separation of mitotic chromosomes in S. pombe. Cell. **50:** 917–925, 1987.

3. Yang, L., Wold, M. S., Li, J. J., Kelly, T. J., and Liu, L. F. Roles of DNA topoisomerase in simian virus 40 DNA replication in vitro. Proc. Natl. Acad. Sci. USA. **84:** 950–954, 1987.

4. Pruss, G. J., and Drlica, K. DNA supercoiling and prokaryotic transcription. Cell. **56:** 521–523, 1989.

5. Wang, J. DNA topoisomerases. Annu. Rev. Biochem. **54:** 665–697, 1985.

6. Wu, H. Y., Shyy, S., Wang, J. C., and Liu, L. F. Transcription generates positively and negatively supercoiled domains in the template. Cell. **53:** 433–440, 1988.

7. Cockerill, P. N. and Garrard, W. T. Chromosomal loop anchorage of the kappa immunoglobulin gene occurs next to the enhancer in a region containing topoisomerase II sites. Cell. **44:** 273–282, 1986.

8. Sperry, A. O., Blasquez, V. C., and Garrard, W. T. Dysfunction of chromosomal loop attachment sites: Illegitimate recombination linked to MAR sequences and topoisomerase II. Proc. Natl. Acad. Sci. USA. **86:** 5491–5501, 1989.

9. Pettijohn, D. E. and Hecht, R. RNA molecules bound to the folded bacterial genome stabilize DNA folds and segregate domains of supercoiling. Cold Spring Harbor Symposia on Quantitative Biology **38:** 31–41, 1973.

10. Worcel, A. and Burgi, E. On the structure of the folded chromosome of Escherichia coli. J. Mol. Biol. **71:** 127–147, 1972.

11. Snyder, M. and Drlica, K. DNA gyrase on the bacterial chromosome: DNA cleavage induced by oxolinic acid. J. Mol. Biol. **131:** 287–302, 1979.

12. Glisson, B. S. and Ross, W. E. DNA topoisomerase II: A primer on the enzyme and its unique role as a multidrug target in cancer chemotherapy. Pharmacol. Ther. **32:** 89–106, 1987.

13. Liu, L. F. DNA topoisomerase poisons as antitumor drugs. Annu. Rev. Biochem. **58:** 351–375, 1989.

14. Tewey, K. M., Rowe, T. C., Yang, L., Halligan, B. D., and Liu, L. F. Adriamycin-induced DNA damage mediated by mammalian DNA topoisomerase II. Science. **226:** 466–468, 1984.

15. Huff, A. C., Leatherwood, J. K., and Kreuzer, K. N. Bacteriophage T4 DNA topoisomerase is the target of antitumor agent 4'-(9-acridinylamino) methane-sulfon-m-anisidide (m-AMSA) in T4 infected Escherichia coli. Proc. Natl. Acad. Sci. USA. **86:** 1307–1311, 1989.

16. Sander, M. and Hsieh, T. Drosophila topoisomerase II double stranded DNA cleavage: Analysis of DNA sequence homology at the cleavage site. Nucleic Acids Res. **13:** 1057–1072, 1985.

17. Spitzner, J. R. and Muller, M. T. A consensus sequence for cleavage by vertebrate DNA topoisomerase II. Nucleic Acids Res. **16:** 5533–5556, 1988.

18. Morrison, A. and Cozzarelli, N. R. Site specific cleavage of DNA by E. coli DNA gyrase. Cell. **17:** 175–184, 1979.

19. Fisher, L. M., Mizuuchi, K., O'Dea, M. H., Ohmori, H., and Gellert, M. Site specific interaction of DNA gyrase with DNA. Proc. Natl. Acad. Sci. USA. **78:** 4165–4169, 1981.

20. Yang, L., Rowe, T. C., Nelson, E. M., and Liu, L. F. In vivo mapping of DNA topoisomerase II-specific cleavage sites on SV40 chromatin. Cell. **41:** 127–132, 1985.

21. Darby, M. K., Herrera, R. E., Vosberg, H., and Nordheim, A. DNA topoisomerase II cleaves at specific sites in the 5' flanking region of c-fos proto-oncogenes in vitro. EMBO J. **5:** 2257–2265, 1986.

22. Riou, J., Multon, E., Vilarem, M., Larsen, C., and Riou, G. In vivo simulation by antitumor drugs of the topoisomerase II induced cleavage sites in c-myc proto-oncogene. Biochem. Biophys. Res. Commun. **137:** 154–160, 1986.

23. Klevan, L., and Wang, J. C. Deoxyribonucleic acid gyrase-deoxyribonucleic acid complex containing 140 base pairs of deoxyribonucleic acid and a protein core. Biochemistry. **19:** 5229–5234, 1980.

24. Hsieh, C. and Griffith, J. D. The terminus of SV40 DNA replication and transcription contains a sharp sequence-directed curve. Cell. **52:** 535–544, 1988.

25. Moore, C. L., Klevan, L., Wang, J. C., and Griffith, J. D. Gyrase·DNA complexes visualized as looped structures by electron microscopy. J. Biol. Chem. **258:** 4612–4617, 1983.

26. Alexeev, D. G., Lipanov, A. A., and Skuratovskii, I. Y. Poly(dA)·poly (dT) is

a B-type double helix with a distinctively narrow minor groove. Nature. **325**: 821–823, 1987.

27. Griffith, J. D. DNA structure: Evidence from electron microscopy. Science. **201**: 525–527, 1978.

28. Peck, L. J. and Wang, J. C. Sequence dependence of the helical *repeat of DNA in solution. Nature. **292**: 375–377, 1981.

29. Rhodes, D. and Klug, A. Sequence-dependent helical periodicity of DNA. Nature. **292**: 378–380, 1981.

30. Satchwell, S. C., Drew, H. R., and Travers, A. A. Sequence periodicities in chicken nucleosome core DNA. J. Mol. Biol. **191**: 659–675, 1986.

31. Rhodes, D., and Klug, A. An underlying repeat in some transcriptional control sequences corresponding to half a double helical turn of DNA. Cell. **46**: 123–132, 1986.

32. Jaworski, A., Hsieh, W. T., Blaho, J. A., Larson, J. E., and Wells, R. D. Left handed DNA in vivo. Science. **238**: 773–777, 1987.

33. Wells, R. D., Collier, D. A., Hanvey, J. C., Shimizu, M., and Wohlrab, F. The chemistry and biology of unusual DNA structures adopted by oligopurineoligopyrimidine sequences. FASEB J. **2**: 2939–2949, 1988.

34. Selsing, E., Wells, R. D., Alden, C. J., and Arnott, S. Bent DNA: Visualization of a base-paired and stacked A-B conformation junction. J. Biol. Chem. **254**: 5417–5422, 1979.

35. Selsing, E., and Wells, R. D. Polynucleotide block polymers consisting of a DNA·RNA hybrid joined to a DNA·DNA duplex. J. Biol. Chem. **254**: 5410–5416, 1979.

36. Marini, J. C., Effron, P. N., Goodman, T. C., Singleton, C. K., Wells, R. D., Wartell, R. M., and Englund, P. T. Physical characterization of a kinetoplast DNA fragment with unusual properties. J. Biol. Chem. **259**: 8974–8979, 1984.

37. Marini, J. C., Levene, S. D., Crothers, D. M., and Englund, P. T. Bent helical structure in kinetoplast DNA. Proc. Natl. Acad. Sci. USA. **79**: 7664–7668, 1982.

38. Wu, H-M. and Crothers, D. M. The locus of sequence-directed and protein-induced DNA bending. Nature. **308**: 509–513, 1984.

39. Koo, H-S., Wu, H-M., and Crothers, D. M. DNA bending at adenine thymine tracts. Nature. **320**: 501–506, 1986.

40. Hagerman, P. Sequence-directed curvature of DNA. Nature. **321**: 449–450, 1986.

41. Trifonov, E. N. Curved DNA. CRC Crit. Rev. Biochem. **19**: 89–106, 1985.

42. Ulanovsky, L. E., and Trifonov, E. N. Estimation of wedge components in curved DNA. Nature. **326**: 720–722, 1987.

43. Yoon, C., Prive, G. G., Goodsell, D. S., and Dickerson, R. E. Structure of an alternating-B DNA helix and its relationship to A-tract DNA. Proc. Natl. Acad. Sci. USA. **85**: 6332–6336, 1988.

44. Griffith, J. D., Hochschild, A., and Ptashne, M. DNA loops induced by cooperative binding of repressor. Nature. **322**: 750–752, 1986.

45. Zahn, K. and Blattner, F. R. Sequence-induced DNA curvature at the bacteriophage origin of replication. Nature. **317**: 451–453, 1985.

46. Zahn, K., and Blattner, R. F. Direct evidence for DNA bending at the lambda replication origin. Science. **236**: 416–422, 1987.

47. Ryder, K., Silver, S., DeLucia, A. L., Fanning, E., and Tegtmeyer, P. An altered DNA conformation in origin region 1 is a determinant for the binding of SV40 large T antigen. Cell. **44**: 719–725, 1986.

48. Stenzel, T. T., Patel, P., and Bastia, D. The integration host factor of Escherichia coli binds to bent DNA at the origin of replication of the plasmid pSC101. Cell. **49**: 709–717, 1987.

49. Snyder, M., Buchman, A. R., and Davis, R. W. Bent DNA at a yeast autonomously replicating sequence. Nature. **324**: 87–89, 1986.

50. Anderson, J. N. Detection, sequence patterns and function of unusual DNA structures. Nucleic Acids Res. **14**: 8513–8533, 1986.

51. Laundon, C. and Griffith, J. Curved helix segments can uniquely orient the topology of supertwisted DNA. Cell. **52**: 545–549, 1988.

52. Kirchhausen, T., Wang, J. C., and Harrison, S. C. DNA gyrase and its complexes with DNA: Direct observation by electron microscopy. Cell. **41**: 933–943, 1985.

53. Lee, M. P., Sander, M., and Hsieh, T. Interactions between Drosophila DNA topoisomerase II and DNA. J. Cell Biol. 107: 402a, 1988.

54. Moore, C. Ph.D. diss., University of North Carolina, 1982.

55. Griffith, J. D., Bleyman, M., Rauch, C. A., Kitchin, P. A., and Englund, P. T. Visualization of the bent helix in kinetoplast DNA by electron microscopy. Cell. **46**: 717–724, 1986.

56. Shore, D. and Baldwin, R. L. Energetics of DNA twisting I. Relation between twist and cyclization probability. J. Mol. Biol. **170**: 957–981, 1983.

Chapter 5

The Role of DNA Topoisomerase I and II in Drosophila Hsp70 Heat-Shock Gene Transcription

PAUL E. KROEGER
AND THOMAS C. ROWE

DNA topoisomerases are an important target for several classes of antitumor drugs. DNA topoisomerase I is a target of camptothecin, while DNA topoisomerase II is a target for anthracyclines, ellipticines, amsacrines, and epipodophyllotoxins (1–5). These drugs interfere with the DNA breakage–reunion reaction of DNA topoisomerases and stabilize a covalent DNA–enzyme intermediate called the "cleavable complex" (6). Treatment of the cleavable complex with a detergent (i.e., SDS) results in either single-stranded (topoisomerase I) or double-stranded (topoisomerase II) DNA breaks with protein coupled to either the 3' (topoisomerase I) or 5' (DNA topoisomerase II) ends of the DNA breaks (3,6). Stabilization of the topoisomerase–DNA cleavable complex is believed to be an important step in the cytotoxic action of these antitumor drugs.

A major consequence of the treatment of cells with topoisomerase-active drugs is a pronounced change in cellular RNA synthesis (7,8). Whether or not these changes are important in the cytotoxic mechanism of these drugs is at present unclear. However, the availability of specific inhibitors of DNA topoisomerase I and II will provide an important tool for probing the cellular functions of these enzymes in gene regulation as well as in DNA replication, recombination, and repair processes. An overall picture of these cellular functions is crucial to understanding the role of DNA topoisomerases as cytotoxic targets of antitumor drugs. This paper will present several studies illustrating how inhibitors of DNA topoisomerases can be used to probe the functions of these enzymes in eukaryotic gene transcription. The significance of these inhibitor studies, with regard to the roles of DNA topoisomerase I and II in the regulation of Drosophila Hsp70 heat-shock gene transcription, will be discussed.

There are two aspects of topoisomerase inhibitors that make them useful for studying the cellular role of topoisomerases in gene transcription. First, since these drugs directly inhibit the catalytic activity of DNA topoisomerases, any drug-induced changes in cellular transcription suggest a catalytic involvement of these enzymes in RNA synthesis. Second, topoisomerase-active antitumor drugs stabilize an enzyme–DNA intermediate termed the cleavable complex. Treatment of this complex with a detergent such as SDS results in the formation of protein-linked DNA breaks. The locations of these DNA breaks can be easily mapped and represent a footprint of topoisomerase-active sites on cellular chromosomes (9). Such footprints are invaluable in ascertaining how topoisomerases might be acting to regulate chromatin function. We have used both approaches to investigate how topoisomerases I and II are involved in the transcription of the Hsp70 heat-shock gene in Drosophila.

RESULTS AND DISCUSSION

Camptothecin-Stimulated Cleavage of Hsp70 Gene by Topoisomerase I

Exposure of cells to temperatures above which they normally grow results in the synthesis of a family of proteins called heat-shock proteins (Hsps) (10,11). Evidence suggests that the presence of these proteins may be important in protecting cells from the cytotoxic effects of high temperature as well as other forms of cytotoxic stress. Synthesis of Hsps is primarily regulated at the level of gene transcription. The Hsp70 gene is the major heat-shock gene in Drosophila and consists of a 2.2 kilobase (kb) conserved transcribed region with a 0.35 kb conserved nontranscribed regulatory region adjoining the 5' end of the gene (Fig. 5.1, and ref. 12). We have mapped the drug-induced topoisomerase I and II cleavage sites on the Hsp70 gene before and after heat-induced activation of

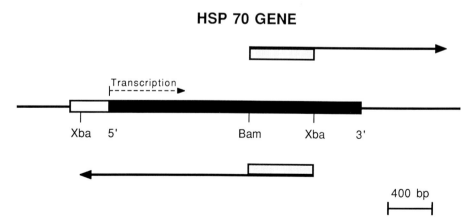

HSP 70 GENE

Figure 5.1. Schematic of Drosophila Hsp70 gene. The gene consists of a nontranscribed regulatory region (open box) adjoining the transcribed region (solid box). The stippled box represents the probe (plasmid pMR4) that was used to map the topoisomerase I and II sites in the 3' (upper solid arrow) or 5' (lower solid arrow) region of the Hsp70 gene when the DNA was restricted with *Bam* HI or Xba I, respectively. The dashed arrow shows the direction of transcription.

Hsp70 transcription using a modification of the indirect-end labeling technique (9,13). Figure 5.2 shows the autoradiographs of Southern blots of DNA isolated from cells treated with camptothecin (Part A) or VM-26 (Part B). The drug-induced cleavage sites in the 5' and 3' regions of the gene were mapped by restricting the DNA with either Xba I or *Bam*HI and then hybridizing the Southern blots to labeled pMR4 DNA which contains the *Bam*HI-Xba I fragment of the Hsp70 gene (see Fig. 5.1). Two striking observations were made concerning camptothecin-induced cleavage of the Hsp70 gene by topoisomerase I: (1) cleavage occurred only when this gene was transcriptionally active

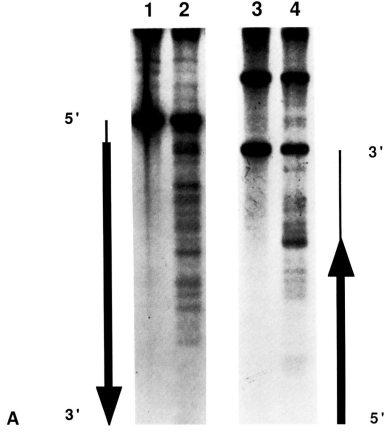

Figure 5.2. Drug-induced cleavage of Drosophila Hsp70 by topoisomerase I and II. Topoisomerase I and II cleavage sites were mapped on the Hsp 70 gene in camptothecin and VM-26–treated cells as described previously using a modification of the indirect end-labeling technique (9,13). **Panel A.** Cells previously incubated for 10 min at 25°C (lanes 1 and 3) or 37°C (lanes 2 and 4) were incubated an additional 10 min at these temperatures in the presence of 20 μM camptothecin before lysis with SDS. The DNA isolated from the cell lysates was restricted with either Xba I (lanes 1 and 2) or *Bam* HI (lanes 3 and 4) to map cleavage sites in the 5' and 3' regions of the gene as illustrated in Figure 5.1. Reproduced with permission from (21).

(Fig. 5.2A, lanes 2 and 4), and (2) cleavage was primarily confined to the transcribed region of the Hsp70 gene (see Fig. 5.3 for summary of cleavage sites). The apparent preferential association of topoisomerase I with transcriptionally active chromatin is not unique to the Hsp70 heat-shock gene. Several other laboratories have also observed that campthothecin-induced cleavage of DNA was localized to actively transcribed genes. Gilmour and Elgin have observed that cleavage of the small Drosophila Hsp genes by topoisomerase I occurred only following heat-induced activation of these genes (14). Similar to our findings with the Hsp70 gene, cleavage was confined to the transcribed region of

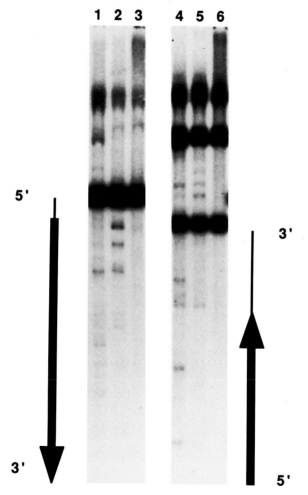

Figure 5.2. Panel B is the same as Panel A except that cells incubated at 25°C (lanes 2,3,5,6) or 37°C (lanes 1 and 4) were placed in drug-free media (lanes 3 and 6) or in media containing 20 μM VM-26 (lanes 1,2,4,5) during the last 10 min of the incubation. The DNA was restricted with either Xba I (lanes 1–3) or *Bam* HI (lanes 4–6). The solid arrows at the sides of Panels A and B represent the region of the Hsp70 gene that was probed in the blots.

these genes. Recent studies on the human ribosomal RNA genes and the rat tyrosine aminotransferase gene have also demonstrated a correlation between transcriptional activity and the level of topoisomerase I cleavage in these genes (15,16). Again, cleavage was primarily localized within the transcribed domains of these genes.

The interaction of topoisomerase I with active regions of chromatin has also been demonstrated using a variety of other approaches. Immunofluorescence staining with topoisomerase I–specific antibodies has been used to delineate the distribution of topoisomerase I on Drosophila polytene chromosomes (17). Fluorescence staining was localized to regions of chromatin that contained transcriptionally active genes. In the case of the heat-shock loci at 87A–87C, staining with topoisomerase I antibody was observed only upon heat-induced activation of these genes. In other studies, nucleosomes isolated from transcriptionally active chromatin were found to contain high levels of topoisomerase I activity signifying an involvement of this enzyme in transcription (18). Photo crosslinking methods have also been used to define the distribution of topoisomerase I on cellular chromosomes in Drosophila cells (19). In these studies, UV light was used to induce crosslinking of topoisomerase I to DNA in cells before and after heat-induced activation of Hsp70 transcription. Chromatin was then isolated, cut into small pieces with DNA restriction enzymes, and the population of DNA fragments crosslinked to topoisomerase I were isolated by immunoprecipitation. The DNA was then analyzed by Southern hybridization using probes specific for different regions of the Hsp70 heat-shock genes. These experiments indicated that topoisomerase I binding to the transcribed region of the Hsp70 gene was stimulated more than 20-fold upon activation of Hsp70 transcription. Binding of topoisomerase I to the flanking nontranscribed regions of Hsp70 genes, however, was not stimulated, suggesting that this enzyme was specifically associated with DNA sequences that were being transcribed by RNA polymerase.

What is the significance of topoisomerase I binding to active regions of cellular chromatin? Evidence suggests that the translocation of the RNA polymerase complex along a segment of the DNA duplex generates positive waves of supercoils ahead and negative supercoils behind the transcription complex (20). If the degree of supercoiling becomes too great, the movement of RNA polymerase can be inhibited. Since topoisomerase I can catalyze the removal of both positive and negative supercoils from DNA, this enzyme may facilitate transcription by relaxing supercoils generated by the movement of the RNA polymerase complex along the DNA double helix. Consistent with this model, we have shown that inhibition of ongoing Hsp70 RNA synthesis by either actinomycin D or 5,6-dichloro-1-β-D-ribofuranosylbenzimidazole abolishes camptothecin-induced topoisomerase I cleavage, suggesting that cleavage is dependent on the movement of the RNA polymerase complex along the Hsp70 gene (21). In addition, *in vitro* experiments have demonstrated that topoisomerase I cleavage is several orders of magnitude greater on a supercoiled versus a relaxed DNA template (22). This latter result also suggests that binding of topoisomerase I to transcribed genes is most likely due to elevated levels of DNA supercoiling that occur during transcription by RNA polymerase.

VM-26 Stimulated Cleavage of the Hsp70 Gene by Topoisomerase II

In contrast to topoisomerase I cleavage, which occurred throughout the transcribed region of the Hsp70 genes, we found that VM-26–induced topoisomerase II cleavage was localized to the ends of the the Hsp70 genes and occurred both before and after gene activation (Fig. 5.2B). Prior to heat-induced gene activation, topoisomerase II cleavage was primarily confined to the 5′ end of the transcribed region (Fig. 5.2B, lanes 2 and 5). However, within 10 min after heat-induced activation of Hsp70 transcription, two of the three major topoisomerase II cleavage sites at the 5′ end of the gene disappeared (compare lanes 1 and 2). Within 20 min following heat-shock, all three sites were gone (data not shown). The loss of topoisomerase II cleavage at the 5′ end of the gene was accompanied by an increase in the intensity of topoisomerase II cleavage at the 3′ end of the gene (compare lanes 4 and 5). A schematic summarizing these results is presented in Figure 5.3. Many of the topoisomerase II cleavage sites were located near or within DNAse I hypersensitive regions of the Hsp70 gene (9). DNAse I hypersensitivity is a property associated with genes that have the potential for transcription (23). The association of topoisomerase II with hypersensitive regions may simply indicate that these areas of the chromatin are more accessible to proteins in general. However, it is also plausible

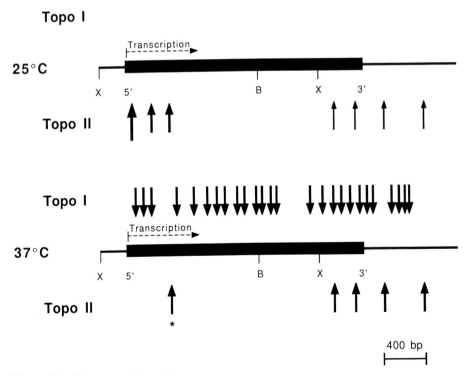

Figure 5.3. Summary of topoisomerase I and II cleavage sites on the Hsp70 gene at 25°C and 37°C. Major and minor cleavage sites are indicated by the size of the arrows. ★This site appears by 20 min post heat-shock.

that topoisomerase II binding to these regions of Hsp70 DNA is related to an important regulatory function of this enzyme in Hsp70 gene expression.

If cells were allowed to recover at 23°C after a brief 37°C heat-shock, Hsp70 RNA synthesis was gradually shut off over a 100 min time period (Fig. 5.4A, lanes 2–5). The decrease in Hsp70 RNA synthesis closely correlated with a return of topoisomerase II cleavage at the 5′ end of the gene (Fig. 5.4B, lanes

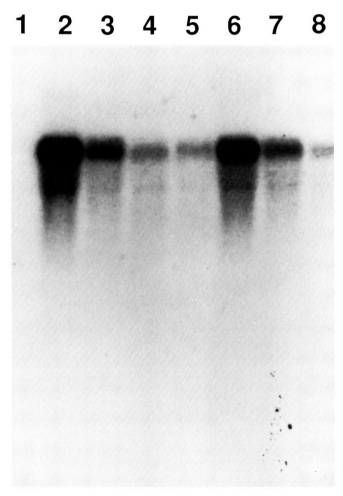

A

Figure 5.4. Correlation between topoisomerase II cleavage and expression of Hsp70 gene. Drosophila K_c cells that had been heat-shocked for 10 min at 37°C were placed at 23°C for an additional 10, 40, 70, or 100 min. (lanes 2–5). At the end of the 100-min recovery period, the cells were given a second 10 min 37°C heat-shock and then returned to 23°C for an additional 10, 70, or 130 min (lanes 6–8). VM-26 (final concentration 20 μM) was added to the culture media during the last 10 min of each incubation to induce topoisomerase II cleavage of the cellular DNA. The RNA or DNA was then isolated and analyzed as described previously (9,35). **Panel A** is an autoradiograph of a Northern blot of total cell RNA hybridized to nick-translated pMR4 DNA.

2–5). If cells were subjected to a second heat-shock at the end of the 100 min recovery period, Hsp70 RNA synthesis was again stimulated (Fig. 5.4A, lane 6) with a simultaneous loss of topoisomerase II cleavage at the 5' end of the gene (Fig. 5.4B, lane 6). During recovery from the second heat-shock there was a subsequent attenuation of Hsp70 RNA synthesis, which again correlated with a return of topoisomerase II cleavage at the 5' end of the gene (Fig. 5.4A, B, lanes 6–8). These results indicate that the association of topoisomerase II with the 5' region of the Hsp70 gene may play a role in the repression of Hsp70 RNA synthesis.

The striking differences between topoisomerase I and II cleavage of the Hsp70 gene indicates that these two enzymes are possibly playing different

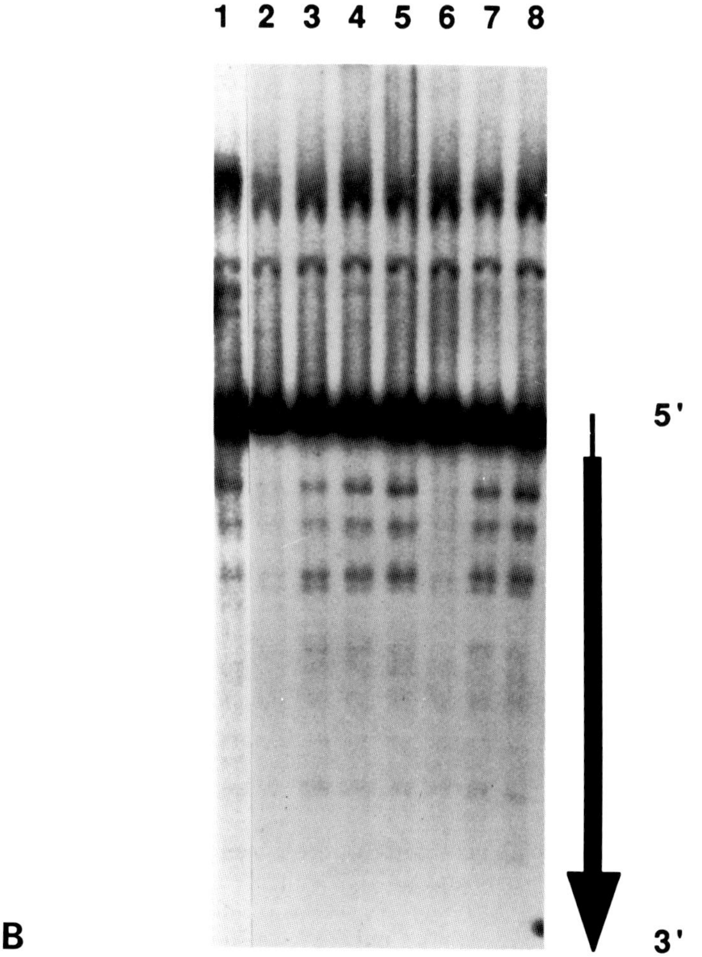

Figure 5.4. Panel B is an autoradiograph of a Southern blot of Xba I restricted cellular DNA that was hybridized to pMR4 probe to map topoisomerase II cleavage in the 5' region of the Hsp 70 gene. The arrow at the side of the autoradiograph schematically depicts the region of the Hsp70 gene in which the cleavage sites are located.

roles in modulating heat-shock gene transcription. As was mentioned previously, topoisomerase I may be required simply to remove topological barriers that arise during transcription. Although topoisomerase II may play a similar role in transcription, there is some evidence that suggests that this enzyme may also be involved in negatively regulating Hsp70 expression. First, treatment of cells at 25°C with VM-26, but not camptothecin, induces Hsp70 transcription 10-fold, suggesting that inhibition of topoisomerase II activity may activate Hsp70 gene expression (9,13). Second, suppression of Hsp70 RNA synthesis is closely linked to topoisomerase II cleavage at the 5' end of the gene (Figs. 5.2B and 5.4B). This region of the Hsp70 gene has previously been shown to negatively regulate Hsp70 transcription (24). A sequence in this region from +82 to +105 is conserved between the different Drosophila heat-shock genes and may be responsible for this negative regulation. The major topoisomerase II cleavage site at the 5' end of the Hsp70 gene has been sequenced and falls within this conserved element (data not shown). Recently, Gilmour and Lis have shown that RNA polymerase is present at the 5' end of the Hsp70 gene prior to transcriptional activation (25,26). However, this enzyme is unable to move beyond nucleotide +65 relative to the start site of transcription. These investigators suggested that RNA polymerase can initiate transcription in the absence of heat-shock but that transcription is then prematurely terminated by some unknown mechanism. Possibly, binding of topoisomerase II to the conserved regulatory element between +82 and +105 prevents the movement of RNA polymerase past the 5' end of the Hsp70 gene. This would also be consistent with the finding that following heat-induced activation of Hsp70 transcription, topoisomerase II binding at this site rapidly disappears (Figs. 5.2B and 5.4B), thus allowing RNA polymerase to then proceed along the Hsp70 gene. The concomitant increase in topoisomerase II cleavage at the 3' end of the gene (Fig. 5.2B), a place where transcription is normally terminated, may indicate that this enzyme also acts to attenuate transcription in this region of the gene as well. Future studies should help to clarify the role of topoisomerase II in Hsp70 transcription.

Drug-induced topoisomerase II cleavage sites have also been mapped on several human genes including the c-myc and c-fos genes (27,28). As was the case for the Hsp70 gene, cleavage was confined to sequences flanking the transcribed region of these genes. Most of the cleavage sites also occurred near DNAse I hypersensitive regions. Studies on the c-fos gene identified a cluster of topoisomerase II cleavage sites that mapped within an enhancer element controlling mitogen-induced c-fos expression, suggesting that topoisomerase II may have an enhancer-associated function (28). An interaction of topoisomerase II with enhancer elements has also been suggested by studies in SV40-virus infected cells (29). These studies showed that the major m-AMSA–induced topoisomerase II cleavage site on SV40 DNA was adjacent to the SV40 enhancer element. The SV40 enhancer potentiates expression of the virally encoded T-antigen gene at early times following infection (30). Paradoxically, topoisomerase II binding near the enhancer region occurs only at late times following infection when T-antigen is not expressed, suggesting that topoisomerase II is not involved in activating T-antigen expression. Perhaps the binding of topoisomerase II to this region inhibits enhancer function. Alternatively, binding of topoisomerase II near the enhancer may reflect a role of this enzyme in the activation of SV40 DNA replication or in the expression of the SV40 late genes.

Effects of Topoisomerase Inhibitors on Hsp70 Transcription

Previous studies have shown that camptothecin and VM-26 have contrasting effects on total cellular RNA synthesis (7,8). Camptothecin was shown to effectively inhibit HeLa cell RNA synthesis greater than 50% at 5 μM. Ribosomal RNA synthesis was particularly sensitive with greater than 80% inhibition at 50 μM camptothecin. In contrast, the topoisomerase II drug VP-16 was found to have a stimulatory effect on total cellular RNA synthesis. At 1 μg/ml VP-16, total RNA synthesis in a murine mastocytoma cell line was increased 36% above control cells.

These drugs cause similar changes in Drosophila Hsp70 RNA synthesis. Heat-induced Hsp70 transcription is highly sensitive to the topoisomerase I inhibitor camptothecin with greater than 95% inhibition at 100 μM (Table 5.1). Camptothecin has also been shown to partially inhibit transcription of the Hsp28 heat-shock gene (14). In both cases, inhibition correlates with the appearance of camptothecin-trapped topoisomerase I–DNA complexes on the transcribed region of these genes, suggesting that these complexes may directly hinder the movement of the transcription complex through these genes. Nuclear run-on transcription studies done on rRNA genes from HeLa cells also suggested that topoisomerase I–DNA complexes might be inhibiting the movement of RNA polymerase (15). Alternatively, camptothecin may block RNA synthesis by inhibiting topoisomerase I–catalyzed changes in DNA topology that are required during transcription. This mode of inhibition has been suggested by *in vitro* transcription studies using extracts from rat mammary adenocarcinoma cells (31). When supercoiled rDNA was used as a template, transcription was almost completely inhibited by 150 μM camptothecin. However, this inhibition could be reversed by adding exogenous topoisomerase I to the reaction, suggesting that the effect of camptothecin on transcription was due to inhibition of DNA topoisomerase I activity rather than the presence of cleavable complexes on DNA. In addition, if linear rDNA was used as a template in the transcription reactions, inhibition by camptothecin was no longer observed.

Table 5.1. Effects of Camptothecin and VM-26 on Hsp70 Transcription[a]

Treatment	Hsp70 RNA (%)
Control—no drug	100
Camptothecin (100 μM)	4
VM-26 (100 μM)	88

[a]Logarithmically growing Drosophila Kc cells were preincubated for 10 min in the presence of camptothecin or VM-26 and then heat-shocked for 10 min at 37°C. The cells were then lysed and the RNA isolated as described previously (9). The RNA was electrophoresed through a 1% agarose gel containing formaldehyde and then transferred onto nitrocellulose by Northern blotting (35). To detect the Hsp70 mRNA, the blot was hybridized to nick-translated pMR4 probe (see Fig. 5.1). The relative levels of Hsp70 RNA were quantitated by densitometry using a BioMed soft laser densitometer.

This result suggested that camptothecin was arresting transcription by inhibiting topoisomerase I–catalyzed changes in DNA topology rather than through the formation of topoisomerase I–DNA complexes that physically impeded the movement of RNA polymerase on DNA.

In contrast to camptothecin, VM-26 does not significantly inhibit Hsp70 RNA synthesis (Table 5.1). Instead, this inhibitor has previously been shown to induce transcription of Hsp70 genes (9). When Drosophila cells incubated at 25°C were treated with 100 μM VM-26, Hsp70 transcription was stimulated ·approximately tenfold, suggesting that inhibition of topoisomerase II by VM-26 may induce the expression of the Hsp70 gene (9). This is consistent with our finding that the major topoisomerase II site at the 5′ end of the Hsp70 gene falls in a region that negatively regulates Hsp70 transcription (Fig. 5.2B).

Although the effects of topoisomerase-active drugs on Hsp70 transcription suggests that these enzymes are important in gene expression, it is possible that these drugs mediate their effects by a different mechanism. In regard to this question, a mutant cell line has recently been identified that has a VM-26–resistant topoisomerase II enzyme. This cell line should be very useful in determining whether or not the VM-26–induced changes in gene expression are mediated through DNA topoisomerase II (32). In addition, temperature-sensitive topoisomerase I and II mutants have been isolated in yeast, and preliminary studies with these mutants indicate that DNA topoisomerases are important in gene expression (33,34). Surprisingly, the yeast studies suggest that DNA topoisomerase I and II have similar and interchangeable roles in regulating overall (poly A$^+$) and (poly A$^-$) RNA synthesis (34). This differs from our findings on the Drosophila Hsp70 heat-shock gene that suggest that the roles of these two enzymes are not necessarily interchangeable. Future investigations should resolve these issues and present a much clearer picture of the role of DNA topoisomerases in gene transcription.

Acknowledgments

The authors wish to acknowledge David Kroll, Jeff Lawrence, and Chris Borgert for their helpful discussions during these studies. This work was supported by Public Health Service grant R29-GM38859 from the National Institutes of Health.

REFERENCES

1. Tewey, K. M., Rowe, T. C., Chen, G. L., Yang, L., Halligan, B. D., and Liu L. F. Adriamycin-induced DNA damage is mediated by mammalian DNA topoisomerase II. Science. 266: 466–468, 1984.

2. Chen, G. L., Yang, L., Rowe, T. C., Halligan, B. D., Tewey, K. M., and Liu, L. F. Nonintercalative antitumor drugs interfere with the breakage-reunion reaction of mammalian DNA topoisomerase II. J. Biol. Chem. 259: 13560–13566, 1984.

3. Hsiang, Y.-H., Hertzberg, R., Hecht, S., and Liu, L. F. Camptothecin induces protein-linked DNA breaks via mammalian DNA topoisomerase I. J. Biol. Chem. 260: 14873–14878, 1985.

4. Ross, W. E. DNA topoisomerase as targets for cancer therapy. Biochem. Pharmacol. 34: 4191–4195, 1985.

5. Drlica, K. and Franco, R. Inhibition of DNA topoisomerases. Biochemistry. 27: 2553–2559, 1988.

6. Nelson, E. M., Tewey, K. M., and Liu, L.F. Mechanism of antitumor drug action: Poisoning of mammalian DNA topoisomerase II on DNA by 4'-(9-acridinylamino)-methanesulfon-m-anisidide. Proc. Natl. Acad. Sci. USA. **81:** 1361–1365, 1984.

7. Horwitz, S. B., Chang, C.-K., and Grollman, A. P. Studies on camptothecin: I. Effect on nucleic acid and protein synthesis. Mol. Pharmacol. **7:** 632–644, 1971.

8. Grieder, A., Maurer, R., and Stahelin, H. Effect of an epipodophyllotoxin derivative (VP 16-213) on macromolecular synthesis and mitosis in mastocytoma cells in vitro. Cancer Res. **34:** 1788–1793, 1974.

9. Rowe, T. C., Wang, J. C., and Liu, L. F. *In vivo* localization of DNA topoisomerase II cleavage sites on Drosophila heat-shock chromatin. Mol. Cell. Biol. **6:** 985–992, 1986.

10. Linquist, S. The heat-shock response. Annu. Rev. Biochem. **55:** 1151–1191, 1986.

11. Lindquist, S. and Craig, E. A. The heat-shock proteins. Annu. Rev. Genet. **22:** 631–677, 1988.

12. Artavanis-Tsakonas, S., Schedl, P., Mirault, M.-E., Moran, L., and Lis, J. Genes for the 70,000 dalton heat-shock protein in two cloned *D. melanogaster* DNA segments. Cell. **17:** 9–18, 1979.

13. Rowe, T. C., Couto, E., and Kroll, D. J. Camptothecin inhibits Hsp70 heat-shock transcription and induces DNA strand breaks in Hsp70 genes in Drosophila. NCI monographs. **4:** 49–53, 1987.

14. Gilmour, D. S. and Elgin, S.C.R. Localization of specific topoisomerase I interactions within the transcribed region of active heat-shock genes by using the inhibitor camptothecin. Mol. Cell. Biol. **7:** 141–148, 1987.

15. Zhang, H., Wang, J. C., and Liu, L. F. Involvement of DNA topoisomerase I in transcription of human ribosomal RNA genes. Proc. Natl. Acad. Sci. USA. **85:** 1060–1064, 1988.

16. Stewart, A. F. and Schutz, G. Camptothecin-induced *in vivo* topoisomerase I cleavages in the transcriptionally active tyrosine aminotransferase gene. Cell. **50:** 1109–1117, 1987.

17. Fleishchmann, G., Pflugfelder, G., Steiner, E. K., Javaherian, K., Howard, G. C., Wang, J. C., and Elgin, S.C.R. Drosophila DNA topoisomerase I is associated with transcriptionally active regions of the genome. Proc. Natl. Acad. Sci. USA. **81:** 6958–6962, 1984.

18. Weisbrod, S. Active chromatin. Nature. **297:** 289–295, 1982.

19. Gilmour, D. S., Pflugfelder, G., Wang, J. C., and Lis, J. T. Topoisomerase I interacts with transcribed regions in Drosophila cells. Cell. **44:** 401–407, 1986.

20. Liu, L. F. and Wang, J. C. Supercoiling of the DNA template during transcription. Proc. Natl. Acad. Sci. USA. **84:** 7024–7027, 1987.

21. Kroeger, P. E. and Rowe, T. C. R. Interaction of topoisomerase I with the transcribed region of the Drosophila hsp70 heat-shock gene. Nucleic Acids Res. **17:** 8495–8509, 1989.

22. Camilloni, G., Di Martino, E., Di Mauro, E., and Caserta, M. Regulation of the function of eukaryotic topoisomerase I: Topological conditions for inactivity. Proc. Natl. Acad. Sci. USA. **86:** 3080–3084, 1989.

23. Gross, D. S. and Garrard, W. T. Nuclease hypersensitive sites in chromatin. Annu. Rev. Biochem. **57:** 159–197, 1988.

24. Corces, V. and Pellicer, A. Identification of sequences involved in the transcriptional control of a Drosophila heat-shock gene. J. Biol. Chem. **259:** 14812–14817, 1984.

25. Gilmour, D. S. and Lis, J. T. RNA polymerase II interacts with the promoter region of the noninduced hsp70 gene in *Drosophila melanogaster* cells. Mol. Cell. Biol. **6:** 3984–3989, 1986.

26. Rougvie, A. E. and Lis, J. T. The RNA polymerase II molecule at the 5' end of the uninduced hsp70 gene of *D. melanogaster* is transcriptionally engaged. Cell. **54:** 795–804, 1988.

27. Riou, J.-F., Vilarem, M.-J., Larsen, C. J., Multon, E., and Riou, G. F. *In vivo* and *in vitro* stimulation by antitumor drugs of the topoisomerase II-induced cleavage sites in c-*myc* proto-oncogene. NCI monographs. **4:** 41–47, 1987.

28. Darby, M. K., Herrera, R. E., Vosberg, P., and Nordheim, A. DNA topoisomerase II cleaves at specific sites in the 5' flanking region of c-*fos* proto-oncogenes *in vitro*. EMBO J. **5:** 2257–2265, 1986.

29. Yang, L., Rowe, T. C., Nelson, E. M., and Liu, L. F. *In vivo* mapping of DNA topoisomerase II-specific cleavage sites on SV40 chromatin. Cell. **41:** 127–132, 1985.

30. Weiher, H., Konig, M., and Gruss, P. Multiple point mutations affecting the Simian virus 40 enhancer. Science. **219:** 626–631, 1983.

31. Garg, L. C., DiAngelo, S., and Jacob, S. T. Role of DNA topoisomerase I in the transcription of supercoiled rRNA gene. Proc. Natl. Acad. Sci. USA. **84:** 3185–3188, 1987.

32. Sullivan, D. M., Latham, M. D., Rowe, T. C., and Ross, W. E. Purification and

characterization of an altered topoisomerase II from a drug resistant Chinese hamster ovary cell line. Biochemistry. **28:** 5680–5687, 1989.

33. DiNardo, S., Thrash, C., Voelkel, K. A., Sternglanz, R. Identification of yeast DNA topoisomerase mutants. In N. R. Cozzarelli, ed. *Mechanisms of DNA Replication and Recombination* New York: Alan R. Liss, 1983, pp. 29–42.

34. Brill, S. J., DiNardo, S., Voelkel-Meiman, K., and Sternglanz, R. Need for DNA topoisomerase activity as a swivel for DNA replication for transcription of ribosomal RNA. Nature. **326:** 434–436, 1987.

35. Maniatis, T., Fritsch, E. F., Sambrook, J. Molecular cloning, a laboratory manual. Cold Spring Harbor, Cold Spring Harbor Laboratory Press, 1982.

Chapter 6

Effect of Inhibitors on Type II Topoisomerase Activity in the Mitochondria of Trypanosomes

THERESA A. SHAPIRO, VIIU A. KLEIN,
AND PAUL T. ENGLUND

The family Trypanosomatidae includes a number of parasitic hemoflagellates pathogenic to man and animals. Each of these protozoa has a single mitochondrion that contains a unique type of DNA called kinetoplast DNA (kDNA; see refs. 1–5 for reviews on kDNA). This DNA is in the form of a single network of thousands of topologically interlocked DNA circles, a structure unique in nature. Two kinds of DNA circles constitute the network. Most abundant are the minicircles, present in several thousand copies per network, that vary in size from 0.5 to 2.8 kilobases (kb) in different species. Their function is not yet known. Networks contain 25–50 maxicircles, and their sizes vary from about 20 to 37 kb in different species. Maxicircles resemble the mitochondrial DNA of other eukaryotes in both structure and genetic function. The electron micrograph in Figure 6.1 shows a portion of an isolated kinetoplast DNA network.

In the replication of a kDNA network, minicircles and maxicircles are synthesized by different mechanisms. Covalently closed minicircles are released from the network, and these free forms replicate as theta structures to produce monomeric progeny circles that contain nicks or small gaps. Daughter minicircles are reattached to the network where they eventually are covalently closed. Maxicircles, on the other hand, are synthesized as network-bound rolling circles. When all the circles have replicated, the double size network splits to yield two progeny that are identical to the parent network, and that segregate into the daughter cells at the time of cell division (see refs. 4 and 5 for reviews of kDNA replication). A simplified scheme for network replication is depicted in Figure 6.2.

The complex nature of kDNA structure and replication creates an unusually high demand for topoisomerase activity. Topoisomerases undoubtedly function at several steps in the minicircle replication process: decatenation of parental circles from networks; unlinking of template strands during fork propagation; segregation of catenated dimers; formation and resolution of knotted

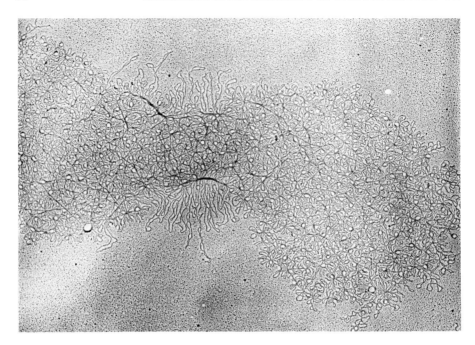

Figure 6.1. Electron micrograph of an isolated, replicating kinetoplast DNA network from *T. equiperdum*. The bulk of the structure is composed of a catenated meshwork of minicircles (small loops at the periphery of the network), of 1 kb each. Maxicircles (23 kb each) are concentrated in the area where the double size network is being separated to form two daughters. Micrograph was provided by Dr. James Ntambi.

free minicircles (6); and recantenation of daughter circles to networks. Topoisomerases probably play an important role in maxicircle replication, and they are likely to be involved in the scission of double size networks. Furthermore, in addition to these enzymatic functions, type II topoisomerases in the mitochondria of trypanosomes might have a structural role (analogous to the topoisomerase in the scaffold of mammalian nuclei [7]), perhaps tethering replicating free circles to the network or constraining the network to one region of the mitochondrion. A type II topoisomerase has been purified from *Crithidia fasciculata,* a related kinetoplastid organism (8). Interestingly, on the basis of immunofluorescence microscopy, this enzyme localizes to two distinct sites at the periphery of the kDNA network but is not detectable in the nucleus (9).

In bacteria and higher eukaryotes, the function and mechanism of topoisomerases have been greatly clarified by inhibitor studies (10). Certain antibacterial agents (11,12) and a variety of intercalative and nonintercalative antitumor agents (13,14) stabilize a "cleavable complex" between the type II topoisomerase and its DNA substrate; a covalent protein–DNA adduct is trapped upon denaturation of the complex with SDS. Furthermore, the catalytic role of type II topoisomerases in the replication of circular DNA molecules is evident from the accumulation of unsegregated daughter circles of SV40 DNA in the presence of type II topoisomerase inhibitors (15).

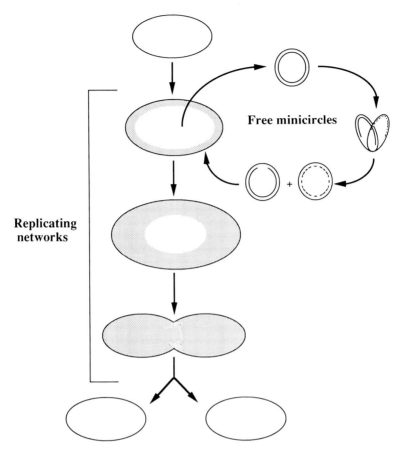

Figure 6.2. Model for replication of kinetoplast DNA. Networks replicate in synchrony with nuclear DNA, in the S-phase of the cell cycle. The dotted region of the network contains reattached progeny minicircles, which have nicks or small gaps. Maxicircles are not depicted. See text for discussion.

VP 16-213 TRAPS A MINICIRCLE DNA–PROTEIN COMPLEX

To explore for a drug-sensitive mitochondrial type II topoisomerase in *Trypanosoma equiperdum*, freshly harvested trypanosomes in tissue culture medium were exposed to VP 16-213 (etoposide; for experimental details see [16]), a potent and highly specific inhibitor of eukaryotic nuclear type II topoisomerases (14). After treatment for 30 min at 37°C, trypanosomes were lysed with SDS. The lysates were digested with proteinase K, phenol extracted, and the purified DNA (which includes nuclear DNA as well as free minicircles and networks) was resolved by agarose gel electrophoresis. To examine minicircle DNA, a Southern blot was probed with [^{32}P]-labeled *T. equiperdum* minicircle DNA. Figure 6.3, lane 1, depicts the normal distribution of DNA among the major components of the free minicircle pool (networks do not enter the gel);

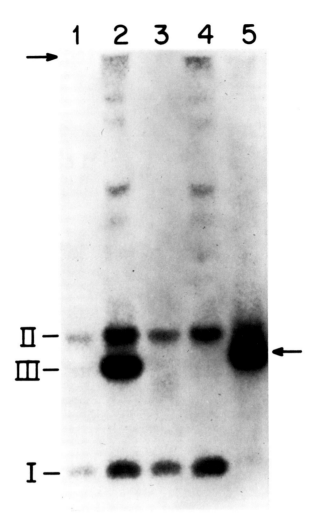

Figure 6.3. VP 16-213 generates protein-bound linearized minicircles. *T. equiperdum* in medium were treated for 30 min at 37°C with VP 16-213 (100 μM) or with vehicle alone as indicated. The SDS lysate was digested with proteinase K as indicated, then with RNase A and RNase T₁. After phenol extraction and ethanol precipitation, the DNA was electrophoresed in a 1.5% agarose gel with buffer containing 1 μg/ml ethidium bromide, transferred to a nylon membrane, and probed with [³²P]-labeled minicircle sequence. Lane 1, cells treated with vehicle; DNA treated with proteinase K (some DNA was lost during processing; form I and II bands should have intensity equal to those in lane 3). Lane 2, cells treated with VP 16-213; DNA treated with proteinase K. Lane 3, cells treated with vehicle; DNA not treated with proteinase K. Lane 4, cells treated with VP 16-213; DNA not treated with proteinase K. Lane 5, interface from phenol extraction of DNA shown in lane 4. II, minicircles containing nicks or small gaps; III, linearized minicircles; I, covalently closed minicircles. Rightward arrow indicates origin; leftward arrow indicates minicircle-protein complex (lane 5).

Table 6.1. Effect of VP 16-213 on *T. equiperdum* Free Minicircles

| Treatment | Minicircle Pool Size (% of Total Minicircles[a]) | | | |
	Form II	Form III	Form I	Sum
No drug[b]	3.4 ± 1.4	1.7 ± 0.8	2.1 ± 0.9	7.2
VP 16-213[c]	9.1 ± 5.5	22.4 ± 9.7	7.1 ± 5.7	38.6

DNA samples from *T. equiperdum* treated in tissue culture medium with no drug or with VP 16-213 (100 μM) (37°C, 30 min) were prepared as described in Figure 6.3. DNA bands were quantitated by densitometry of autoradiographs like that in Figure 6.3. Values are mean ± standard deviation. Smaller increases in minicircle pool sizes are seen in samples from trypanosomes treated in rat blood (16).
[a]Total minicircle DNA (network-bound plus free) was estimated by densitometry of autoradiographs of *Bgl* II digests of total cell DNA (*Bgl* II cleaves all minicircles once).
[b]Data from four experiments.
[c]Data from six experiments.

the predominant free forms are nicked or uniquely gapped circles (II), linearized circles (III), and covalently closed circles (I). VP 16-213 perturbed this distribution, causing an increase in the mass of the free minicircle DNA population, most strikingly in the linearized form (Fig. 6.3, lane 2 and Table 6.1). There was no detecable formation of fragments smaller than 1 kb, indicating the minicircles were cleaved only once.

The drug-induced linearized minicircles are protein-linked. If proteinase K treatment was omitted, the aqueous phase after phenol extraction contained essentially no linear forms (Fig. 6.3, lane 4). During phenol extraction of the VP 16-213–treated samples that had not been treated with proteinase K, a copious interface formed between the phenol and aqueous phases. Analysis of the interface revealed minicircle DNA with a mobility intermediate between that of nicked and linearized forms (Fig. 6.3, lane 5). When treated with proteinase K, this DNA was converted to a form that comigrated with form III minicircles (data not shown).

Exonuclease treatment demonstrates that the protein trapped from the mitochondria of VP 16-213–treated cells is linked to both 5′ ends of the linearized minicircles. DNA purified from drug-treated trypanosomes was digested with exonuclease III (a 3′ to 5′ exonuclease) or lambda exonuclease (a 5′ to 3′ exonuclease). The VP 16-213–induced linearized minicircles (Fig. 6.4, lane 1; form III) were completely digested by exonuclease III (Fig. 6.4, lane 2) but were impervious to lambda exonuclease (Fig. 6.4, lane 3). An internal monitor of nuclease activity included in these reactions (pBR322 DNA linearized by *Hin*d III) was fully digested by lambda exonuclease.

TIME COURSE OF VP 16-213 TREATMENT

Linearization of minicircles by SDS lysis of intact trypanosomes treated with VP 16-213 was evaluated as a function of time. The minicircle DNA–protein complex reached a maximum within 5 min of drug exposure (Fig. 6.5, lane 2).

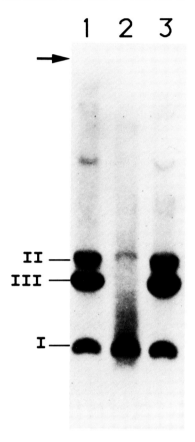

Figure 6.4. Exonuclease treatment of linearized minicircles. Trypanosomes in medium were treated with VP-16-213 (100 μM, 37°C, 30 min), and lysed with SDS. The lysate was digested with proteinase K and the DNA was processed as described in Figure 6.3. DNA from 4.5 × 10⁷ cells, containing 120 ng of control *Hin*d III-linearized pBR322 DNA, was digested (30 min, 37°C) with exonuclease III or with lambda exonuclease and electrophoresed in 1.5% agarose with buffer containing 1 μg/ml ethidium bromide. After visualization of the control pBR322 DNA by photography, the DNA was transferred to a nylon membrane and probed with [³²P]-labeled minicircle sequence. Lane 1, no nuclease treatment. Lane 2, exonuclease III digest. Lane 3, lambda exonuclease digest. I, II, III as defined in Figure 6.3 legend.

At saturation, about 12% of the total (network-bound plus free) minicircle population is linearized. In an asynchronous population of untreated *T. equiperdum*, only about 5% of the minicircles are free for the purpose of replication (Table 6.1); therefore, most drug-promoted form III minicircles must derive from networks. In further support of this notion, the free minicircle population from VP 16-213–treated cells also contains increased amounts of form I and II minicircles (Fig. 6.5, lanes 2–6 and Table 6.1), which may be released from networks when neighboring circles are linearized. In contrast, some of the bands migrating slower than form II are probably multimeric minicircle repli-

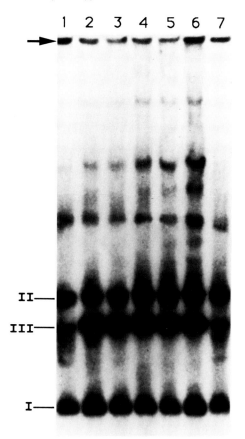

Figure 6.5. Time course of VP 16-213 treatment. Trypanosomes in rat blood were treated at 37°C with VP 16-213 (100 μM) or with vehicle for the indicated times, and lysed with SDS. The lysate was digested with proteinase K and the DNA further processed as described in Figure 6.3. Each lane contains DNA from 7.5 × 10⁶ cells, which was electrophoresed in a 1.5% agarose gel with buffer containing 1 μg/ml ethidium bromide. Lane 1, vehicle control, treated 5 min. Lanes 2 to 6, treated with VP 16-213 for 5, 10, 20, 30, and 45 min, respectively. Lane 7, vehicle control, treated 45 min. By densitometry, Form III minicircles in lanes 1–7 constitute <1, 11.3, 13.6, 12.0, 10.9, 12.0 and <1 percent of the total minicircle population, respectively.

cation intermediates that accumulate with time owing to inhibition of type II topoisomerase catalytic activity (Fig. 6.5, lanes 2–6).

Assuming each cell has 5000 minicircles (17) (of 1 kb each), if 12% are linearized after VP 16-213 treatment, there must be at least 600 copies of mitochondrial type II topoisomerase in each cell, or about 1 enzyme per 8 kb of minicircle DNA. This value is higher than the estimated 1 per 23 kb ratio for type II topoisomerase in the cells of rapidly dividing *Drosophila* embryos (18), but is comparable to the 1 per 5 kb ratio in transformed chicken erythroblasts (19). The relatively high topoisomerase:minicircle DNA ratio may be required for replication and maintenance of the topologically complex kDNA network.

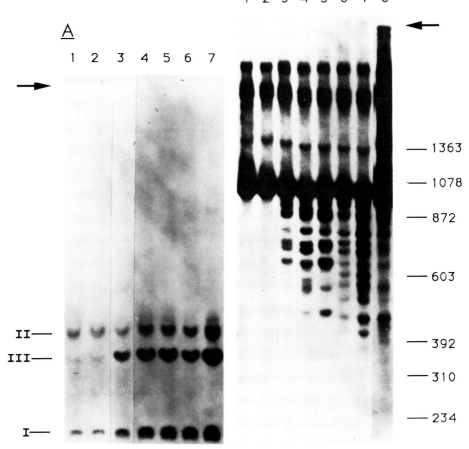

Figure 6.6. Treatment of trypanosomes with various type II topoisomerase inhibitors. Trypanosomes in medium were treated for 30 min at 37°C with drug or with solvent. The DNA was processed as in Figure 6.3. DNA from 3×10^7 cells was electrophoresed directly in a 1.5% agarose gel with buffer containing 1 μg/ml ethidium bromide (Panel A). An equal quantity of each sample was digested with *Bgl*II before electrophoresis in a 2% agarose gel with buffer containing 1 μg/ml ethidium bromide. **Panel A.** Lane 1, DNA from control cells. Lane 2, from cells treated with nalidixic acid (400 μM). Lane 3, from cells treated with acriflavine (50 μM). Lane 4, from cells treated with MHE (5 μM). Lane 5, from cells treated with *m*-AMSA (6 μM). Lane 6, from cells treated with VM-26 (100 μM). Lane 7, from cells treated with VP 16-213 (100 μM). Samples from cells treated with dimethyl sulfoxide or with vehicle were identical to control DNA (lane 1). **Panel B.** Lanes 1 to 7, *Bgl*II digests of DNA as described in Panel A (the autoradiograph was exposed for 3 h). Lane 8, same as lane 1 except autoradiograph was exposed for 16 h.

SUSCEPTIBILITY TO OTHER TYPE II TOPOISOMERASE INHIBITORS

Live trypanosomes were exposed to various compounds known to affect type II topoisomerases. These compounds included inhibitors of gyrase (oxolinic and nalidixic acids) (11,12), agents active against eukaryotic type II topoisomerases (the epipodophyllotoxins, 2-methyl-9-hydroxyellipticine (MHE), 4'-(9-acridinylamino)-methanesulfon-*m*-anisidine (*m*-AMSA), and acriflavine) (14,20,21), and novobiocin (which competes with ATP for binding to both prokaryotic and eukaryotic type II topoisomerases, but does not stabilize cleavable complexes) (21,22). The compounds were tested at concentrations reported to be effective against intact cells in culture or in animals. Like VP 16-213 (Fig. 6.6A, lane 7), the other inhibitors of eukaryotic type II topoisomerases promote minicircle cleavage (Fig. 6.6A, lanes 3–6). However, novobiocin (at concentrations up to 4mM) or compounds known to generate DNA–protein complexes with gyrase (nalidixic and oxolinic acids, at concentrations up to 400 μM and 50μM, respectively) (Fig. 6.6A, lane 2, and data not shown) do not cause detectable cleavage of *T. equiperdum* minicircles.

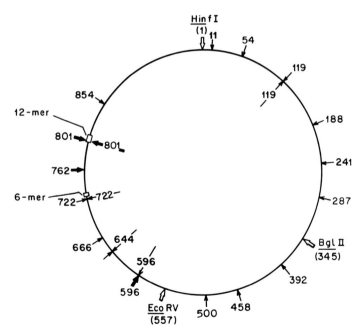

Figure 6.7. Map of cleavage sites induced in *T. equiperdum* kDNA minicircles by VP 16-213. This map is based on the published nucleotide sequence (1012 base pairs); numbering begins at the *Hin*f I site (34). "Natural" sites (produced by SDS lysis in the absence of drug) are indicated by outward pointing arrows. VP 16-213–induced breaks are depicted with inward pointing arrows; heavy arrows represent major cleavage points.

MAPPING THE CLEAVAGE SITES

The sites of minicircle cleavage were mapped by digesting DNA samples from control or drug-treated cells with *Bgl* II (an enzyme that cuts minicircles once at nucleotide 345, see map Fig. 6.7). The fragments were separated by agarose gel electrophoresis, transferred to GeneScreen and probed with [^{32}P]-labeled minicircle sequence. The linearized minicircles naturally present in samples not treated with drug create a distinct pattern of bands (Fig. 6.6B, lane 8; these bands are not detectable in the shorter exposure shown in lane 1). More complex patterns are generated by drug treatment (Fig. 6.6B, lanes 3–7). As anticipated, digests of DNA from cells treated with compounds that do not generate linearized minicircles (nalidixic acid, Fig. 6.6B, lane 2 and longer exposures) display only the "natural" cleavage pattern like that in lane 8. As has been reported previously for other cell types and with purified nuclear type II topoisomerases *in vitro,* drugs of different chemical classes generate strikingly different cleavage patterns (23,24). Interestingly, within the resolution of agarose electrophoresis, drugs appear to enhance the "natural" cut sites, perhaps by stabilizing type II topoisomerase at these preferred locations. Figure 6.7 is a map of naturally occurring and VP 16-213–induced cleavage sites in *T. equiperdum* minicircles.

DISCUSSION

Treatment of intact *T. equiperdum* with compounds known to be active against mammalian type II topoisomerases results in DNA cleavage after SDS lysis. Because minicircle DNA is present in the cleaved complex, the type II topoisomerase that has been trapped must be mitochondrial in origin. As is characteristic of the type II topoisomerase–DNA complexes that have been evaluated, the enzyme from *T. equiperdum* mitochondria binds to both 5' ends of the substrate DNA. Furthermore, prior to cell lysis, VP 16-213 inhibits catalytic activity of the enzyme, resulting in an accumulation of multimeric replicating minicircle forms. Gyrase inhibitors, even at concentrations 25 times greater than those effective against *Escherichia coli* (25,26), do not promote minicircle linearization or give evidence of type II topoisomerase inhibition. In terms of inhibitor susceptibility, the mitochondrial type II topoisomerase of *T. equiperdum* would appear to resemble most closely the type II topoisomerase in the nuclei of higher eukaryotes, rather than gyrase, the type II topoisomerase of prokaryotes.

Mitochondrial type II topoisomerase activity has been partially purified from human leukemia cells (27) and from rat liver (28), and purified to homogeneity from *C. fasciculata* (8). Nalidixic acid inhibits catalytic activity of the isolated enzyme from *C. fasciculata,* but not of those from rat liver or human leukemia cells. These differences in susceptibility to gyrase inhibitors may reflect isofunctional enzyme differences, or they may be an artifact of differences in DNA substrate, assay conditions, or, in the case of *T. equiperdum,* perhaps in drug transport.

Treatment of kinetoplastid protozoa with dyes such as acriflavine results in selective interference with the structure and division of kinetoplast (rather than nuclear) DNA (29,30). In time, the population of dividing cells with one nucleus and one kinetoplast is replaced by cells with one nucleus and no kinetoplast. This phenotype is stable only in bloodstream forms of trypanosomes, which do not rely on oxidative phosphorylation as a source of energy. "Dyskinetoplastic" cells retain mitochondrial membranes (31,32), but the characteristic densely staining kDNA disc is absent on light or electron microscopy, and no DNA homologous to minicircle or maxicircle sequences is detectable (17). Acriflavine promotes minicircle DNA–type II topoisomerase complexes (Fig. 6.6A, lane 3) and inhibits the catalytic activity of isolated type II topoisomerase from trypanosomes (20). It therefore seems likely that the genesis of dyskinetoplastic trypanosomes by acriflavine is mediated, at least in part, by interference with kinetoplast type II topoisomerase activity. The basis for the selectivity of this effect against kDNA replication is an interesting and unexplained phenomenon. Preliminary results indicate that in trypanosomes, acriflavine (unlike its structural analog, *m*-AMSA) causes cleavage of mitochondrial, but not nuclear DNA (Shapiro and Englund, unpublished). A number of antitrypanosomal drugs also promote the selective cleavage of minicircle DNA (33). These data suggest that the nuclear and mitochondrial type II topoisomerases of trypanosomes may be different.

The type II topoisomerase inhibitors will undoubtedly prove important in understanding the role of type II topoisomerases in trypanosomes, and may also provide a much needed new approach to antitrypanosomal chemotherapy.

REFERENCES

1. Englund, P. T., Hajduk, S. L., and Marini, J. C. The molecular biology of trypanosomes. Annu. Rev. Biochem. **51:** 695, 1982.

2. Stuart, K. Kinetoplast DNA, mitochondrial DNA with a difference. Mol. Biochem. Parasitol. **9:** 93, 1983.

3. Simpson, L. The mitochondrial genome of kinetoplastid protozoa: Genomic organization, transcription, replication, and evolution. Annu. Rev. Microbiol. **41:** 363, 1987.

4. Ray, D. S. Kinetoplast DNA minicircles: High-copy-number mitochondrial plasmids. Plasmid. **17:** 177, 1987.

5. Ryan, K. A., Shapiro, T. A., Rauch, C. A., and Englund, P. T. The replication of kinetoplast DNA in trypanosomes. Annu. Rev. Microbiol. **42:** 339, 1988.

6. Ryan, K. A., Shapiro, T. A., Rauch, C. A., Griffith, J. D., and Englund, P. T. A knotted free minicircle in kinetoplast DNA. Proc. Natl. Acad. Sci. USA. **85:** 5844, 1988.

7. Earnshaw, W. C., Halligan, B., Cooke, C.

A., Heck, M. M. S., and Liu, L. F. Topoisomerase II is a structural component of mitotic chromosome scaffolds. J. Cell Biol. **100:** 1706, 1985.

8. Melendy, T. and Ray, D. S. Novobiocin affinity purification of a mitochondrial type II topoisomerase from the Trypanosomatid Crithidia fasciculata. J. Biol. Chem. **264:** 1870, 1989.

9. Melendy, T., Sheline, C., and Ray, D. S. Localization of a type II DNA topoisomerase to two sites at the periphery of the kinetoplast DNA of Crithidia fasciculata. Cell. **55:** 1083, 1988.

10. Drlica, K. and Franco, R. J. Inhibitors of DNA topoisomerases. Biochemistry. **27:** 2253, 1988.

11. Sugino, A., Peebles, C. L., Kreuzer, K. N., and Cozzarelli, N. R. Mechanism of action of nalidixic acid: Purification of Escherichia coli nalA gene product and its relationship to DNA gyrase and a novel nicking-closing enzyme. Proc. Natl. Acad. Sci. USA. **74:** 4767, 1977.

12. Gellert, M., Mizuuchi, K., O'Dea, M. H.,

Itoh, T., and Tomizawa, J-I. Nalidixic acid resistance: A second genetic character involved in DNA gyrase activity. Proc. Natl. Acad. Sci. USA. **74**: 4772, 1977.

13. Tewey, K. M., Chen, G. L., Nelson, E. M., and Liu, L. F. Intercalative antitumor drugs interfere with the breakage-reunion reaction of mammalian DNA topoisomerase II. J. Biol. Chem. **259**: 9182, 1984.

14. Chen, G. L., Yang, L., Rowe, T. C., Halligan, B. D., Tewey, K. M., and Liu, L. F. Nonintercalative antitumor drugs interfere with the breakage-reunion reaction of mammalian DNA topoisomerase II. J. Biol. Chem. **259**: 13560, 1984.

15. Yang, L., Wold, M. S., Li, J. J., Kelly, T. J., and Liu, L. F. Roles of DNA topoisomerases in simian virus 40 DNA replication in vitro. Proc. Natl. Acad. Sci. USA. **84**: 950, 1987.

16. Shapiro, T. A., Klein, V. A., and Englund, P. T. Drug promoted cleavage of kinetoplast DNA minicircles: Evidence for type II topoisomerase activity in trypanosome mitochondria. J. Biol. Chem. **264**: 4173, 1989.

17. Riou, G. F. and Saucier, J.-M. Characterization of the molecular components in kinetoplast-mitochondrial DNA of Trypanosoma equiperdum. J. Cell Biol. **82**: 248, 1979.

18. Fairman, R. and Brutlag, D. L. Expression of the Drosophila type II topoisomerase is developmentally regulated. Biochemistry. **27**: 560, 1988.

19. Heck, M.M.S. and Earnshaw, W. C. Topoisomerase II: A specific marker for cell proliferation. J. Cell Biol. **103**: 2569, 1986.

20. Riou, G., Douc-Rasy, S., and Kayser, A. Inhibitors of trypanosome topoisomerases. Biochem. Soc. Trans. **14**: 496, 1986.

21. Nelson, E. M., Tewey, K. M., and Liu, L. F. Mechanism of antitumor drug action: Poisoning of mammalian DNA topoisomerase II on DNA by 4'-(9-acridinylamino)-methanesulfon-*m*-anisidine. Proc. Natl. Acad. Sci. USA. **81**: 1361, 1984.

22. Hsieh, T-S. and Brutlag, D. ATP-dependent DNA topoisomerase from D. melanogaster reversibly catenates duplex DNA rings. Cell. **21**: 115, 1980.

23. Tewey, K. M., Rowe, T. C., Yang, L.,

Halligan, B. D., and Liu, L. F. Adriamycin-induced DNA damage mediated by mammalian DNA topoisomerase II. Science. **226**: 466, 1984.

24. Snapka, R. M. Topoisomerase inhibitors can selectively interfere with different stages of simian virus 40 DNA replication. Mol. Cell. Biol. **6**: 4221, 1986.

25. Wolfson, J. S. and Hooper, D. C. The fluoroquinolones: Structures, mechanisms of action and resistance, and spectra of activity in vitro. Antimicrob. Agents Chemother. **28**: 581, 1985.

26. Goss, W. A., Deitz, W. H., and Cook, T. M. Mechanism of action of nalidixic acid on Escherichia coli. J. Bacteriol. **89**: 1068, 1965.

27. Castora, F. J. and Lazarus, G. M. Isolation of a mitochondrial DNA topoisomerase from human leukemia cells. Biochem. Biophys. Res. Commun. **121**: 77, 1984.

28. Castora, F. J., Vissering, F. F., and Simpson, M. V. The effect of bacterial DNA gyrase inhibitors on DNA synthesis in mammalian mitochondria. Biochim. Biophys. Acta. **740**: 417, 1983.

29. Simpson, L. The kinetoplast of the hemoflagellates. Int. Rev. Cytol. **32**: 139, 1972.

30. Hajduk, S. L. Influence of DNA complexing compounds on the kinetoplast of trypanosomatids. Prog. Mol. Subcell. Biol. **6**: 158, 1978.

31. Mühlpfordt, V. H. Über die bedeutung und feinstruktur des blepharoplasten bei parasitischen flagellaten. Z. Tropenmed. Parasitol. **14**: 357, 1963.

32. Trager, W. and Rudzinska, M. A. The riboflavin requirement and the effects of acriflavin on the fine structure of the kinetoplast of Leishmania tarentole. J. Protozool. **11**: 133, 1964.

33. Shapiro, T. A. and Englund, P. T. Selective cleavage of kinetoplast DNA minicircles promoted by anti-trypanosomal drugs. Proc. Natl. Acad. Sci. USA. **87**: 950, 1990.

34. Barrois, M., Riou, G., and Galibert, F. Complete nucleotide sequence of minicircle kinetoplast DNA from Trypanosoma equiperdum. Proc. Natl. Acad. Sci. USA. **78**: 3323, 1981.

Chapter 7
Yeast as a Genetic System in the Dissection of the Mechanism of Cell Killing by Topoisomerase-Targeting Anticancer Drugs

JOHN L. NITISS
AND JAMES C. WANG

A number of antitumor drugs are known to target the DNA topoisomerases (reviewed in 1–4). For example, the plant alkaloid camptothecin has been shown to act on eukaryotic DNA topoisomerase I, a type I topoisomerase, and a number of epipodophyllotoxin and anilinoacridine derivatives have been shown to act on eukaryotic DNA topoisomerase II, a type II topoisomerase (for recent reviews on DNA topoisomerases see 5–8).

We have previously reported the use of permeability mutants of the yeast *Saccharomyces cerevisiae* in the study of such drugs (9). There is ample evidence that the yeast enzymes resemble their counterparts in other eukaryotes, including human. Functional similarity of topoisomerase II from different eukaryotes has been demonstrated by showing that the Drosophila *TOP2* gene encoding the enzyme can complement the lethal phenotype of a deletion of the yeast *TOP2* gene (10); complementation of a yeast *TOP2* deletion has also been achieved by the expression of human *TOP2* (M. Tsai-Pflugfelder, C. Kanik-Ennulat, and J. C. Wang, unpublished). A comparison of sequences of DNA topoisomerases I and II from a variety of eukaryotes also shows a high degree of conservation of each of the enzymes (11–13).

The genetic tools that are available for yeast provide distinct advantages in the use of this microorganism for studies of the topoisomerase-targeting drugs. The ease with which targeted gene replacement can be carried out in yeast is particularly advantageous in the construction of isogenic strains that differ only in defined characters; comparative studies of drug actions in these isogenic strains provide important clues in deducing the mechanisms of cell killing by these drugs. A recent example of this approach is the demonstration that in yeast the only cellular target of the drug camptothecin is DNA topoisomerase I; *top1* mutants of yeast in which the enzyme is inactivated are resistant to the drug (9,14). Furthermore, the expression of human *TOP1* gene in yeast *top1* mutants confers again camptothecin sensitivity, which makes it possible to study interactions between camptothecin and human DNA topoisomerase I in yeast (15).

We and others (9,14) have also reported previously that the yeast *RAD52* recombinational repair pathway is likely to be involved in the processing of camptothecin-induced lesions; mutations in *RAD52* greatly increase sensitivity of cells to camptothecin.

In the present communication, we show that the *RAD52* pathway appears to be involved in the processing of lesions induced by both type I and type II DNA topoisomerase-targeting drugs. The effects of mutations in two other repair pathways were also tested. Neither mutations in *RAD2*, a member of the epistatic group involved in excision repair, nor mutations in *RAD6*, which encodes a ubiquitin conjugating enzyme (19) and is a member of the epistatic group involved in the repair, has significant effect on cytotoxicity of topoisomerase-targeting drugs (for review on recombination pathways in yeast see 16–18). We show also that when yeast mutants permeable to both type I and type II DNA topoisomerase-targeting drugs are used, simultaneous treatment of cells with a DNA topoisomerase I drug and a DNA topoisomerase II drug results in a higher level of cytotoxicity than that caused by either drug alone. These results demonstrate further the potential of yeast as a genetic system in the study of antitumor drugs. Some implications of the results are discussed.

RESULTS

Purified Yeast DNA Topoisomerases Are Similar to Their Mammalian Counterparts in Their Interactions with Camptothecin, 9-Anilinoacridines and the Epipodophyllotoxin Derivatives Etoposide and Teniposide

Purified yeast and mammalian DNA topoisomerase I are similar in their response to the antitumor drug camptothecin. In the presence of this alkaloid, the yield of the covalent complex between tyrosine 727 of *Saccharomyces cerevisiae* DNA topoisomerase I and a DNA 3' phosphoryl group is much increased when the DNA-bound enzyme is exposed to sodium dodecyl sulfate (SDS) (11). As proposed previously for mammalian DNA topoisomerase I, this increase in covalent adduct formation is indicative of the trapping of a complex by the drug, termed the "cleavable complex," in which the reformation of the DNA phosphodiester linkage is prevented (20).

Purified yeast and mammalian DNA topoisomerase II are again similar in their response to a number of antitumor drugs that appear to act by blocking the DNA rejoining step. In the presence of the epipodophyllotoxin derivative teniposide (VM-26), for example, covalent complex formation between *S. cerevisiae* DNA topoisomerase II and DNA is nearly quantitative when the DNA–enzyme mixture is treated with sodium dodecyl sulfate (21); similar treatment in the absence of the drug yields little covalent complex.

In the experiments depicted in Figure 7.1, samples of a unique 3' end-labeled restriction fragment were incubated with purified yeast DNA topoisomerase II in the absence or presence of an anilinoacridine drug *m*-AMSA (amsacrine), or an epipodophyllotoxin derivative teniposide (VM-26), or etoposide (VP-16). Sodium dodecyl sulfate was then added to each incubation mixture to effect the breakage of the DNA, and the products were analyzed by gel electrophoresis following the removal of DNA-linked topoisomerase by exhaustive digestion with proteinase K. In the absence of the topoisomerase II–targeting drugs, little topoisomerase II–mediated DNA cleavage was observed (Figs. 7.1B,C, lane 2). The presence of *m*-AMSA (Fig. 7.1A,B, lanes 3–5), teniposide (Fig. 7.1B, lanes 6–8), or etoposide (Fig. 7.1A, lanes 6–9; Fig. 7.1B, lanes 9–11) greatly increases the extent of DNA cleavage. As reported previously for the mammalian enzyme, the sites of enhanced cleavage in the presence of *m*-AMSA and those in the presence of teniposide or etoposide form overlapping but nonidentical sets. Because some of the drug stock solutions were in DMSO, control samples were also done in which no drug but the maximal amount of DMSO was present. DMSO itself stimulates slightly the DNA topoisomerase II–mediated reaction at one major site in the particular restriction fragment used (Fig. 7.1 A,B, rightmost lanes). This stimulation of DNA topoisomerase II–mediated cleavage of DNA by DMSO was also observed previously for the mammalian enzymes. For all of the drug-containing samples shown in Figure 7.1, only the sample run in lane 9 of Figure 7.1A contained 10% DMSO; all other contained less than 2% DMSO, and the drug-enhanced cleavage patterns were little affected by the presence of DMSO in most of the incubation mixtures.

A similar experiment was carried out with three 9-anilinoacridine derivatives in addition to *m*-AMSA. In analogs A, B, and C, the 1' hydrogen of 9-anilinoacridine is substituted by -$NHSO_2CH_3$, -NH_2, and -$NHSO_2C_6H_4NH_2$, respectively (compound 10, 4, and 13, respectively, in Table 1 of reference 23; analog A is *m*-AMSA without the 3' or meta-position methoxy group). In Figure 7.1C, lane 1 contained the sample in which neither yeast DNA topoisomerase II nor drug was present, and lane 2 contained the sample with enzyme but no drug. Lanes 3–5 contained samples in which the end-labeled 2 kb DNA fragment was incubated with yeast DNA topoisomerase II in the presence of, respectively, 0.5, 2.5, and 10 µg/ml of analog A; lanes 6–8 and 10–12, respectively, contained similar sets of samples with analogs B and C. Lane 9 contained 0.1 µg/ml of analog C. The extents of DNA cleavage in the presence of comparable concentrations of analogs A and B are similar, and analog C is the most effective among the 9-anilinoacridines tested in enhancing DNA cleavage by the yeast enzyme.

Yeast Cells Can Be Sensitized to Topoisomerase-Targeting Anticancer Drugs by the Introduction of Mutations That Affect Drug Permeability

We have reported previously that although ordinary laboratory strains of *S. cerevisiae* are relatively insensitive to topoisomerase-targeting drugs, their sensitivity can be increased by the introduction of mutations that most likely affect cell permeability to the drugs (9). The recessive mutation *ise1* sensitizes cells to the alkaloid camptothecin but not *m*-AMSA or teniposide, as illustrated by

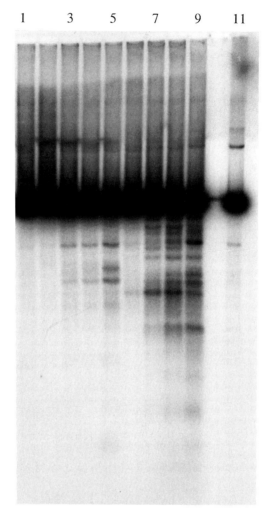

Figure 7.1. Enhancement of yeast DNA topoisomerase II–mediated cleavage of DNA by the anticancer drugs teniposide, etoposide, *m*-AMSA, and analogs of *m*-AMSA. The 3′ ends of *EcoRI* cut pHC624 were [^{32}P]-labeled by incubating the DNA with the Klenow fragment of *E. coli* DNA polymerase I, first in the presence of α-[^{32}P]-dATP, and then in the presence of all four unlabeled deoxynucleoside triphosphates. The DNA polymerase was heat inactivated; *Hind* III restriction endonuclease, which cuts pHC624 once at a site very close to *EcoRI*, was added to yield a unique end-labeled fragment about 2 kb in length, and a very short labeled fragment. The DNA was phenol extracted and dialyzed. The labeled DNA was mixed with *S. cerevisiae* DNA topoisomerase II, purified according to Goto and Wang (22), in a medium containing 20 mM Tris-HCl, pH 7.4, 7 mM MgCl$_2$, 50 mM KCl, 10 mM 2-mercaptoethanol, 0.5 mM ATP, and 50 μg/ml bovine serum albumin. The mixture was divided into 19 μl aliquots in Eppendorf centrifuge tubes, and 2 μl of H$_2$O, DMSO, or stock solutions of drugs (in H$_2$O or DMSO as specified below), were added to each. Following mixing and incubation at 37°C for 30 min, 2 μl of 10% sodium dodecyl sulfate was added to each sample to effect topoisomerase II–mediated DNA cleavage. Proteinase K was then added to 100 μg/ml, and the mixtures were incubated at 50°C for 30 min before loading on 1% agarose gel slabs.

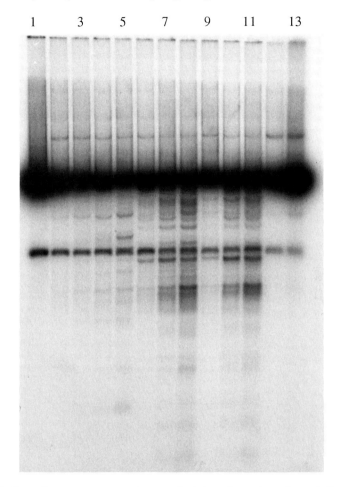

Figure 7.1B. Lane 1, no enzyme, no drug control; lane 2, no drug; lanes 3–5, *m*-AMSA, 0.1, 0.3, and 1.0 μg/ml, respectively; lanes 6–8, teniposide, 0.1, 0.3, and 1.0 μg/ml, respectively; lanes 9–11, same as lanes 6–8 but with etoposide instead of teniposide; lanes 12, no drug, twice the amount of topoisomerase II; lane 13, no drug, 10% DMSO. (Figure 7.1C follows, on page 82.)

(Figure 7.1C follows, on page 82.)

Control samples without the topoisomerase were similarly treated and analyzed. The gels were run in 50 mM Tris-borate, 1 mM Na₂ EDTA, and 0.6 μg/ml ethidium, photographed to view the DNA size markers, then dried and autoradiographed; only the autoradiograms are shown here. All labeled DNA fragments in the autoradiograms were derived from the 2 kb end-labeled fragment; the other very short end-labeled fragment had run off the gel. **A.** The final concentrations of drugs in the various incubation mixtures prior to the addition of sodium dodecyl sulfate were: lanes 1 and 2, ethidium bromide, 0.3 μg/ml and 1 μg/ml, respectively; lanes 3–5, *m*-AMSA, 0.1 μg/ml, 0.3 μg/ml, and 1 μg/ml, respectively; lanes 6–9, etoposide, 0.5 μg/ml, 2.5 μg/ml, 10 μg/ml, and 50 μg/ml, respectively. Rightmost lane: no drug, 10% DMSO (by volume).

C   1   3   5   7   9   11   13

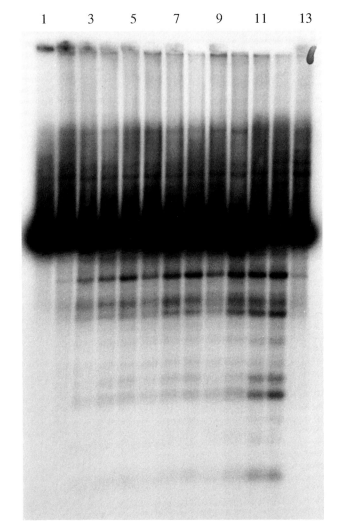

Figure 7.1C. Lane 1, no enzyme, no drug control; lane 2, no drug; lanes 3–5, 0.5, 2.5, and 10 μg/ml, respectively, of an *m*-AMSA analog A; lanes 6–8, 0.5, 2.5, and 10 μg/ml, respectively, of an *m*-AMSA analog B; lanes 9–12, 0.12, 0.5, 2.5, and 10 μg/ml, respectively, of an *m*-AMSA analog C; lane 13, no drug, 10% DMSO. The amount of DMSO in the incubation mixture run in lane 9 of Figure 7.1(A) was 10%; in all other mixtures less than 2% DMSO was present during incubation.

data shown in Figure 7.2. Strain FL599 *(ise1)* is also insensitive to etoposide (data not shown).

One mutation that particularly sensitizes cells to both camptothecin and agents affecting topoisomerase II is the semidominant mutation *ISE2*. *ISE2* strains are sensitive to camptothecin (9) as well as antitopoisomerase II agents such as amsacrine and etoposide (Fig. 7.3). Strains that are heterozygous for *ISE2* remain sensitive to amsacrine and camptothecin, but are insensitive to etoposide and teniposide (J. Nitiss and J. C. Wang, unpublished data).

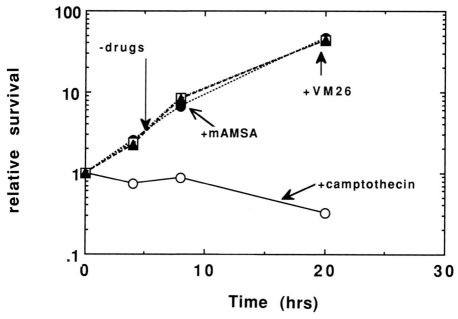

Figure 7.2. Sensitivity of an *ise1* strain to various topoisomerase-targeting drugs. Strain FL599 was treated with either 50 μg/ml camptothecin (lactone form), 100 μg/ml *m*-AMSA, or 100 μg/ml teniposide. Camptothecin was dissolved in DMSO at a concentration of 5 mg/ml, and the other agents were dissolved in DMSO at a concentration of 10 mg/ml. The sample without topoisomerase inhibitors had an equivalent volume of DMSO added. Logarithmically growing yeast cells were diluted in YPDA medium (2% Bacto-peptone, 2% dextrose, 1% yeast extract, 4 mg adenine sulfate per liter) and inhibitors or DMSO were added at time 0. Samples were obtained at the times indicated, diluted, and plated on YPDA solidified with 15 g/l agar to determine viability. The *ise1* strain is inhibited by camptothecin (open circles); *m*-AMSA and teniposide have no detectable effect on growth (other symbols).

Sensitivity of Yeast Cells to Both Type I and Type II Topoisomerase-Targeting Drugs is Strongly Affected by the *RAD52*, but not the *RAD2* or *RAD6* DNA Repair Pathways

It has been shown previously that the inactivation of the *RAD52* repair pathway greatly increases the sensitivity of yeast cells to camptothecin (9,14). To test the possibility that the *RAD52* gene product might diminish the cytotoxicity of camptothecin by a mechanism unrelated to the action of the drug on DNA topoisomerase I, we constructed strain 2-232 (*ise1 rad52 Δtop1;* see Table 7.1 for a list of strains used in this work). As shown in Figure 7.4, the inactivation of DNA topoisomerase I in an *ise1 rad52* background confers resistance to camptothecin, which is no different from the results previously obtained in an *ise1 RAD52* isogenic strain (9). As an additional control, *ise1 rad52 top1-1* cells were transformed back to TOP1[+] with a plasmid borne *TOP1* gene, and sensitivity of the transformed cells to camptothecin was restored (result not shown). These experiments suggest that the *RAD52* gene product is normally

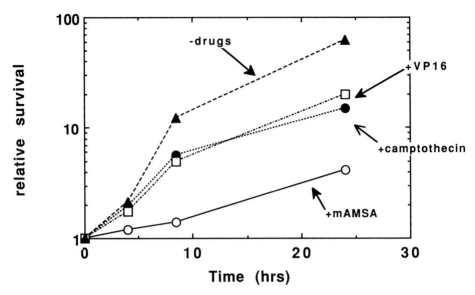

Figure 7.3. Sensitivity of an *ISE2* strain to various antitopoisomerase inhibitors. Cells were treated as described in the legend to Figure 7.2 and plated for viability. Cells carrying *ISE2* mutations are sensitive to camptothecin (filled circles) as well as to the topoisomerase II inhibitors teniposide (open squares) and *m*-AMSA (open circles). Viability of cells grown in the absence of drug is also shown (filled triangles). *ISE2* strains are insensitive to *o*-AMSA (data not included in the figure).

involved in the repair of lesions introduced by camptothecin, and that the production of lesions that require the *RAD52* gene product requires an active topoisomerase I.

Significantly, the inactivation of *RAD52* also enhances sensitivity of yeast cells toward drugs that target DNA topoisomerase II. When strain JN362a (*ISE2 RAD52*) is converted to JN394 (*ISE2 rad52*) by insertional inactivation of the *RAD52* gene, sensitivity of the cells to teniposide and *m*-AMSA is greatly increased (Fig. 7.5A,B; compare data shown in Fig. 7.5B to those shown in Fig. 7.3). JN394 (*ISE2 rad52*) is also sensitive to VP16 (data not shown). As shown in Figure 7.5B, *o*-AMSA, the inactive analog of *m*-AMSA, exhibits little cytotoxicity in JN394 (*ISE2 rad52*).

We have also tested the effects of two additional *RAD* mutations on drug sensitivity. *ISE2* strains that carry a *rad2* mutation are no more sensitive to

Table 7.1. Genotypes of Yeast Strains

FL599	*a ise1*
JN362a	*a ISE2 ura3-52 leu2-3,112 trp1-289 ade1 his7*
JN2-232	*a top1-△:URA3 rad52::LEU2 ura3-52*
JN392	*a rad52::LEU2 ise1*
JN394	JN362a converted to *rad52::LEU2*
JN362R2	JN362a converted to *rad2::URA3*
JN362R6	JN362a converted to *rad6::LEU2*

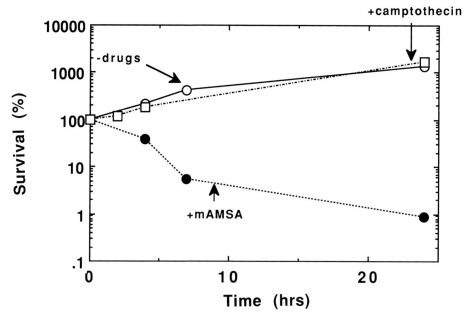

Figure 7.4. Resistance of *rad52 top1⁻* cells to camptothecin. Strain 2-232 was treated with 50 μg/ml of the lactone form of camptothecin (open squares) or 100 μg/ml *m*-AMSA (filled circles), as described in the legend to Figure 7.2. This strain remains fully sensitive to *m*-AMSA, indicating that drug permeability is unaltered.

either camptothecin or *m*-AMSA than their RAD⁺ parents. Similarly, *rad6* deletions are only slightly more sensitive to *m*-AMSA, and are no more sensitive to camptothecin, in comparison with their *RAD⁺* parents.

A Combination of a DNA Topoisomerase I–Targeting Drug with a DNA Topoisomerase II–Targeting Drug Exhibits Higher Cytotoxicity Than Can Be Achieved with Either Drug Alone

Figure 7.6 depicts data on the survival of strain 362a (*ISE2* RAD⁺) cells treated with camptothecin, *m*-AMSA, and both camptothecin and *m*-AMSA. Whereas either drug alone exhibits only a low level of cytotoxicity in the RAD⁺ background, a combination of the drugs induces a high level of cell killing when the cells were exposed to the drug over long periods of time. A series of experiments were also performed with a diploid strain JN173 (*ISE2 RAD⁺/ise2 rad52*) reported previously (9), and similar results were obtained (data not shown).

DISCUSSION

It is now well established that in yeast cells, toxicity of camptothecin requires the presence of active DNA topoisomerase I. This provides strong support to the hypothesis that cytotoxicity of many of the topoisomerase-targeting anti-

A

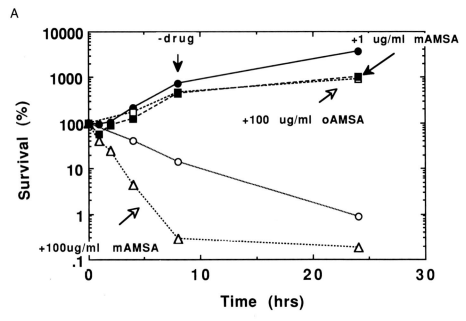

Figure 7.5. *rad52* mutants are hypersensitive to topoisomerase II inhibitors. Strain JN394 was treated with various concentrations of either *m*-AMSA, *o*-AMSA, or teniposide as described in the legend to Figure 7.2. **A.** Cells were treated with 0 (filled circles), 1 (filled squares), 10 (open circles) or 100 (open triangles) μg/ml *m*-AMSA, or 100 μg/ml *o*-AMSA (open squares).

cancer drugs is due to the conversion of the topoisomerases to cellular poisons in the presence of these drugs (reviewed in references 1–4).

Data presented in the Results section for purified yeast DNA topoisomerase II provide further evidence that biochemically this enzyme is remarkably similar to its mammalian counterpart in its interactions with amsacrines and epipodophyllotoxins. In a previous report, etoposide was found to be ineffective against the yeast enzyme (24), a conclusion that contradicted the present findings; the same authors also reported that novobiocin was a good inhibitor of the yeast enzyme, while an earlier report from this laboratory showed that it was not (22). The reasons for these discrepancies are obscure.

The similarity between yeast and mammalian DNA topoisomerase II as drug targets is probably not surprising in view of the sequence homologies that have been noted for type II DNA topoisomerases from bacteriophage T4, *E. coli, B. subtilis, Trypanosoma brucei, Drosophila melanogaster,* the two distantly related yeasts *S. cerevisiae* and *Schizosaccharomyces pombe,* and human (12,13,25,26). On the other hand, some differences in the active site structures and DNA binding domains of the enzymes from various organisms are likely, and these differences are expected to be manifested in interactions between these enzymes and various drugs. The drug *m*-AMSA, for example, is ineffective in trapping the cleavable complexes between DNA and bacterial gyrases; similarly, nalidixic acid acts effectively on bacterial gyrases but is ineffective against eukaryotic DNA topoisomerase II (see the reviews previously

B

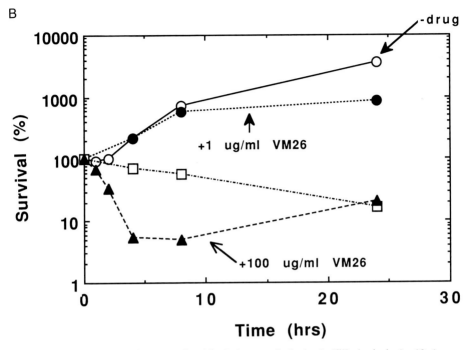

Figure 7.5B. JN394 cells treated with 0 (open circles), 1 (filled circles), 10 (open squares) or 100 (filled triangles) μg/ml VM-26.

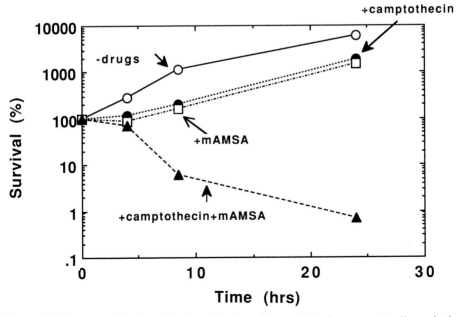

Figure 7.6. The combined effect of *m*-AMSA and camptothecin on yeast cell survival. Strain JN362a cells were treated without antitopoisomerase agents (open circles), with 50 μg/ml of the lactone form of camptothecin (filled circles), with 100 μg/ml *m*-AMSA (open squares), or with 50 μg/ml camptothecin (lactone) and 100 μg/ml *m*-AMSA (filled triangles).

cited and ref. 24). As an additional example, Drosophila topoisomerase II is highly sensitivite to epipodophyllotoxins, but much less so to *m*-AMSA (T.-S. Hsieh, personal communication). Pharmacologically, it will be important to explore the similarities as well as differences in interactions between the various drugs and topoisomerases of different organisms.

We have shown previously that for yeast strains permeable to the drug camptothecin, the cytotoxicity of the drug is much enhanced by the inactivation of the *RAD52* repair pathway (9; see also 14). Because *rad52 top1* cells remain resistant to the drug, it is most likely that *RAD52* is involved in the repair of lesions induced by the formation of the camptothecin–DNA–protein ternary complex. Interestingly, *rad52* not only increases cell sensitivity to camptothecin, which acts solely on DNA topoisomerase I, but also increases cell sensitivity to *m*-AMSA, teniposide, and etoposide, drugs that act on DNA topoisomerase II. Significantly, *o*-AMSA remains inactive in *rad52* cells, as it is in *RAD*$^+$ cells. The simplest interpretation of these results is that cytotoxicity of all drugs trapping the cleavable complexes of DNA topoisomerases is related to a common cellular pathway involving *RAD52*. Because *RAD52* function is required in the recombinational repair of DNA double-stranded breaks, it is tempting to infer that the formation of enzyme–drug–DNA ternary complexes may lead to double-stranded DNA breakage. Additional cellular processes are almost surely involved in between the formation of the ternary complex and the action of the *RAD52* product. In a separate communication, we will report studies in yeast that implicate DNA replication as one of such processes (see also 27,28 for studies in mammalian cells).

In contrast to the strong dependence of cytotoxicity of topoisomerase-targeting drugs on *RAD52*, inactivation of *RAD2*, which is involved in excision repair pathway (29,30), or *RAD6*, which is involved in a separate repair pathway (31,32), has but little effect. It is premature to infer, however, that other repair genes in the *RAD2* and *RAD6* epistatic groups are also unimportant in the processing of lesions produced by topoisomerase-targeting drugs. We have carried out preliminary screens to identify yeast mutants that are hypersensitive to either camptothecin or etoposide. Among the mutants identified, several are hypersensitive only to ultraviolet (UV) light, and several are hypersensitive to both UV and methyl methanesulfonate (MMS). These preliminary observations hint that other genes involved in the *RAD2* and *RAD6* epistatic groups might be important in the repair of lesions caused by topoisomerase-targeting drugs.

In view of our finding that cell killing by drugs targeting either DNA topoisomerase I or II may share a common pathway involving *RAD52*, it is surprising that treatment of cells simultaneously with camptothecin and *m*-AMSA induces a level of cytotoxicity higher than that achievable with either drug alone. We do not know the cause of this compounded effect. Extensive cell killing becomes evident, however, only when the cultures have been exposed to both drugs over a long period of time (relative to the generation time). It is plausible that cells treated with both drugs might be arrested at a point in the cell cycle different from the point(s) of arrest when cells are treated with either drug alone. A number of topoisomerase-targeting drugs, similar to many other DNA-damaging agents, are known to effect arrest at G_2 (33). When both DNA topoisomerases I and II are inactivated, cell-cycle progression to G_2 might be prevented (8).

The wealth of biochemical and genetic information that has been accumulated for yeast makes it potentially a powerful system for elucidating the mechanisms of topoisomerase-targeting drugs. Recent successes in expressing functional human DNA topoisomerases I and II in yeast have also made it possible to study interactions between anticancer drugs and their human enzyme targets in yeast, so as to take full advantage of the powerful genetic techniques that are applicable in this unicellular organism. The results that have been obtained so far in yeast are encouraging, and we believe that the development and further perfection of such a genetic system is likely to open new avenues in the study of topoisomerase-targeting therapeutics.

Acknowledgments

We thank Dr. Louise Prakash and Dr. Satya Prakash for *rad2* and *rad6* interruption plasmids, Dr. Leroy Liu for antitopoisomerase drugs, and Drs. Leroy Liu and Tao Hsieh for communicating results prior to publication. This work was supported by a grant from the National Cancer Institute, and a postdoctoral fellowship to J.N. from the American Cancer Society.

REFERENCES

1. Ross, W. E. DNA topoisomerases as targets for cancer therapy. Biochem. Pharmacol. **34:** 4191–4195, 1985.
2. Chen, G. L. and Liu, L. F. DNA topoisomerases as the therapeutic targets in cancer chemotherapy. Annu. Rep. Med. Chem. **21:** 257–262, 1986.
3. Drlica, K. and Franco, R. J. Inhibitors of DNA topoisomerases, Biochemistry. **27:** 2253–2259, 1988.
4. Liu, L. F. DNA topoisomerase poisons as antitumor drugs, Annu. Rev. Biochem. **58:** 351–375, 1989.
5. Wang, J. C. DNA topoisomerases, Annu. Rev.Biochem. **54:** 665–697, 1985.
6. Vosberg, P.-H. DNA topoisomerase enzymes that control DNA conformation, Curr. Top. Microbiol. Immunol. **114:** 19–102, 1985.
7. Wang, J. C. Recent studies of DNA topoisomerases, Biochim. Biophys. Acta. **909:** 1–9, 1987.
8. Yanagida, M. and Wang, J. C. Yeast DNA topoisomerases and their structural genes. In F. Eckstein and D.M.J. Lilley, eds. *Nucleic Acids and Molecular Biology,* vol. 1, Berlin: Springer-Verlag, 1987, pp. 196–209.
9. Nitiss, J. and Wang, J. C. DNA topoisomerase-targeting antitumor drugs can be studied in yeast, Proc. Natl. Acad. Sci. USA. **85:** 7501–7505, 1988.
10. Wyckoff, E. and Hsieh, T. Functional expression of a *Drosophila* gene in yeast: Genetic complementation of DNA topoisomerase II. Proc. Natl. Acad. Sci. USA. **85:** 6262–6276, 1988.
11. Lynn, R. M., Bjornsti, M. A., Caron, P., and Wang, J. C. Peptide sequencing and site-directed mutagenesis identify tyrosine 727 as the active site tyrosine of *Saccharomyces cerevisiae* DNA topoisomerase I. Proc. Natl. Acad. Sci. USA. **86:** 3559–3563, 1989.
12. Wyckoff, E., Natalie, D., Nolan, J. M., Lee, M., and Hsieh, T. Structure of the *Drosophila* DNA topoisomerase II gene: Nucleotide sequence and homology among topoisomerase II. J. Mol. Biol. **205:** 1–14, 1989.
13. Strauss, P. R., and Wang, J. C. The *TOP2* gene of *Trypanosoma brucei:* A single-copy gene that shares extensive homology with other *TOP2* genes encoding eukaryotic DNA topoisomerase II. Mol. Biochem. Parasitol. **38:** 141–150, 1990.
14. Eng, W.-K., Faucette, L., Johnson, R. K., and Sternglanz, R. Evidence that

DNA topoisomerase I is necessary for the cytotoxic effects of camptothecin. Mol. Pharmacol. **34**: 755–760, 1988.

15. Bjornsti, M. A., Benedetti, P., Viglianti, G. A., and Wang, J. C. Expression of human topoisomerase I in yeast cells lacking yeast DNA topoisomerase I: restoration of sensitivity of the cells to the antitumor drug camptothecin. Cancer Res. **49**: 6318–6323, 1989.

16. Haynes R. and Kunz B. DNA repair and mutagenesis in yeast. In J. N. Strathern, E. W. Jones, and J. R. Broach, eds. *Molecular Biology of the Yeast Saccharomyces.* vol. 1. *Life Cycle and Inheritance.* Cold Spring Harbor, N.Y.: Cold Spring Harbor Laboratory, 1981, pp. 371–414.

17. Friedberg E. C. *DNA Repair,* San Francisco: W. H. Freeman, 1985.

18. Game, J. Radiation sensitivity and repair in yeast. In J.F.T. Spencer, D. M. Spencer, and A.R.W. Smith, eds. *Yeast Genetics: Fundamental and Applied Aspects.* Berlin: Springer-Verlag, 1983, pp. 109–137.

19. Jentsch, S., McGrath, P., and Varshavsky, A. The yeast DNA repair gene *RAD6* encodes a ubiquitin-conjugating enzyme. Nature. **329**: 131–134, 1987.

20. Hsiang, Y.-H., Hertzberg, R., Hecht, S., and Liu, L. R. Camptothecin induces protein-linked DNA breaks via mammalian DNA topoisomerase I. J. Biol. Chem. **260**: 14873–14878, 1985.

21. Worland, S. T. and Wang, J. C. Inducible overexpression, purification, and active site mapping of DNA topoisomerase II from the yeast *Saccharomyces cerevisiae.* J. Biol. Chem. **264**: 4412–4416, 1989.

22. Goto, T. and Wang, J. C. Yeast DNA topoisomerase II. J. Biol. Chem. **257**: 5866–5872, 1982.

23. Baguley, B. C. and Nash, R. Antitumor activity of substituted 9-anilinoacridines: Comparison of in vivo and in vitro testing systems. Eur. J. Cancer. **17**: 671–679, 1981.

24. Figett, D. P., Danyer, S. P., Dewick, P. M., Jackson, D. E., and Williams, P. Topoisomerase II: A potential target for novel anti-fungal drugs. Biochem. Biophys. Res. Commun. **160**: 257–262, 1989.

25. Tsai-Pflugfelder, M., Liu, L. F., Liu, A. A., Tewey, K. M., Whang-Pheng, J., Knutsen, T., Huebner, K., Croce, C. M., and Wang, J. C. Cloning and sequencing of cDNA encoding human DNA topoisomerase II and localization of the gene to chromosome region 17q21–22, Proc. Natl. Acad. Sci. USA. **85**: 7177–7181, 1988.

26. Lynn, R., Giaever, G., Swanberg, S. L., and Wang, J. C. Tandem regions of yeast DNA topoisomerase II share homology with different subunits of bacterial gyrase. Science. **233**: 647–649, 1986.

27. Snapka, R. M. Topoisomerase inhibitors can selectively interfere with different stages of Simian virus 40 DNA replication. Mol. Cell. Biol. **6**: 4221–4227, 1986.

28. Avemann, K., Knippers, R., Koller, T., and Sogo, J. Camptothecin, a specific inhibitor of type I DNA topoisomerases, induces DNA breakage at replication forks. Mol. Cell. Biol. **8**: 3026–3034, 1988.

29. Naumovski, L. and Friedberg, E. C. *Saccharomyces cerevisiae RAD2* gene: Isolation, subcloning and partial characterization. Mol. Cell. Biol. **4**: 290–295, 1984.

30. Madura, K. and Prakash, S. Nucleotide sequence, transcript mapping, and regulation of the *RAD2* gene of *Saccharomyces cerevisiae.* J. Bacteriol. **166**: 914–923, 1986.

31. Reynolds, P., Weber, S. C., and Prakash, L. *RAD6* gene of *Saccharomyces cerevisiae* encodes a protein containing a tract of 13 consecutive aspartates. Proc. Natl. Acad. Sci. USA. **82**: 168–172, 1985.

32. Morrison, A., Miller, E., and Prakash, L. Domain structure and functional analysis of the carboxyl-terminal polyacidic sequence of the *RAD6* protein of *Saccharomyces cerevisiae.* Mol. Cell. Biol. **8**: 1185–1190, 1988.

33. Yang, L., Rowe, T., and Liu, L. F. Identification of DNA topoisomerase II as an intracellular target of anti-tumor epipodophyllotoxins in Simian virus 40 infected monkey cells. Cancer Res. **45**: 5872–5876, 1985.

PART II

INHIBITORS OF TOPOISOMERASE I

Chapter 8
Chemistry and Antitumor Activity of Camptothecins

MONROE E. WALL

AND MANSUKH C. WANI

Camptothecin **1** was first isolated from the wood, bark, and fruits of *Campto-theca acuminata,* DECAISNE (Nyssaceae) (1). The taxonomy, occurrence, and the interesting manner in which the seeds of this Chinese tree were collected from Szechwan Province and sent to the United States many years ago have been reported (2). The structure of camptothecin, an alkaloid that has been shown to be derived from the commonly occurring indole alkaloid group (3) is shown in Figure 8.1. It will be noted that the compound has a pentacyclic ring structure with only one asymmetric center in ring E with the 20(*S*) configuration. Other notable features are the presence of the α-hydroxy lactone system in ring E, the pyridone ring D moiety, and the conjugated system that links rings ABCDE. Because of its noteworthy antitumor activity on murine L1210 leukemia, camptothecin was of great interest from the time of its initial isolation. The compound demonstrated this antitumor activity between 0.25 mg to 3.0 mg/kg with T/C values frequently in excess of 200. It is one of the few antineoplastic alkaloids that has shown consistent high activity on the above L1210 murine leukemia. In addition, **1** has great activity in inhibition of the growth of solid tumors in rodents. In the form of its water-soluble salt **2** (Fig. 8.1) the compound received early clinical trial but was not effective (4,5). It was not realized until much later that the sodium salt of camptothecin is only about *1/10 as potent* as the parent compound (6).

INITIAL CAMPTOTHECIN STRUCTURE ACTIVITY RELATIONSHIP STUDIES (SAR)

Initial activity studies quickly revealed some interesting structure activity relationships (SAR) (7). These are outlined in Figure 8.2, and several important features were noted. Hydroxylation of ring A of camptothecin is compatible with activity, and indeed this compound, 10-hydroxycamptothecin **3**, has greater activity than camptothecin (6,7) (cf. Table 8.1). Camptothecin reacts

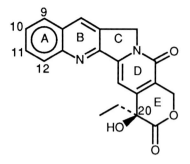

Camptothecin (1)   Camptothecin Sodium (2)

Figure 8.1. Structures of camptothecin and camptothecin sodium.

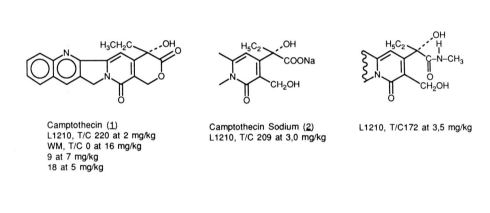

Camptothecin (1)
L1210, T/C 220 at 2 mg/kg
WM, T/C 0 at 16 mg/kg
9 at 7 mg/kg
18 at 5 mg/kg

Camptothecin Sodium (2)
L1210, T/C 209 at 3,0 mg/kg

L1210, T/C172 at 3,5 mg/kg

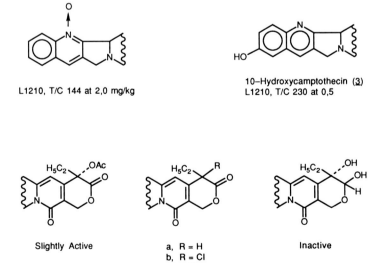

L1210, T/C 144 at 2,0 mg/kg

10–Hydroxycamptothecin (3)
L1210, T/C 230 at 0,5

Slightly Active

a, R = H
b, R = Cl
Inactive

Inactive

Figure 8.2. Structure activity relationships in the camptothecin series.

Table 8.1. Comparison of *In Vivo* and *In Vitro* Activity of Camptothecin and Analogs

Name of Camptothecin (CPT) Analogs	*In Vivo* L1210[a] T/C (mg/kg)	9KB[b] 9PS[b] ED_{50} (μ/ml)
20(S)-CPT	197 (8)	10^{-2} 10^{-2}
20(R)-CPT	132 (10)	10^{-1} 10^{0}
10-hydroxy-20(S)-CPT	230 (24)	10^{-2}
10-methoxy-20(S)-CPT	167 (2)	10^{-2}
10,11-dimethoxy-20(RS)-CPT	Inactive (50)	10^{-1}
10,11-methylenedioxy-20(RS)-CPT	325 (2)	10^{-2}
12-nitro-20(S)-CPT	151 (40)	
12-amino-20(S)-CPT	Inactive	
11-nitro-20(RS)-CPT	147 (80)	10^{0}
11-amino-20(RS)-CPT	147 (40)	10^{-1}
10-nitro-20(RS)-CPT	219 (16)	10^{-1}
10-amino-20(RS)-CPT	365 (4)	10^{-2}
9-nitro-20(S)-CPT	348 (10)	10^{-2}
9-amino-20(S)-CPT	361 (3)	10^{-2}
20(RS)-amino-CPT	Inactive	10^{0}
20(RS)-lactam-CPT	Inactive	10^{1}

[a]Antitumor activity on murine L1210 leukemia (15).
[b]Inhibition of cell growth in 9KB or 9PS as defined in reference 15, expressed as ED_{50} μg/ml.

readily with bases or amines to give water-soluble salts or amides, formed by reaction with the lactone moiety with concomitant opening of ring E (7). Reaction of the lactone moiety with nitrogenous bases analogous to amide formation may possibly be involved in the antitumor activity and potency of **1**. The water-soluble sodium salt **3** has a potency 8–10 times less than that of the natural product (6).

Major reduction of antineoplastic activity was noted as a result of reactions involving the hydroxyl or lactone moiety in ring E (7) (cf. Fig. 8.2). After acetylation of camptothecin, the resultant acetate is virtually inactive. Other reactions also point to the absolute requirement of the α-hydroxyl group as shown by the fact that after replacement of this group by chlorine, both the resultant chloro-analog and the corresponding reduction product, desoxycamptothecin, are inactive in L1210 and PS leukemia. Reduction of the lactone under mild conditions to give the lactol also results in complete loss of activity. Our early studies have clearly indicated the absolute requirement for the α-hydroxy lactone moiety. It is thus quite clear that the activity of the sodium salt is due entirely to the ability of **2** to recyclize to **1** at least to a limited extent under physiological conditions.

RECENT SYNTHETIC STUDIES

Improved procedures for the total synthesis of camptothecin and analogs involving the Friedlander reactions of a properly substituted ortho aminobenzaldehyde with a tricyclic synthon have permitted studies of the effects of modifications in both rings A and E (Fig. 8.3) (6, 8–11).

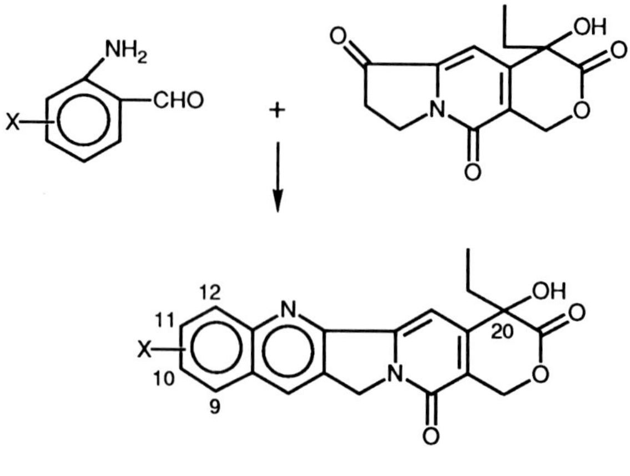

X = Ring A substituents, cf references 6, 8-10.

Figure 8.3. Synthesis of camptothecin analog.

Our early work discussed previously (7) clearly demonstrated the need for the α-hydroxy lactone moiety. More recent studies have given even greater information on the specificity required in this system (11). Thus, we have been able to synthesize the 20(S) and 20(R)-hydroxy forms of camptothecin (11), the former having the stereochemistry of that of the naturally occurring alkaloid. The 20(R) form is virtually inactive in L1210 *in vivo* and *in vitro* assays (11). Thus, not only is the hydroxyl moiety required, but specific stereochemistry at 20(S) is also an absolute necessity for *in vitro* cytotoxicity, inhibition of topo-isomerase I activity and *in vivo* antitumor activity (11,12).

Recent studies from our laboratory have shown that not only must the correct C20 stereochemistry be present for activity, but that the oxygen of the C20 hydroxyl moiety and the oxygen in the lactone ring cannot be replaced by nitrogen. Thus, 20(RS)-aminocamptothecin **4** and the 20(S)-lactam analog of camptothecin **5** are inactive compounds *in vitro* and *in vivo* (Fig. 8.4).

The lack of activity of the amino-(20) analog may be due to the fact that hydro-gen bonding to the C21 carbonyl moiety in ring E is stronger with the C20 hydroxyl moiety than with the corresponding C20 amino group. As a conse-quence the C21 carbonyl in the amino analog is less susceptible to nucleophilic attacks. The inactivity of the lactam is more readily explicable, since lactams are much more sluggishly reactive than lactones. It seems increasingly apparent

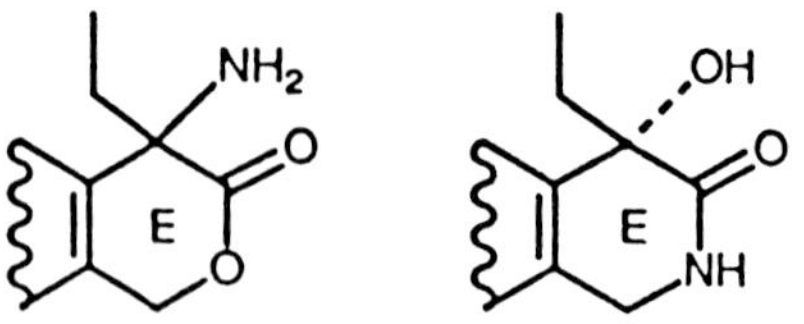

Figure 8.4. Structure of 20(RS)-amino and 20-(RS)-lactam.

that one of the major features of the biological activity of the camptothecin molecule is the chemical reactivity of the lactone moiety which is readily attacked by nucleophiles, forming a carboxylic salt in the presence of bases or amides by reaction with amines (1,7). The reactions are reversible, and hence one can postulate a readily reversible reaction involving the lactone carbonyl with a nucleophilic group on an enzyme or enzyme–DNA complex.

EFFECT OF RING SIZE AND RING SHAPE ON ACTIVITY

In order to determine whether the α-hydroxy lactone was the only moiety required for biological activity in camptothecin, we have prepared simple monocyclic ring E, bicyclic DE, tricyclic CDE, and tetracyclic BCDE analogs containing the α-hydroxy lactone (Fig. 8.5). We found that all the compounds were completely inactive *in vitro,* and, with the exception of the tetracyclic compound, which has yet to be tested, all of the compounds are inactive *in vivo.* Thus, it would seem that there is also a minimum requirement for a conjugated ring system such as is found in camptothecin. The pentacyclic ring structure of **1** has a very specific molecular shape that is undoubtedly required for binding, possibly to the DNA topoisomerase I complex. Activity can be retained with a larger number of rings. Thus a hexacyclic analog (6) has activity comparable to that of camptothecin. There are other specific characteristics that are inherent for activity in the camptothecin series.

Although the shape of the camptothecin molecule is important, analogs very similar in shape can be active or inactive. Replacement of carbon by nitrogen in ring A at positions 12 or 10 (9) (Fig. 8.6) gives compounds with shapes superimposable on each other and on camptothecin. Yet the 12-aza-analog is inactive, whereas the 10-aza-analog is of the same order of activity as camptothecin (9). As will be shown in a subsequent section, structural changes at

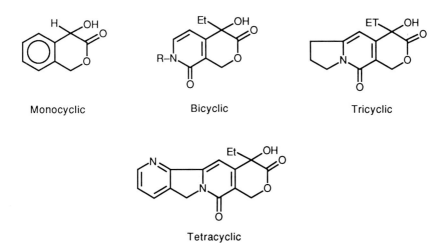

Monocyclic   Bicyclic   Tricyclic

Tetracyclic

Figure 8.5. Monocyclic, bicyclic, tricyclic, and tetracyclic analogs of camptothecin.

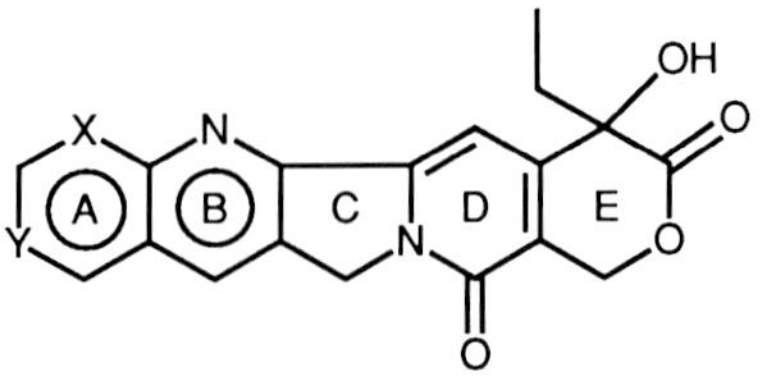

12- and 10–20(RS)-azacamptothecin
12 aza : X = N, Y = CH
10 aza: X = CH, Y = N

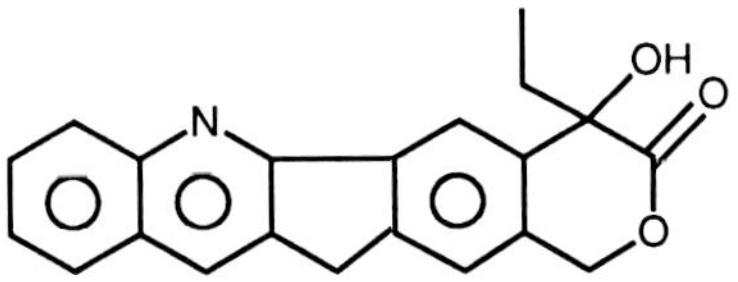

Ring D–Benzo–Analog

Figure 8.6. Structure of ring A-aza and ring D-benzo camptothecin analogs.

C-12 invariably lead to inactivation. In another instance exemplifying specificity of shape, the pyridone moiety present in ring D of camptothecin was replaced by an aromatic benzene ring (13) (Fig. 8.6). This compound has a shape
that superimposes almost exactly on that of camptothecin. While it is not inactive, its activity is much lower than that of camptothecin, again showing the
rigorous requirements for activity.

RING A-ANALOGS

The synthetic scheme shown in Figure 8.3 for the synthesis of camptothecin
has also permitted us to prepare many ring A-analogs by suitable manipulation
of the orthoaminobenzaldehyde synthon (6, 8–10). Most of these analogs have
the 20(RS) stereochemistry (i.e., they are racemic and have only one half the
potency of the naturally occurring 20(S) form). Since we can now synthesize
pure 20(S) analogs (11), the potency for 20(RS) analogs shown in Table 8.1 can
in most cases be doubled by the synthesis of the pure 20(S) form. Modification
of ring A results in a wide gamut of compounds with an equally large gradient
of activity from inactive through exceptionally active (9,10). As we will show,
the inactivity or loss of activity can result from steric factors. Moreover, substitution at positions 11 and 12 are virtually prohibited if one wishes to obtain
active compounds.

The effect of steric hindrance is shown in Table 8.1 in which 10-hydroxy-20(S)-camptothecin is compared with its naturally occurring 10-methoxy-20(S) analog and the synthetic 10,11-dimethoxy-20(RS) analog. As is readily apparent, the 10-hydroxy analog has excellent activity in L1210 mouse leukemia. The 10-methoxy analog is active but the activity is considerably reduced, and the 10,11-dimethoxy compound is totally inactive. Molecular models show considerable steric interaction of the 10,11-methoxy groups. Interestingly however, the 10,11-methylenedioxy-20(RS) analog is highly active. Models show that in this compound the methylenedioxy moiety is co-planer with ring A and hence steric hindrance does not occur. However, Dreiding models show that the bond angles of the 10,11-methylenedioxy analog in ring A are not identical with camptothecin (Fig. 8.7). Further molecular modelling studies are underway.

Substitutions at 9 or 10 by an amino group lead to compounds with considerably greater *in vivo* activity than is found with the corresponding parent compound (cf. Table 8.1). Thus 9-amino-20(S)-camptothecin is a very active compound in the assay for antitumor activity on murine L1210 leukemia. Interestingly, the corresponding 9-nitro analog also has excellent activity, although a considerably higher dose level is required. In this case the 9-nitro moiety is undoubtedly a prodrug for the 9-amino group. 10-Amino-20(RS)-camptothecin also shows excellent activity at low dose levels and the 10-nitro analog has good activity but is of a lower order of potency. Substitutions of amino or hydroxyl group at positions 9 or 10 in ring A (10-chloro and 10-methyl analogs are also quite active) do not lead to undesirable steric or electronic interactions. These groups may possibly permit better penetration of cell walls or membranes. However, when the same groups are substituted at C11 or C12, reduced biological activity is found. Thus, 12-aminocamptothecin is inactive and the 12-nitro analog shows only modest activity at very high dose levels and is virtually nontoxic. It is evident that substitution at C12 is a prohibitive feature.

Most 11-substituted camptothecin analogs also show poor or no activity (10). For example 11-amino-20(RS)-camptothecin in contrast to the 9- and 10-amino analogs is of very low activity. The only exception to this is 11-hydroxy-20(RS)-camptothecin, which shows an excellent T/C of 357% but at a very high dose level of 60 mg/kg. Hence, it has very low potency. More recently we have synthesized 9-hydroxy and 9-methoxy analogs of camptothecin and as would be expected they show considerable activity *in vitro*. Their *in vivo* activity is being evaluated.

Conceivably camptothecin may be reacting with an enzyme or enzyme–DNA complex (14) on the face proximal to the C11 and particularly the C12

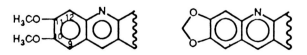

Figure 8.7. Structure of 10,11-dimethoxy-20(RS) and 10,11-methylenedioxy-20(RS).

region. Hence, groups substituted in these positions may cause unfavorable steric or stereoelectronic interactions. Substituents at positions 9 and 10 are more distant from this region. Hence, substitution at these locations does not cause problems.

COMPARISON OF *IN VIVO* AND *IN VITRO* DATA

All of the compounds that have been discussed in the previous section have been tested for cytotoxicity in cell culture screening, 9KB and/or 9PS (15). In general there is an excellent correlation between the *in vitro* and *in vivo* activities of the compounds (10). Most of the highly active hydroxy or amino-camptothecin analogs that have been discussed (cf. Table 8.1) have cell cytotoxicity (9KB) ED_{50} values of the order of 10^{-2} µg/ml; compounds of intermediate activity have values of the order of 1×10^{-1}, and inactive compounds show values of the order of 1×10^{0}. Thus, for 10-nitro-20*(RS)*-camptothecin, which is less active than the 10-amino-20*(RS)* analog, the comparable values are respectively 3×10^{-1} versus 3×10^{-2}. Similar results have been obtained for the *in vitro* 9PS (lymphocytic leukemia) assay. Many of these same compounds have been tested for their topoisomerase I inhibition. Since the relationship between camptothecin structure and topoisomerase I inhibition is described in Chapter 10, we will state only that in general there is also an excellent correlation between antitumor activity on murine L1210 leukemia and topoisomerase I inhibitionin the camptothecin series.

WATER-SOLUBLE ANALOGS

With the exception of water-soluble sodium salt of camptothecin, most of the compounds that we have discussed are water insoluble. Even the simple 9- or 10-amino compounds are not sufficiently basic to form stable hydrochloride salts. In order to facilitate clinical use of camptothecin analogs, some of our most recent studies deal with the possibility of forming water-soluble salts at positions that in most cases are other than the lactone. A notable exception, however, is the sodium salt of 10,11-methylenedioxy-20*(RS)*-camptothecin (Fig. 8.8). This compound is 10–12 times more potent in the 9KB cell culture growth inhibition assay (15) than camptothecin and seems to be of a similar order of potency in topoisomerase I inhibition. Another type of water-soluble compound we have developed is the 9-glycinamide hydrochloride-20*(RS)* analog of camptothecin. This compound (Fig. 8.8) is of the same order of activity as camptothecin in 9KB and 9PS and also in inhibition of topoisomerase I. Other water-soluble compounds derived from 9- or 10-hydroxy-camptothecin or the corresponding 9- and 10-amino analogs are now under study. We are also seeking ways to make the 10,11-methylenedioxy compound water soluble without hydrolysis of the lactone.

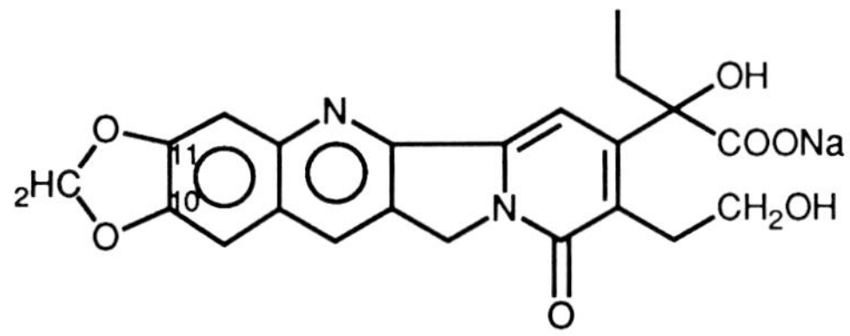

10,11–Methylenedioxy–20(RS)-camptothecin, Sodium Salt

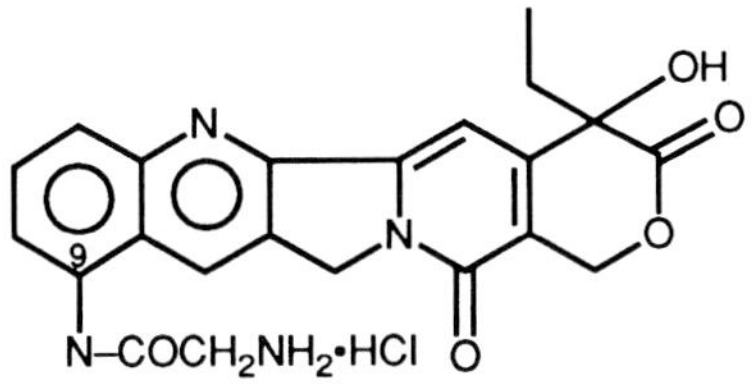

9–aminoglycinamide-20(RS)-camptothecin hydrochloride

Figure 8.8. New water-soluble camptothecin analogs.

Acknowledgments

This work was supported in part by National Cancer Institute Grant CA 38996.

REFERENCES

1. Wall, M. E., Wani, M. C., Cook, C. E., Palmer, K. H., McPhail, A. T., and Sim, G. A. Plant antitumor agents. I. The isolation and structure of camptothecin, a novel alkaloidal leukemia and tumor inhibitor from *Camptotheca acuminata*. J. Am. Chem. Soc. **88:** 3888–3890, 1966.

2. Perdue, R. E., Jr., Smith, R. L., Wall, M. E., Hartwell, J. L., and Abbott, B. J. *Camptotheca acuminata* Decaisne (Nyssaceae). Source of camptothecin. U.S. Dept. Agr., Agr. Research Service, Technical Bulletin No. 1415, 1–26, 1970.

3. Heckendorf, A. H., Mattes, K. C., Hutchinson, C. R., Hagaman, E. W., and Wenkert, E. Stereochemistry and conformation of biogenetic precursors of indole alkaloids. J. Org. Chem., **41:** 2045–2047, 1976.

4. Moertel, C. G., Schutt, H. J., Reitmerer, R. J., and Hahn, R. G. Phase II study of camptothecin (NSC-100880) in the treatment of advanced gastrointestinal cancer. Cancer Chemother. Rep. Part 1. **56:** 95, 1972.

5. Gottleib, J. A. and Luce, J. K. Treatment of malignant melanoma with camptothecin (NSC-100880). Cancer Chemother. Rep. **56:** 103, 1972.

6. Wani, M. C., Ronman, P. E., Lindley, J. T., and Wall, M. E. Plant antitumor agents. 18. Synthesis and biological activity of camptothecin analogs. J. Med. Chem. **23:** 554–560, 1980.

7. Wall, M. E. Plant antitumor agents. V. Alkaloids with antitumor activity. Symposiumberichtes, 4. Internationales Symposium, Biochemie und Physiologie der Alkaloide, K. Mothes, K. Schreiber, and

H. R. Schutte, eds. Berlin: Akademie-Verlag, 1969, pp. 77–87.

8. Wall, M. E., Wani, M. C., Natschke, S. M., and Nicholas, A. W. Plant antitumor agents. 22. Isolation of 11-hydroxycamptothecin from *Camptotheca acuminata* Decne: Total synthesis and biological activity. J. Med. Chem. **29:** 1553, 1986.

9. Wani, M.C., Nicholas, A. W., and Wall, M. E. Plant antitumor agents. 23. Synthesis and antileukemic activity of camptothecin analogues. J. Med. Chem. **29:** 2358, 1986.

10. Wani, M. C., Nicholas, A. W., Manikumar, G., and Wall, M. E. Plant antitumor agents. 25. Total synthesis and antileukemic activity of ring A-substituted camptothecin analogs, structure activity. J. Med. Chem. **30:** 1774, 1987.

11. Wani, M. C., Nicholas, A. W., and Wall, M. E. Plant antitumor agents. 28. Resolution of a key tricyclic synthon. 5'-(RS)-1,5-dioxo-(5'-ethyl-5'-hydroxy-2'H, 5'H, 6'H-6-oxopyrano) [3',4'-f]Δ⁶,⁸-tetrahydroindolizine: Total synthesis and antitumor activity of 20(S)- and 20(R)-camptothecin. J. Med. Chem. **30:** 2317, 1987.

12. Jaxel, C., Kohn, K. W., Wani, M. C., Wall, M. E., and Pommier, Y. Structure activity study of the actions of camptothecin derivatives on mammalian topoisomerase I: Evidence for a specific receptor site and for a relation to antitumor activity. Cancer Res. **49:** 1465, 1989.

13. Nicholas, A. W., Wani, M. C., Manikumar, G., Wall, M. E., Kohn, K. W., and Pommier, Y. Plant antitumor agents. 29. Synthesis and biological activity of ring D and ring E modified analogs of camptothecin. J. Med. Chem. **33:** 972, 1990.

14. Hsiang, Y. H., Hertzberg, R., Hecht, S., and Liu, L. R. Camptothecin induced protein linked DNA breaks via mammalian DNA topoisomerase I. J. Biol. Chem. **260:** 14873–14878, 1985.

15. Geran, R. I., Greenberg, N. H., MacDonald, M. M., Schumacher, A. M., and Abbott, B. J. Protocols for screening chemical agents and natural products against animal tumors and other biological systems. Cancer Chemother. Rep. **3(2):**1, 1972.

Chapter 9
The Biochemistry of Camptothecin– Topoisomerase I Interaction

ROBERT P. HERTZBERG, MARY JO CARANFA,
WILLIAM D. KINGSBURY, BRIAN SMITH,
RANDALL K. JOHNSON, AND SIDNEY M. HECHT

Camptothecin, a cytotoxic alkaloid with significant antitumor activity in animal tumor models, has a unique mechanism of action: it produces DNA damage mediated by topoisomerase I (1–5). Three compelling lines of evidence argue that the antitumor activity of camptothecin derives from the stabilization of a covalent binary complex formed by DNA and topoisomerase I. First, yeast cells in which the gene for topoisomerase I has been deleted are completely resistant to camptothecin (6,7). This suggests that camptothecin subverts the activity of topoisomerase I in a manner that leads to cytotoxic DNA lesions, since deletion of the target enzyme confers camptothecin resistance. Second, two different mammalian cell lines resistant to camptothecin were shown to contain a qualitatively different form of the target enzyme (3,4). Topoisomerase I from the resistant cells, when isolated and studied in purified systems, did not produce increased DNA strand breaks in the presence of camptothecin. Third, camptothecin analogs that do not inhibit topoisomerase I have no antitumor activity (8–10). These findings strongly implicate topoisomerase I as the primary cellular target for camptothecin and related derivatives.

The details of camptothecin–topoisomerase I–DNA interaction that lead to inhibition of DNA unwinding by topoisomerase I have been clarified. In the absence of inhibitors, topoisomerase I binds to DNA and introduces a transient single-strand break, alters DNA topology by mediating strand passage, and subsequently reseals the break before dissociating (11). One characterized intermediate consists of an enzyme–DNA complex in which one strand of the DNA has been broken and linked covalently to topoisomerase I. While this protein-linked DNA break is normally resealed, camptothecin stabilizes the covalent DNA–topoisomerase I complex and temporarily prevents religation (1, 12–15). The available evidence suggests that camptothecin binds reversibly to the DNA–topoisomerase I complex subsequent to the DNA cleavage step.

Herein, we present evidence that supports this mechanism of inhibition. Further, data are presented on the importance of the lactone ring of camptothecin for topoisomerase I inhibition.

THE LACTONE RING OF CAMPTOTHECIN AND TOPOISOMERASE I INHIBITION

Prior to the discovery that camptothecin acts as an inhibitor of topoisomerase I, Wall and coworkers defined some of the structural features that are important for cytotoxicity and antitumor activity (16,17). In particular, it was shown that the α-hydroxy lactone ring is critical for biological activity, since 20-deoxycamptothecin, 20-chlorocamptothecin, and camptothecin lactol are inactive as antitumor agents (16). We have shown that camptothecin derivatives lacking the intact α-hydroxy lactone ring are markedly less active than camptothecin with respect to the stabilization of DNA cleavage mediated by topoisomerase I (10). Further, these compounds do not affect topoisomerase I–mediated DNA relaxation, unlike camptothecin, which reduces the rate of enzyme catalysis. That the α-hydroxy lactone ring of camptothecin is necessary for inhibition of topoisomerase I, as well as for cytotoxicity and antitumor activity in whole cells and animals, is consistent with the hypothesis that topoisomerase I is the relevant target for these drugs.

The production of DNA cleavage mediated by topoisomerase I in the presence of camptothecin derivatives was measured by agarose gel electrophoresis and densitometry (see Fig. 9.2). Compounds 2 and 4 contain modified lactone rings, in that the 20-hydroxy group is absent; compounds 3 and 4 contain substituents on the A-ring that increase water solubility (camptothecin is not water soluble above 10 μM, but 3 and 4 are fully soluble even at 100 μM). The 20-deoxy derivatives (2 and 4) were significantly less active than their 20-hydroxylated counterparts (1 and 3). The 20-hydroxy group may be important for DNA cleavage because it alters the chemical reactivity of the lactone ring, or because it produces a key hydrogen bond in the enzyme–DNA complex. In this context, we thought it possible that compound 4 might bind to the enzyme–DNA complex but, due to the absence of the 20-OH group, be incapable of stabilizing the covalent DNA–topoisomerase I complex. We tested to see if 4 could bind in a nonproductive manner, thus preventing 3 from stabilizing the covalent binary complex. We found, however, that a 50-fold excess of 4 had little effect on the activity of 3 (see Fig. 9.2a, inset), suggesting that 4 has little affinity for the complex. The slight increase in DNA cleavage in the presence of large concentrations of 4 was likely due to a 1% impurity of 3 in the sample.

Consistent with its importance in stabilization of the DNA–topoisomerase I covalent complex, the stereochemistry of the OH group at position 20 was shown to be important for enzyme inhibition and for cytotoxicity (9,18). Other functional groups in the E ring are also important for activity. For example, the lactam analog of camptothecin (5), which contains the 20-hydroxy group but lacks the lactone functionality and would be expected to be less reactive chemically, did not stabilize the DNA–topoisomerase I complex (10). Similarly, the α-hydroxy thiolactone and hemilactol derivatives of camptothecin were shown to be inactive (10). So the 20-hydroxy group is necessary, but not sufficient; each of the oxygen atoms within the α-hydroxy lactone ring are required for inhibition of topoisomerase I and for antitumor activity.

While six-membered lactones are usually quite stable at neutral pH, the lactone moiety of camptothecin is unusually reactive. It partially hydrolyzes at pH 7.4, and an equilibrium is established between the open-ring and closed-ring forms (Fig. 9.1). Sodium camptothecin (6, sodium salt), in which the lactone ring is hydrolyzed, had antitumor activity similar to 1 but was found to be about 10-fold less potent with respect to therapeutic dosage range (17). In *in vitro* assays, however, 6 appears to be equivalent to 1; for example, both forms inhibit isolated topoisomerase I at similar concentrations and both are cytotoxic to mammalian cells with equal potency *in vitro* (10). In animals, the difference in potency of the two administered forms most likely reflects different pharmacokinetic properties such as serum protein binding or clearance. *In vitro*, the similarity between 1 and 6 suggests that 6 is converted to 1 in aqueous buffered solutions during the course of the assays.

To study the intrinsic activities of these interconvertible forms of camptothecin, we have investigated the inhibition of topoisomerase I at several pH values. As shown in Figure 9.2b, when either 1 or 6 was added to a reaction mixture containing DNA and topoisomerase I, DNA cleavage was observed at pH values below 9. With either form, more enzyme-mediated DNA cleavage occurred at lower pH values than at higher pH values. Since acidic pH is known to induce the formation of camptothecin lactone from sodium camptothecin (19), this observation suggests that the lactone form of the drug is more potent than the open-ring form. That no cleavage was produced above pH 8.5, even though topoisomerase I is catalytically active in this pH range, suggests that the open-ring form is completely inactive (10). The DNA cleavage observed in drug-free reaction mixtures at pH values between 6 and 7 was most likely the result of pH-dependent conformational changes in the DNA or topoisomerase I.

It was not possible to measure the equilibrium quantities of 1 and 6 in aqueous solution, since 1 precipitated from solution and influenced the equilibrium. Compound 3, however, is more water soluble and we have been able to demonstrate the pH-dependent interconversion between 3 and its open-ring form by HPLC and NMR measurements (data not shown). When either form of 3 was incubated at pH 5 and allowed to come to equilibrium, only the lactone form was detected. At pH 6.8, both forms were present in approximately equal amounts; at pH 8.5, none of the lactone form remained and only the open-ring form was present. It took from 30 min to several hours to reach equilibrium, depending on conditions. The diminution of topoisomerase I inhibition by 3 paralleled the extent of lactone hydrolysis, demonstrating that only the lactone form of 3 was capable of stabilizing the covalent topoisomerase I–DNA complex. Reports of topoisomerase I inhibition in experiments using the open-ring form of camptothecin are probably due to lactone formation *in situ* and should be interpreted in the context of the reaction pH and time.

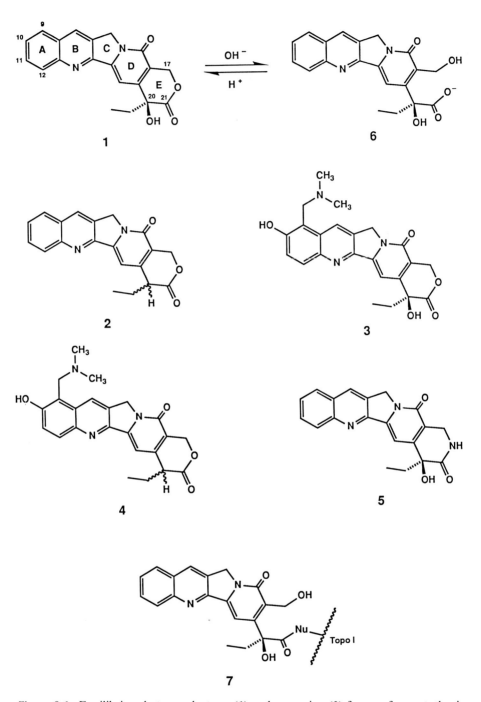

Figure 9.1. Equilibrium between lactone (**1**) and open-ring (**2**) forms of camptothecin (CPT); structures of CPT analogs.

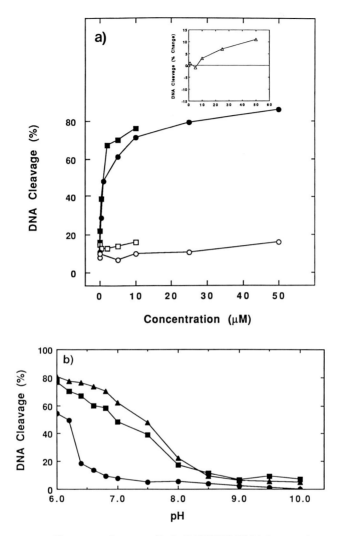

Figure 9.2. Panel a. Cleavage of supercoiled pDPT2789 DNA by topoisomerase I (topo I) in the presence of CPT congeners. Form I DNA was treated with 10 nM topo I in the presence of CPT (**1**, filled box), 20-deoxycamptothecin (**2**, open box), compound **3** (filled circle), or compound **4** (open circle). **Panel a, inset.** DNA was treated with topo I, 1 µM compound **3**, and varying concentrations of compound **4** (open triangle). The samples were treated with SDS/proteinase K, and DNA cleavage was measured by agarose gel electrophoresis and densitometry as described (12). **Panel b.** Effect of pH on the cleavage of supercoiled pDPT2789 DNA by 17 ng topo I in the presence of 5 µM CPT (**1**, filled triangle), 5 µM sodium CPT (**6**,filled box), or in the absence of drug (filled circle). Panel (b) was reprinted with permission from *J. Med. Chem.* (10), copyright 1989, American Chemical Society.

In addition to the E-ring derivatives of camptothecin described before, we have synthesized several camptothecin derivatives with modifications in the A-ring. To summarize our findings, we have found that camptothecin has a reasonably large degree of bulk-tolerance at position 9; most 9-substituted derivatives inhibited topoisomerase I and had good antitumor activity. Bulk-tolerance at the 10-position is somewhat limited; derivatives with flexible side chains that can occupy space in the plane of the A-ring were able to produce enzyme-mediated DNA cleavage, but derivatives with side chains that protrude above or below the plane of the A-ring were found to be much less active. The 11-position does not tolerate large substituents, and the 12-position does not tolerate any of the substituents that we have investigated, including those as small as a hydroxyl or primary amino group. In general, A-ring modified camptothecins that did not inhibit topoisomerase I were not cytotoxic and had no antitumor activity. These findings are consistent with those reported by Pommier and coworkers (Chapter 10) and by Wall and Wani (Chapter 8).

REVERSIBILITY OF CAMPTOTHECIN-STABILIZED TOPOISOMERASE I–DNA COVALENT COMPLEX FORMATION

The covalent DNA–topoisomerase I intermediate contains a phosphotyrosine bond that is broken concomitant with ligation of the phosphodiester backbone of DNA (11,20). Experimentally, one can observe the disappearance of the enzyme–DNA covalent intermediate, concomitant with DNA resealing, by altering the reaction conditions to effect a reduction in the apparent enzyme–DNA binding affinity. The most commonly used method to effect this change is to increase the salt concentration. The enhanced formation of the enzyme–DNA covalent complex that occurs in the presence of camptothecin is also reversed by the addition of high concentrations of NaCl (1, 12, 13, Fig. 9.3a). Supercoiled plasmid DNA (form I) was rapidly converted to open-circular DNA (form II) after the addition of topoisomerase I and camptothecin (lanes 4–6). After 0.5 M NaCl was added virtually all of the cleavage was reversed, resulting in covalently closed circular relaxed DNA (form I^r) (lanes 7–10).

The reversal of DNA cleavage by the addition of high salt was probably caused by enzyme–DNA dissociation from a noncovalent binary complex, which perturbs a set of equilibria resulting in diminution of the amount of enzyme–DNA covalent complexes (1,12,13). However, high salt can change DNA conformation (or enzyme conformation), and so this experiment did not establish conclusively that camptothecin inhibition is reversible under physiological conditions. Therefore, we have used other methods to examine the reversibility of DNA cleavage induced by camptothecin. For example, the addition of a large molar excess of linear DNA to a camptothecin–topoisomerase I–plasmid DNA mixture resulted in complete reversal of plasmid cleavage (12). Similarly, when a reaction mixture containing preformed enzyme–DNA complexes are diluted with buffer, DNA cleavage was rapidly reduced to a level equivalent to the amount present in a prediluted reaction (Fig. 9.3b). Since topoisomerase I cleavage of DNA can be represented by a

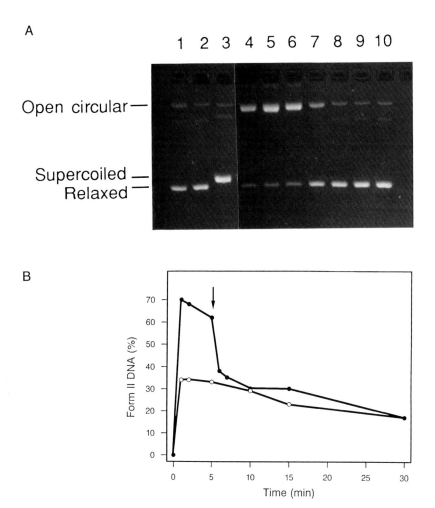

Figure 9.3. Reversal of covalent complex formation by addition of NaCl or dilution. **Panel a.** Form I DNA was treated with 10 nM topo I and 5 μM CPT for 30.5 min and then NaCl was added to 0.5 M, final concentration. Aliquots were removed at varying times and DNA cleavage was measured as described (12). Lane 1, topo I, 30 min; lane 2, topo I for 30.5 min, then NaCl for 90 min; lane 3, untreated DNA; lane 4, topo I and CPT, 1 min; lane 5, topo I and CPT, 15 min; lane 6, topo I and CPT, 30 min; lane 7, topo I and CPT for 30.5 min, then NaCl for 1.5 min; lane 8, topo I and CPT for 30.5 min, then NaCl for 4.5 min; lane 9, topo I and CPT for 30.5 min, then NaCl for 14.5 min; lane 10, topo I and CPT for 30.5 min, then NaCl for 89.5 min. **Panel b.** Form I DNA was treated with 50 nM topo I and 5 μM CPT (filled circle). After 5 min (arrow) the reaction was diluted 10-fold with buffer and BSA. A second reaction mixture contained 5 nM topo I and 0.5 μM CPT (open circle).

set of equilibria involving noncovalent and covalent DNA–topoisomerase I complexes (12), these results suggest that camptothecin perturbs the equilibria by binding reversibly to an intermediate enzyme–DNA complex. Dilution of the reaction mixture establishes a new equilibrium that reflects the lower concentrations of reactants (12).

As a consequence of binding to the DNA–topoisomerase I complex, camptothecin inhibits the catalytic activity of topoisomerase I (1,3,4,9,12). The relaxation of supercoiled DNA, which is the most common assay for topoisomerase I catalysis, involves a number of discrete steps: (1) DNA binding, (2) DNA single-strand cleavage concomitant with covalent enzyme–DNA binding, (3) unwinding of the free DNA strand, (4) resealing of the DNA phosphodiester linkage concomitant with breakage of the phosphotyrosine bond, and (5) dissociation of the enzyme from the DNA (11,21). Camptothecin has been shown to reduce the initial rate of enzyme catalysis, but consistent with reversible inhibition, DNA relaxation eventually proceeds to completion (12). Camptothecin does not alter the apparent processive behavior of topoisomerase I at low KCl concentrations, or the apparent distributive behavior at high KCl concentrations, implying that the drug does not affect noncovalent enzyme–DNA association (12,15).

Among camptothecin derivatives synthesized in our laboratories, the structural requirements for inhibition of DNA relaxation closely matched those found for DNA–enzyme covalent complex stabilization (data not shown). For example, several E-ring modified derivatives that were incapable at stabilizing covalent complex (10) also failed to inhibit DNA relaxation. These results are consistent with those reported by Pommier and coworkers (Chapter 10) and by Wall and Wani (Chapter 8). This suggests that prevention of DNA resealing is the mechanism by which camptothecin derivatives inhibit topoisomerase I catalysis.

BINDING OF [³H]CAMPTOTHECIN TO A DNA–TOPOISOMERASE I COMPLEX

Regarding the molecular details of topoisomerase I inhibition by camptothecin, most of the available evidence suggests that the drug binds reversibly to a covalent complex formed when topoisomerase I cleaves DNA (1, 12–15). We have used radiolabeled camptothecin and equilibrium dialysis to measure this interaction (12). As shown in Table 9.1, the binding of camptothecin to isolated calf thymus DNA or supercoiled DNA was negligible. Similar experiments, which used camptothecin at concentrations up to 50 μM, single-stranded DNA, or buffers containing $MgCl_2$, showed no detectable DNA binding. Similarly, camptothecin was found not to bind to 2.1 μM topoisomerase I in the absence of DNA (Table 9.1). Under the same experimental conditions, however, the retention of camptothecin was increased in a dialysis chamber containing both topoisomerase I and calf thymus DNA. Further, the amount of bound camptothecin increased with increasing enzyme concentration (12). That campto the-

Table 9.1. Binding of [³H]Camptothecin to a DNA–Topoisomerase I Complex as Determined by Equilibrium Dialysis[a]

Linear DNA[b]	Denatured DNA[c]	Supercoiled DNA[d]	Topo I	Total CPT[e]	Bound CPT (mole %)
1.1 mM	—	—	—	22.4 nM	0.4
1.1 mM	—	—	—	0.98 μM	0.3
1.1 mM	—	—	—	9.94 μM	0.6
1.1 mM	—	—	—	49.1 μM	0.1
—	1.1 mM	—	—	24.0 nM	0.2
—	—	0.66 mM	—	21.6 nM	0
—	—	—	2.1 μM	22.9 nM	0
1.1 mM	—	—	2.1 μM	23.9 nM	17
1.1 mM	—	—	2.1 μM	22.7 nM	0[f]

[a]The binding assay was carried out and analyzed as described (12); the volume was 0.4 ml.
[b]Sonicated calf thymus DNA.
[c]Heat-denatured sonicated calf thymus DNA.
[d]pDPT2789 plasmid DNA.
[e]Total of bound and free CPT present at the end of dialysis.
[f]Bound CPT remaining after 24 h dialysis vs. 1 liter of cleavage buffer.

cin did not bind until topoisomerase I and DNA were combined suggests that a drug binding site was created as the enzyme–DNA covalent complex was formed. Both camptothecin–enzyme and camptothecin–DNA interactions within the ternary complex are implied, but we cannot exclude the possibility that a binding site is produced entirely within the DNA helix or topoisomerase I molecule as the two macromolecules come together.

The chemical nature of the E-ring of camptothecin (see Fig. 9.1) suggests the possibility that stabilization of the enzyme–DNA complex by camptothecin could involve a chemical reaction between an enzyme nucleophile and the α-hydroxy lactone to form an intermediate such as 7. This intermediate, if formed, is likely to be labile, since C-21 ester or amide derivatives of campto-thecin revert to camptothecin via intramolecular attack of the C-17 primary alcohol on the electrophilic C-21 carbonyl (22). We therefore studied the chemical nature of the enzyme–DNA–camptothecin ternary complex to test the possibility of covalent drug binding. [³H]Camptothecin (25 nM) was incubated with either topoisomerase I (2.1 μM), calf thymus DNA (1.1 mM bp), or a mixture of enzyme and DNA. After 30 min at 37°C, the mixture was dialyzed to remove unbound camptothecin and analyzed for the presence of irreversibly bound camptothecin. No significant amount of [³H]camptothecin remained associated with DNA or topoisomerase I (Table 9.1). Another reaction mixture containing supercoiled DNA, topoisomerase I, and labeled camptothecin was treated with SDS and dialyzed; no [³H]camptothecin remained associated with either macromolecule. These results fail to provide support for the thesis that camp-tothecin may bind covalently to topoisomerase I or to DNA, but we cannot rule out the possible existence of a transient drug–enzyme (–DNA) covalent complex that was not stable under the conditions used for this study. The lability of such a complex, if it exists, may hamper its detection.

ANALYSIS OF DNA–TOPOISOMERASE I COMPLEXES
BY FILTER BINDING

Topoisomerase I and DNA form both covalent and noncovalent binary complexes. The observation that [³H]camptothecin binds to an enzyme–DNA complex raises the issue of which binary complex is bound. The covalent complex is stoichiometric with DNA cleavage (11) and is usually measured by gel electrophoresis (Figs. 9.2 and 9.3). The noncovalent enzyme–DNA complex can be quantified by a nitrocellulose filter binding assay, which is often used to study protein–DNA interactions (23–25). While double-stranded DNA binds

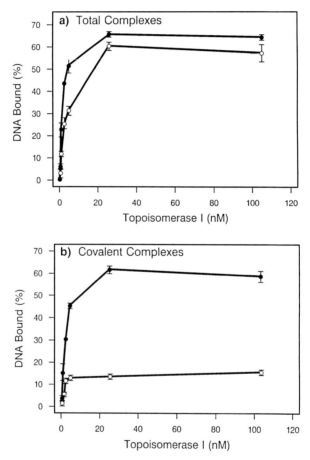

Figure 9.4. Quantitation of the binding of topoisomerase I to a 381 bp fragment of pBR322 DNA as analyzed by nitrocellulose filter binding (12). Reaction mixtures contained [³²P] labeled DNA, topo I, and 5 μM CPT (filled circle) or no CPT (open circle). **Panel a.** Reaction mixtures were filtered before the addition of SDS. **Panel b.** Reaction mixtures were filtered after the addition of SDS. Values represent the mean ± SD (n = 2). Reprinted with permission from *Biochemistry* (12), copyright 1989, American Chemical Society.

very poorly to nitrocellulose, many proteins (including topoisomerase I) bind quite strongly. Protein–DNA complexes are quantified by measuring the retention by the nitrocellulose filter of radiolabeled DNA bound to topoisomerase I. We determined the effect of camptothecin on the binding of topoisomerase I to a 381 bp 3'-[^{32}P]end-labeled DNA fragment (Fig. 9.4).

Reaction mixtures were filtered: (1) without SDS addition (Fig. 9.4a), to measure the percentage of DNA molecules bound either covalently or noncovalently to topoisomerase I, and (2) after SDS addition (Fig. 9.4b), to measure the percentage of DNA molecules bound covalently to topoisomerase I. In the presence or absence of camptothecin, the proportion of DNA molecules bound to topoisomerase I increased as the enzyme concentration was raised (Fig. 9.4a). Significant quantities of enzyme-bound DNA were detected when reaction mixtures were filtered without SDS addition, even in the absence of camptothecin (Fig. 9.4a). In contrast, very few DNA molecules were bound covalently to enzyme in the absence of camptothecin, even at relatively high topoisomerase I concentrations (Fig. 9.4b). The addition of camptothecin significantly increased the proportion of DNA molecules that were covalently bound to topoisomerase I. These results imply that in the absence of camptothecin, topoisomerase I binds tightly, but usually noncovalently, to DNA. In the presence of camptothecin, the equilibrium appears to shift such that most of the enzyme–DNA complexes are covalent. These results are consistent with the conclusion that the drug binds with higher affinity to the covalent enzyme–DNA complex.

EFFECT OF CAMPTOTHECIN ON TOPOISOMERASE I CLEAVAGE OF SINGLE-STRANDED DNA

Topoisomerase I can introduce nicks into single-stranded DNA (ssDNA) as well as double-stranded DNA (dsDNA). Unlike the case with duplex DNA, where the detection of a nick requires the addition of protein denaturants, the breakage of ssDNA by eukaryotic topoisomerase I can be observed under native conditions (26,27). This is because after DNA cleavage, the strand with the 5' hydroxy group is not held in place by a complementary strand and is free to diffuse away from the cleavage site. The 5' hydroxy end of ssDNA is not bound to enzyme since it can be phosphorylated by polynucleotide kinase, in contrast to the situation in dsDNA (27). In addition, the amount of cleavage observed with ssDNA is greater than the amount observed with dsDNA, since the resealing reaction involves attack by a free DNA end rather than an end held in place by base pairing.

We examined the effect of camptothecin on the cleavage of ssDNA mediated by topoisomerase I. While camptothecin enhanced the cleavage of double-stranded supercoiled SV40 DNA, it had no effect on the cleavage of single-stranded circular ϕX174 DNA (Fig. 9.5a). Similarly, camptothecin had no effect on the reversal of single-stranded DNA cleavage (recircularization of linear ϕX174; Fig. 9.5b), which is induced by the addition of 10 mM MgCl$_2$ (28). Neither the rate nor the extent of ssDNA cleavage or ligation was affected

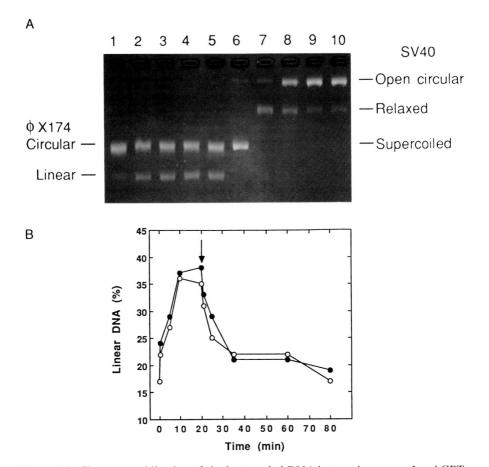

Figure 9.5. Cleavage and ligation of single-stranded DNA by topoisomerase I and CPT. **Panel a.** 400 ng single-stranded circular φX174 DNA (lanes 1–5) was treated with 21 nM topo I and CPT in a buffer containing 10 mM Tris-HCl, pH 7.5, 50 mM KCl, 1 mM EDTA, and 0.25 mM DTT. In lanes 6–10, 100 ng supercoiled SV40 DNA was treated with topo I and CPT as described (12). After SDS and proteinase K treatment, the samples were electrophoresed on a 1.6% agarose gel; the gel was soaked in ethidium bromide and electrophoresis was continued to separate all forms of DNA. Lane 1, untreated φX174 DNA; lane 2, φX174 and topo I; lane 3, φX174, topo I, and 1 μM CPT; lane 4, φX174, topo I, and 5 μM CPT; lane 5, φX174, topo I, and 10 μM CPT; lane 6, untreated SV40 DNA; lane 7, SV40 and topo I; lane 8, SV40, topo I, and 1 μM CPT; lane 9, SV40, topo I, and 5 μM CPT; lane 10, SV40, topo I, and 10 μM CPT. **Panel b.** The time course of cleavage and ligation of single-stranded φX174 by topoisomerase I was followed by agarose gel electrophoresis and densitometry. Recircularization of linear φX174 DNA was induced after 20 min (arrow) by the addition of $MgCl_2$ to 10 mM, final concentration (28). Cleavage and ligation was carried out without (filled circle) or with 10 μM camptothecin (open circle).

by camptothecin (Fig. 9.5b). The cleavage of ssDNA by topoisomerase I has been reported to occur at regions with the potential for intramolecular base pairing (29). The lack of effect by camptothecin on these reactions may be the result of a different enzyme–DNA conformation at the putative hairpinlike cleavage sites that does not bind the drug, or may simply reflect the inability of camptothecin to preclude dissociation of the free 5′ end of the DNA from the formed ternary complex. Alternatively, the DNA sequences at which ssDNA cleavage and resealing occur on φX174 DNA may not be preferred sites for camptothecin interaction; camptothecin has been shown to enhance cleavage at some DNA sites much more efficiently than at other sites (13–15, 30).

EFFECT OF CAMPTOTHECIN ON DNA STRAND TRANSFER MEDIATED BY TOPOISOMERASE I

Topoisomerase I has been shown to mediate intermolecular DNA strand transfer; enzyme-linked ssDNA fragments (donors) can be joined to dsDNA possessing a terminal 5′ hydroxy group (acceptors) (28,31). Competent dsDNA acceptors include nicked circles and linear DNA fragments bearing either flush, 5′ protruding, or 5′ recessed ends. The only requirement for the acceptor is a 5′ hydroxy terminus, since the donor DNA fragment contains a 3′ phosphate linked to a tyrosine residue on topoisomerase I.

We have investigated the effect of camptothecin on the strand-transferase activity of topoisomerase I. The covalent [^{32}P]DNA–topoisomerase I complex (donor) was prepared by first annealing a 17-nucleotide primer to single-stranded M13 DNA and extending the primer with [^{32}P]dCTP and Klenow polymerase (Fig. 9.6). The resultant product was denatured to yield a nonradioactive M13 circle and a series of uniformly labeled linear ssDNA fragments; topoisomerase I was added to form enzyme–DNA complexes. The acceptor, a

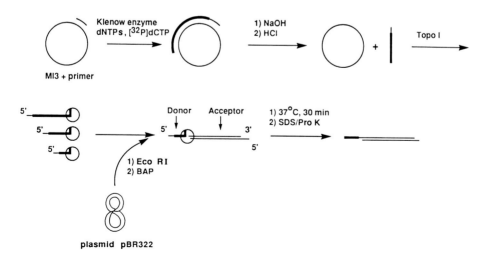

Figure 9.6. DNA strand transfer mediated by topoisomerase.

| 1 | 2 | 3 | 4 | 5 | 6 | 7 |

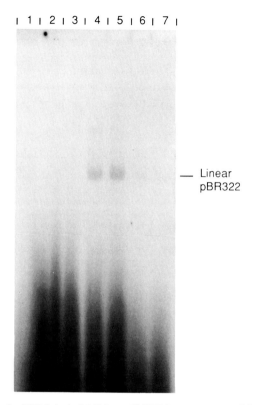

— Linear
pBR322

Figure 9.7. Uniformly [³²P]-labeled M13mp 18 DNA was prepared by primer extension using a 17-nucleotide sequencing primer, Klenow polymerase, and [α-³²P]dCTP as described (32). The DNA was denatured with 0.11 N NaOH at 37°C for 10 min and then neutralized with a predetermined titrated amount of 1 N HCl. The strand transferase reaction was carried out as described (31). Denatured M13 DNA (100,000 cpm) and 85 ng of topo I were incubated at 37°C for 30 min; CPT (when present) was added to the mixture followed by acceptor DNA (Eco RI-digested pBR322 DNA, dephosphorylated unless noted). The mixture was incubated at 37°C for 30 min, treated with SDS/proteinase K for 1 h, and electrophoresed on a 0.8% agarose gel at 40 V overnight. The gel was dried *in vacuo* and autoradiographed at −70°C with an intensifying screen. Lane 1, M13 DNA only; lane 2, M13 DNA and topo I; lane 3, M13 DNA, topo I, and 1 μg 5′ phosphorylated acceptor DNA; lane 4, M13 DNA, topo I, and 1 μg acceptor DNA; lane 5, M13 DNA, topo I, and 0.5 μg acceptor DNA; lane 6, M13 DNA, topo I, 0.5 μg acceptor DNA, and 5 μM CPT; lane 7, M13 DNA, topo I, 0.5 μg acceptor DNA, and 10 μM CPT.

linear DNA fragment with 5′ protruding ends, was prepared by cleaving pBR322 DNA with Eco RI and dephosphorylating the 5′ ends with bacterial alkaline phosphatase (BAP). The donor and acceptor were mixed, and the transfer of radioactive DNA fragments to the acceptor was examined by agarose gel electrophoresis and autoradiography.

Radioactive DNA fragments linked to topoisomerase I were transferred to the Eco RI/BAP–treated DNA acceptor (Fig. 9.7). There was no strand transfer when the acceptor was omitted from the reaction mixture (lane 2), or when the acceptor carried a 5′ phosphoryl group (lane 3). The presence of 5 or 10 μM camptothecin significantly reduced the intensity of the radioactive band (lanes 6 and 7), indicating that the drug inhibited the DNA ligation reaction associated with strand-transferase activity. Inhibition by camptothecin of DNA ligation in this system is similar to the enhancement of DNA cleavage observed with camptothecin and double-stranded DNA (see Figs. 9.2 and 9.3). The findings that camptothecin inhibits strand transfer mediated by topoisomerase I but has no effect on the cleavage or ligation of single-stranded φX174 DNA could reflect conformational differences between the respective enzyme–DNA complexes. Differences in DNA sequence and/or strandedness may influence these putative conformational changes and affect camptothecin inhibition (13–15, 30).

EFFECT OF CAMPTOTHECIN ON REPAIR-DEFICIENT PERMEABLE YEAST CELLS

Camptothecin shows minimal activity against wild-type *Saccharomyces cerevisiae* (6), producing only a minimal zone of inhibition surrounding a well containing 1 mg/ml of drug. We have increased the sensitivity of *S. cerevisiae* to camptothecin by inducing a mutation that increases permeability of the fungal cell membrane; a similar effect was demonstrated by Nitiss and Wang (7) with another permeability mutation. As shown in Figure 9.8, camptothecin had an IC_{12} (concentration producing a 12 mm zone of inhibition) of 98 μg/ml in the permeable mutant. The zone size did not increase at concentrations of >200

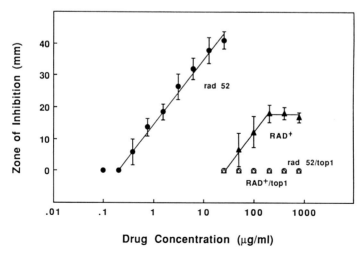

Figure 9.8. Evidence that topoisomerase I is the target for camptothecin. The *S. cerevisiae* strains contained a mutation that increased permeability of the fungal cell membrane. In addition, strains were either RAD+ (filled triangle), deleted inn the RAD52 gene (*rad52*, filled circle), deleted in the topoisomerase I gene (RAD+/*top1*, open triangle), or deleted in the RAD52 gene and the topoisomerase I gene, (*rad52/top1*, open circle). The assay is described in Eng et al. (6).

µg/ml owing to the insolubility of camptothecin. Deletion of the *RAD52* gene in the permeable strain increased sensitivity to camptothecin 145-fold (IC_{12} of 0.67 µg/ml), indicating that toxicity of camptothecin is due to induction of DNA damage that is repaired by recombination. Congenic DNA repair-proficient (*RAD+*) and DNA repair-deficient (*rad52*) strains in which the topoisomerase I gene has been deleted (6) are completely insensitive to camptothecin, even at a concentration of 800 µg/ml (Fig. 9.8), demonstrating that topoisomerase I is the cellular target for the drug. Drug resistance in the topoisomerase I deletion mutants is seen for analogs of camptothecin but is not evident for other classes of DNA damage-inducing drugs.

We have also constructed a strain of yeast with inducible expression of the yeast topoisomerase I gene on a plasmid transfected into an *S. cerevisiae* mutant in which the chromosomal topoisomerase I gene was deleted (6). Upon induction of topoisomerase I, this strain regained sensitivity to camptothecin. Overexpression of topoisomerase I resulted in hypersensitivity to camptothecin, indicating that drug toxicity is related to the quantity of target enzyme within the cell.

CONCLUSIONS

Chemistry and Structure–Activity Relationships

The lactone ring of camptothecin is a critical structural feature for enzyme inhibition; each of the oxygens in the hydroxylactone moiety are required. The lactone ring of a water-soluble camptothecin analog hydrolyzes in aqueous solution in a pH dependent manner. At neutral pH, about half of the lactone form hydrolyzes to the open-ring form, which does not inhibit topoisomerase I. The A-ring of camptothecin is more tolerant of substitution, with the 9 position displaying the largest degree of bulk-tolerance with respect to topoisomerase I inhibition. There is partial bulk-tolerance at the 10-position, and little tolerance at the 11 and 12 positions of camptothecin. Compounds that do not stabilize the enzyme–DNA covalent complex do not inhibit enzyme catalytic activity, are generally not cytotoxic, and have no antitumor activity.

Biochemistry

Enzyme-mediated cleavage of supercoiled plasmid DNA in the presence of camptothecin is reversible. Consistent with reversible inhibition, camptothecin decreases the initial velocity of supercoiled DNA relaxation mediated by catalytic quantities of topoisomerase I, but does not prevent relaxation. The alkaloid binds reversibly to a DNA–topoisomerase I complex, but not to isolated enzyme or isolated DNA. It is likely that camptothecin binds to covalent enzyme–DNA complexes more tightly than to noncovalent complexes. Camptothecin does not inhibit the cleavage and ligation of single-stranded ϕX174 DNA, but does inhibit the ligation reaction associated with DNA strand transfer mediated by topoisomerase I.

Pharmacology

That topoisomerase I is the target for camptothecin is supported by the finding that yeast lacking the enzyme is totally resistant to camptothecin. Transfection of topoisomerase I–deficient yeast with an inducible topoisomerase I gene, followed by gene induction, restores camptothecin sensitivity. In addition, repair-deficient yeast cells are hypersensitive to camptothecin, indicating that toxicity of the drug is due to induction of DNA damage that is repaired by recombination.

REFERENCES

1. Hsiang, Y.-H., Hertzberg, R., Hecht, S., and Liu, L. F. Camptothecin induces protein-linked DNA breaks via mammalian DNA topoisomerase I. J. Biol. Chem. **260:** 14873–14878, 1985.

2. Mattern, M. R., Mong, S.-M., Bartus, H. F., Mirabelli, C. K., Crooke, S. T., and Johnson, R. K. Relationship between the intracellular effects of camptothecin and the inhibition of DNA topoisomerase I in cultured L1210 cells. Cancer Res. **47:** 1793–1798, 1987.

3. Andoh, T., Ishii, K., Suzuki, Y., Ikegami, Y., Kusunoki, Y., Takemoto, Y., and Okada, K. Characterization of a mammalian mutant with a camptothecin-resistant DNA topoisomerase I. Proc. Natl. Acad. Sci. USA. **84:** 5565–5569, 1987.

4. Gupta, R. S., Gupta, R., Eng, B., Lock, R. B., Ross, W. E., Hertzberg, R. P., Caranfa, M. J., and Johnson, R. K. Camptothecin-resistant mutants of Chinese hamster ovary cells containing a resistant form of topoisomerase I. Cancer Res. **48:** 6404–6410, 1988.

5. Hsiang, Y.-H. and Liu, L. F. Identification of mammalian DNA topoisomerase I as an intracellular target of the anticancer drug camptothecin. Cancer Res. **48:** 1722–1726, 1988.

6. Eng, W.-K., Faucette, L., Johnson, R. K., and Sternglanz, R. Evidence that DNA topoisomerase I is necessary for the cytotoxic effects of camptothecin. Mol. Pharmacol. **34:** 755–760, 1988.

7. Nitiss, J. and Wang, J. C. DNA topoisomerase-targeting antitumor drugs can be studied in yeast. Proc. Natl. Acad. Sci. USA. **85:** 7501–7505, 1988.

8. Hertzberg, R. P., Holden, K. G., Hecht, S. M., Mattern, M. R., Faucette, L. F., and Johnson, R. K. Characterization of the structural features of camptothecin essential for topoisomerase I interaction and for induction of protein-linked DNA breaks in cells. Proc. Am. Assoc. Cancer Res. **28:** 27, 1987.

9. Pommier, Y., Jaxel, C., Covey, J. M., Kerrigan, D., Wani, M. C., Wall, M. E., and Kohn, K. W. Structure-activity study of the relation between topoisomerase I inhibition and antitumor activity of camptothecin. Proc. Am. Assoc. Cancer Res. **29:** 1080, 1988.

10. Hertzberg, R. P., Caranfa, M. J., Holden, K. G., Jakas, D. R., Gallagher, G., Mattern, M. R., Mong, S.-M., O'Leary Bartus, J., Johnson, R. K., and Kingsbury, W. D. Modification of the hydroxylactone ring of camptothecin: Inhibition of mammalian topoisomerase I and biological activity. J. Med. Chem. **32:** 715–720, 1989.

11. Maxwell, A. and Gellert, M. Mechanistic aspects of DNA topoisomerases. Adv. Protein Chem. **38:** 69–107, 1986.

12. Hertzberg, R. P., Caranfa, M. J., and Hecht, S. M. On the mechanism of topoisomerase I inhibition by camptothecin: Evidence for binding to an enzyme-DNA complex. Biochemistry. **28:** 4629–4638, 1989.

13. Kjeldsen, E., Mollerup, S., Thomsen, B., Bonven, B., Bolund, L., and Westergaard, O. Sequence-dependent effect of camptothecin on human topoisomerase I DNA cleavage. J. Mol. Biol. **202:** 333–342, 1988.

14. Thomsen, B., Mollerup, S., Bonven, B. J., Frank, R., Blocker, H., Nielsen, O. F., and Westergaard, O. Sequence specificity of DNA topoisomerase I in the presence and absence of camptothecin. EMBO J. **6:** 1817–1823, 1987.

15. Champoux, J. J. and Aronoff, R. The effects of camptothecin on the reaction and the specificity of the wheat germ type I topoisomerase. J. Biol. Chem. **264:** 1010–1015, 1989.

16. Wall, M. E. and Wani, M. C. Antineo-plastic agents from plants. Annu. Rev. Pharmacol. Toxicol. **17:** 117–132, 1977.

17. Wani, M. C., Ronman, P. E., Lindley, J. T., and Wall, M. E. Plant antitumor agents. 18. Synthesis and biological activity of camptothecin analogues. J. Med. Chem. **23:** 554–560, 1980.

18. Wani, M. C., Nicholas, A. W., and Wall, M. E. Plant antitumor agents. 28. Resolution of a key tricyclic synthon, 5'(RS)-1,5-dioxo-5'-ethyl-5'-hydroxy-2'H,5'H,6'H-6',-oxopyrano[3'4'-f]$\Delta^{6,8}$-tetrahydroin-dolizine: Total synthesis and antitumor activity of 20(S)- and 20(R)-camptothecin. J. Med. Chem. **30:** 2317–2319, 1987.

19. Wall, M. E., Wani, M. C., Cook, C. E., Palmer, K. H., McPhail, A. T., and Sim, G. A. Plant antitumor agents. I. The isolation and structure of camptothecin, a novel alkaloidal leukemia and tumor inhibitor from *Camptotheca acuminata.* J. Am. Chem. Soc. **88:** 3888–3890, 1966.

20. Champoux, J. J. DNA is linked to the rat liver DNA nicking-closing enzyme by a phosphodiester bond to tyrosine. J. Biol. Chem. **256:** 4805–4809, 1981.

21. Wang, J. C. DNA topoisomerases. Annu. Rev. Biochem. **54:** 665–697, 1985.

22. Adamovics, J. A. and Hutchinson, C. R. Prodrug analogues of the antitumor alkaloid camptothecin. J. Med. Chem. **22** 310–314, 1979.

23. Riggs, A. D., Suzuki, H., and Bourgeois, S. Lac repressor-operator interaction. I. Equilibrium studies. J. Biol. Chem. **48:** 67–83, 1970.

24. Melancon, P., Burgess, R. R., and Record, M. T. Nitrocellulose filter binding studies of the interactions of Escherichia coli RNA polymerase holoenzyme with deoxyribonucleic acid restriction fragments: Evidence for multiple classes of nonpromoter interactions, some of which display promoter-like properties. Biochemistry. **21:** 4318–4331, 1982.

25. Woodbury, C. P. and von Hippel, P. H. On the determination of deoxyribonucleic acid-protein interaction parameters using the nitrocellulose filter-binding assay. Biochemistry. **22:** 4730–4737, 1983.

26. Prell, B. and Vosberg, H.-P. Analysis of covalent complexes formed between calf thymus DNA topoisomerase and single-stranded DNA. Eur. J. Biochem. **108:** 389–398, 1980.

27. Been, M. D. and Champoux, J. J. Breakage of single-stranded DNA by rat liver nicking-closing enzyme with the formation of a DNA-enzyme complex. Nucleic Acids Res. **8:** 6129–6142, 1980.

28. Been, M. D. and Champoux, J. J. DNA breakage and closure by rat liver type 1 topoisomerase: Separation of the half-reactions by using a single-stranded DNA substrate. Proc. Natl. Acad. Sci. USA. **78:** 2883–2887, 1981.

29. Been, M. D. and Champoux, J. J. Breakage of single-stranded DNA by eukaryotic type 1 topoisomerase occurs only at regions with the potential for base-pairing. J. Mol. Biol. **108:** 515–531, 1984.

30. Jaxel, C., Kohn, K. W., and Pommier, Y. Topoisomerase I interaction with SV40 DNA in the presence and absence of camptothecin. Nucleic Acids Res. **16:** 11157–11170, 1988.

31. Halligan, B. D., Davis, J. L., Edwards, K. A., and Liu, L. F. Intra- and intermolecular strand transfer by HeLa DNA topoisomerase I. J. Biol. Chem. **257:** 3995–4000, 1982.

32. Chow, K.-C., Johnson, T. L., and Pearson, G. D. A novel method for the detection and quantitation of eukaryotic topoisomerase I. BioTechniques. **3:** 290–297, 1985.

Chapter 10
Structure–Activity Relationship of Topoisomerase I Inhibition by Camptothecin Derivatives: Evidence for the Existence of a Ternary Complex

YVES POMMIER, CHRISTINE JAXEL, CAROLINE R. HEISE,
DONNA KERRIGAN, AND KURT W. KOHN

DNA topoisomerase I is a nuclear enzyme that can relieve the DNA torsional tension that accumulates as a result of DNA replication, transcription, or repair (1–3). DNA relaxation can be monitored *in vitro* by using duplex DNA circles (Fig. 10.1). The key reaction for this enzyme activity is the transfer of a co-valent bond from a phosphate in the DNA backbone to the OH group of a topoisomerase I tyrosine residue (black dots, step 2, Figs. 10.1 and 10.2; see also Fig. 10.8). Tyrosine-727 has been identified as the active tyrosine of *Saccharomyces cerevisiae* DNA topoisomerase I (4). The DNA linking number (Lk) changes by one as a result of the passage of the intact DNA strand through the gap made in the complementary strand (step 2, Figs. 10.1 and 10.2), and the resealing of this strand on the other side (step 3, Figs. 10.1 and 10.2). In the absence of drug, the intermediate represented in step 2 is usually not detectable because it is very transient. It has been identified as a "cleavable complex" (5), because after protein denaturation (by sodium dodecylsulfate [SDS]) and/or pH denaturation (by NaOH), it can be isolated as one DNA–protein crosslink (DPC) and one DNA single-strand break (SSB) (step 4, Figs. 10.2). This type of DNA strand break is specific for topoisomerase I. Cleavable complexes have also been described for topoisomerase II (6,7). However, in the latter case, the enzyme is covalently linked to the 5′ termini of a DNA single- or double-strand break and each strand passage reaction changes DNA linking number by steps of two (1–3). The human DNA topoisomerase I gene has been isolated and mapped on chromosome 20q12-13.2 (8,9).

Camptothecin (Fig. 10.3), an alkaloid isolated from *Camptotheca acuminata* (10), inhibits topoisomerase I by stabilizing the cleavable complex intermediate of the topoisomerase reactions (step 2, Fig. 10.2) (5,11,12). This can be inferred from the observations that (1) both inhibition of DNA relaxation

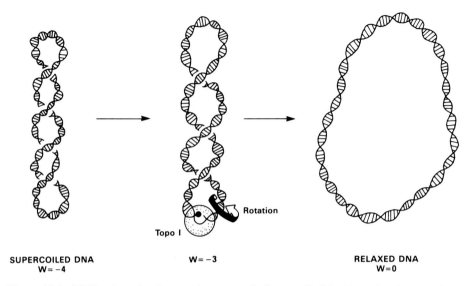

SUPERCOILED DNA   W= -3   RELAXED DNA
W= -4   W=0

Figure 10.1. DNA relaxation by topoisomerase I. Supercoiled DNA (**1**) is relaxed (**3** by topoisomerase I in steps of one. The middle panel (**2**) represents the first step of the reaction (one superturn being removed). The black dot in the middle panel indicates the covalent linkage between the enzyme (topo I) and the 3′ DNA terminus during the catalytic reaction. Topoisomerase I activity is processive under normal conditions.

and induction of DNA single-strand breaks occur at similar drug concentrations (5,12,13); (2) the potency of camptothecin derivatives to induce DNA cleavage correlates with their ability to inhibit DNA relaxation (13), and (3) the sites of DNA cleavage induced by camptothecin correspond to sites that are cleaved in the absence of the drug (12,14,15).

Camptothecin is used as an anticancer agent in China and exhibits anti-tumor activity in a number of screening systems (10,16). The sodium salt of camptothecin has undergone clinical trial in the United States, but severe toxicity has limited its utility (17,18). Current drug development efforts are focused on the synthesis of water-soluble analogs of camptothecin that could be used in cancer chemotherapy (19,20).

The present study summarizes the structure–activity of 30 camptothecin analogs synthesized in the laboratory of Dr. M. E. Wall (Research Triangle Institute, Research Triangle Park, NC). Inhibition of DNA relaxation and induction of DNA single-strand breaks by mouse leukemia L1210 topoisomerase I were used to compare the derivatives.

TOPOISOMERASE I ASSAYS

Two types of assays can be used with purified topoisomerase I: inhibition of DNA relaxation, and induction of DNA cleavage. The optimum experimental conditions are different for each assay (Table 10.1). In the relaxation assay, maximum enzyme activity is obtained at physiological ionic strength (100–200

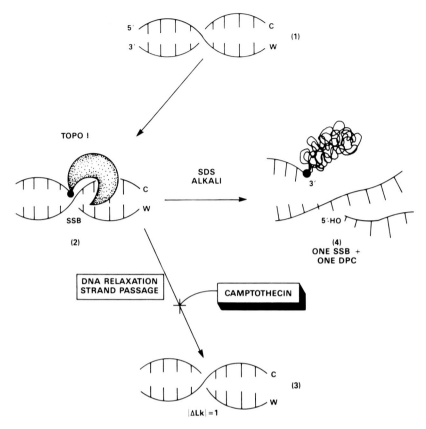

Figure 10.2. Topoisomerase I–mediated DNA break. One helical turn of duplex DNA is represented (**1**); the Watson strand (W) is above the Crick strand (C). The intermediate (**2**) represents topoisomerase I (topo I) covalently linked (black dot) to the 3' terminus of the W strand; the covalent bond has been transferred by the enzyme from the phosphodiester DNA backbone to a tyrosine enzyme residue. Passage of the C strand through the DNA single-strand break (SSB) relaxes the DNA, and topoisomerase I reseals the break and dissociates from the DNA (**3**). The cleavage intermediate (**2**) can be detected after denaturation with sodium dodecyl sulfate (SDS) and alkali (cleavable complex) (**4**). Camptothecin stabilizes the intermediate (**2**).

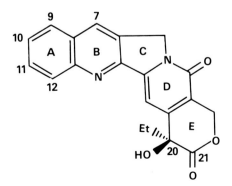

Figure 10.3. Structure of natural camptothecin (20(*S*)-camptothecin).

Table 10.1. Differential Reaction Conditions for Topoisomerase I Assays with Purified Mammalian Topoisomerase I

DNA	Inhibition of Relaxation Supercoiled	Induction of DNA Cleavage Supercoiled or linear ($[^{32}P]$ labeled)
Monovalent cations	100–150 mM NaCl or KCl	<50 mM NaCl or KCl
Topo I (per reaction)	Low (~1 unit)	Excess (>10 units)

mM NaCl or KCl), and inhibition of enzyme activity is best detectable under first order kinetics conditions with limiting topoisomerase I concentrations (approximately one unit enzyme per reaction) (12). In the topoisomerase I–induced DNA cleavage assay, maximum cleavage is achieved at low ionic strength (<50 mM NaCl or KCl) and in the presence of excess enzyme (>10 units enzyme/µg DNA). The latter assays can be performed either with supercoiled DNA or with linear $[^{32}P]$end-labeled DNA. Since the topoisomerase I molecule is covalently bound to the 3' terminus (21) (Fig. 10.2), the $[^{32}P]$ label has to be at the 3' terminus of the DNA fragment (labeling with Klenow polymerase). This avoids the retardation of DNA fragments covalently linked to polypeptide residues and allows an accurate determination of the cleavage sites. The advantages of using $[^{32}P]$end-labeled DNA fragments instead of supercoiled DNA are that (1) sensitivity is greater, since a few nanograms of DNA are sufficient to detect DNA cleavage bands by autoradiography, and (2) the cleavage sites can be mapped, since the DNA fragment is uniquely end labeled (12–15).

It is also possible to quantify topoisomerase I–induced DNA single-strand breaks (SSB) in whole cells and in isolated nuclei. Alkaline elution remains the method of choice because it is relatively simple, sensitive, allows the quantification of the associated DNA protein crosslinks (DPC), and demonstrates the protein linkage of the topoisomerase I–mediated DNA breaks (22,23). Two characteristics of camptothecin-induced DNA breaks have to be considered when performing assays in whole cells: (1) the camptothecin-induced DNA lesions can form and reverse at 0°C, and (2) approximately twofold fewer lesions are detected after lysis with sarkosyl than with SDS (23). Therefore, camptothecin-induced SSB and DPC have to be assayed without removing the drug prior to lysis, and lysis must include a strong detergent, such as SDS. Mapping of camptothecin-induced DNA breaks in selected genes has also been examined (24–26; see also Kroeger and Rowe, this volume). Although these studies have given important information on the location of topoisomerase I in chromatin, they are technically impractical for testing the potency of a large number of compounds.

The 30 camptothecin derivatives were prepared by Drs. M. E. Wall, M. C. Wani, and colleagues (Research Triangle Institute, Research Triangle Park, NC). Semisynthetic derivatives were obtained from natural camptothecin (20(S)stereoisomer) and synthetic derivatives consisted of a racemic mixture of 20(S)- and 20(R)-camptothecin.

Camptothecin derivatives were compared in two assays, inhibition of relaxation and induction of cleavage of SV40 DNA. Both assays were performed with purified mouse leukemia L1210 topoisomerase I (12,13,27). The parent compounds, camptothecin *(S)* for the semisynthetic derivatives, and camptothecin *(RS)* for the synthetic derivatives, were used as references in all experiments. Results are expressed as relative potencies, which represent the ratio of the concentration of the parent compound to that of the derivative giving similar topoisomerase I inhibition. Thus, compounds with relative potencies greater than 1 were more active than camptothecin. Compounds were identified as inactive when no significant topoisomerase I inhibition could be found at 200 μM concentrations. For all derivatives, comparable results were obtained in the DNA relaxation and cleavage assays.

In order to simplify the presentation of the results, compounds were divided into three groups according to substitution positions (Figs. 10.3–10.6). The data are summarized in Figures 10.4–10.6. The relative potency of each compound has been indicated in parenthesis under its name.

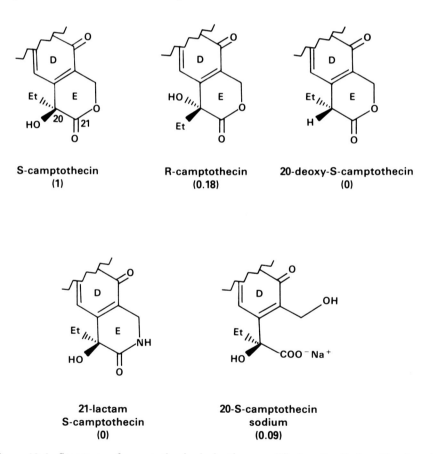

Figure 10.4. Structure of camptothecin derivatives modified on the E-ring. Numbers in parentheses indicate the potency of the derivatives as inhibitors of purified topoisomerase I, relative to that of camptothecin. No change can be made in the E-ring without losing activity.

CAMPTOTHECIN DERIVATIVES MODIFIED ON THE E-RING

Camptothecin has a single asymmetric carbon at position 20. The natural derivative, 20(S)-camptothecin, has the hydroxyl above the plane (Fig. 10.4). Synthetic camptothecin is a racemic mixture of 20(S)- and 20(R)-camptothecin (camptothecin-[RS]), and is approximately twofold less potent than 20(S)-camptothecin. This is explained by the fact that 20(R)-camptothecin (Fig. 10.4) is a very weak topoisomerase I inhibitor. This critical observation indicates that camptothecin interacts with a stereospecific site on the topoisomerase I–DNA "cleavable complex" (Fig. 10.3).

An interaction of the E-ring, in the vicinity of position 20, with a specific binding site is further supported by the loss of activity resulting from substitution of the 20-OH group by $OCOCH_2NH_3+$, or from the loss of the hydroxyl group (20-deoxycamptothecin). In addition, replacement of the 21-lactone by a 21-lactam (Fig. 10.4) also resulted in a loss of activity. The 20-hydroxy-21-lactone structure undergoes facile ring opening and closure reactions under mild conditions, and ring opening does not occur easily in the lactam or in 20-deoxycamptothecin (Dr. Wall, personal communication and this volume; 28, 29). This suggests that opening of the lactone may be an essential part of the drug action mechanism. Possibly, the ring-opened drug may form a reversible covalent bond with the enzyme via an ester exchange reaction, which might be facilitated by hydrogen bonding of the 20-hydroxyl to an electronegative atom on the enzyme.

CAMPTOTHECIN DERIVATIVES MODIFIED ON THE A-RING

Substitution on the 12 position with an amino or a nitro group caused inactivation, whereas similar substitutions on positions 9 increased activity (Fig. 10.5). Similarly, substitutions on the 11 position with bulky groups (NO_2, CN) reduced camptothecin activity. These results suggest that substituents that encroach upon space in the vicinity of position 12 block interaction with its DNA binding site.

This hypothesis is supported by the results with the 10,11-dimethoxy and 10,11-methylenedioxy derivatives (Fig. 10.5). Whereas the former is inactive, the latter has enhanced activity. Steric repulsion between the two methoxy groups at positions 10 and 11 may cause the 11-methoxy to encroach upon a critical region in the vicinity of position 12. In the came of methylenedioxy-camptothecin, which has substitutions that are chemically very similar to those of 10,11-dimethoxycamptothecin, the substituent atoms are tied together in a ring, which prevents encroachment upon the critical region.

The observation that 10,11-methylenedioxycamptothecin was 10-fold more potent than camptothecin, while 9,10-methylenedioxycamptothecin and camptothecin were equipotent (Fig. 10.5), suggests that the additional ring system opposite the B-ring may stabilize the camptothecin molecule through hydrophobic interactions with the topoisomerase I–DNA complex.

Substitution on the 9 position generally increased drug activity. 9-Hydroxycamptothecin was 10-fold more potent than camptothecin and 9-meth-

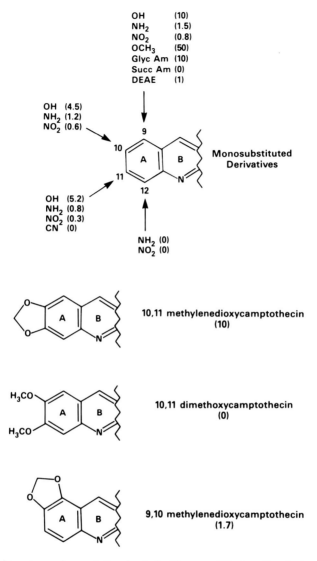

Figure 10.5. Structure of camptothecin derivatives modified on the A-ring. Numbers in parentheses indicate the potency of the derivatives as inhibitors of purified topoisomerase I, relative to those of the parent compound (20S- or 20RS-camptothecin for the semisynthetic and synthetic compounds, respectively). Substitutions around position 12 cannot be made without losing activity. Substitutions on the other positions can be used to synthesize active camptothecin derivatives.

oxycamptothecin was 50-fold more potent (Fig. 10.5). Bulky substitutions in the 9 position did not affect activity since 9-glycinaminocamptothecin was approximately tenfold more potent than camptothecin (Fig. 10.5). These results indicate that no close interaction seems to take place between camptothecin and the topoisomerase I–DNA complex via the 9 position. Thus, substitutions on the 9 position with water-soluble groups could be used to synthesize camptothecin derivatives useful as anticancer agents. This is the case of 9-glycin-aminocamptothecin in the present study and of 9-dimethylaminomethyl-10-hydroxy-20(S)-camptothecin. The latter compound was developed by SmithKline & French laboratories and is currently in phase I clinical trials (19).

SYNTHETIC COMPOUNDS RELATED TO CAMPTOTHECIN

The five rings of camptothecin are coplanar and are not aligned but curved (Figs. 10.3 and 10.6). A synthetic derivative was made by replacing the D-ring by a benzene ring (ring D-benzo-20(RS)-camptothecin; Fig. 10.6). Although its overall shape is superimposable with that of camptothecin, it was five- to ten-fold less potent than camptothecin in inhibiting topoisomerase I. An isomer of the latter compound was also made (ring D-isobenzo-20(RS)-camptothecin; Fig. 10.6). This compound was inactive. Thus, the curved shape of campto-thecin may be required for bringing rings A to C into proper orientation for interaction with the topoisomerase I–DNA complex. The additional finding that tricyclic–ketone–camptothecin, which lacks the A and B rings, was inac-tive (Fig. 10.6) indicates also the importance of rings A to C for camptothecin action.

CONCLUSION

The structure–activity relationship of some 30 camptothecin derivatives sug-gests that camptothecin interacts with the topoisomerase I–DNA complex via stereospecific binding. The binding site probably accommodates the whole drug molecule, since the two most distant rings of camptothecin (rings A and

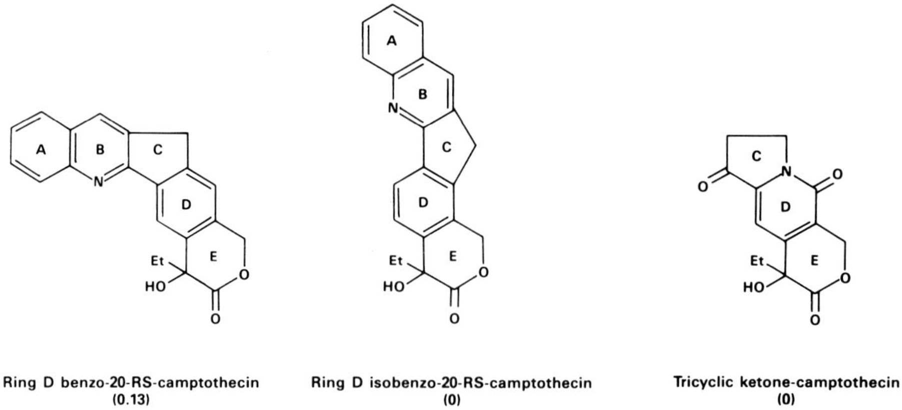

Ring D benzo-20-RS-camptothecin   Ring D isobenzo-20-RS-camptothecin   Tricyclic ketone-camptothecin
(0.13)   (0)   (0)

Figure 10.6. Structure of synthetic compounds related to camptothecin. Numbers in parentheses indicate the potency of the compounds to inhibit purified topoisomerase I, relative to that of 20(RS)-camptothecin. The arched shape of camptothecin conferred by the positioning of the A to C rings is critical for activity.

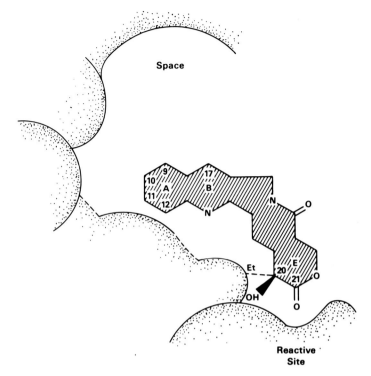

Figure 10.7. Hypothetical interactions between camptothecin and its topoisomerase I–DNA binding site. Camptothecin is represented by the hatched area, with relevant positions and rings indicated. The five rings of camptothecin are in the plane of the figure, the 20-OH is above the plane, and the 20-ethyl below. The topoisomerase I–DNA receptor site is represented by the shaded area.

E) are critical for topoisomerase I inhibition (Fig. 10.7). Near the E-ring, a reactive site possibly forms a hydrogen bond with the 21-hydroxy of a ring-opened camptothecin, and that reaction may be critical for drug action. In ring A, no bulky group may be added to positions 12 or 11 without loss of drug activity. This implies that steric hindrance in this region inactivates campto-thecin (Fig. 10.7). Also, a space probably exists outside of positions 9 and 17 of the A- and B-rings (Fig. 10.7), since camptothecin derivatives substituted on these positions with bulky groups retain activity (19,20). This space seems cru-cial for the synthesis of water-soluble derivatives that could be developed as anticancer agents.

The camptothecin binding site probably involves the topoisomerase I mol-ecule, since camptothecin does not bind significantly to purified DNA (30). The camptothecin association could be either on the enzyme or at the interface of the enzyme–DNA complex (Fig. 10.8). The observation that camptothecin in-duces DNA cleavage at sites that represent a subset of those cleaved by topo-isomerase I in the absence of drug (12,14,15) suggests that camptothecin inter-acts both with the enzyme and the DNA (29) (Fig. 10.8). Therefore, it is likely that camptothecin forms a *ternary complex* with topoisomerase I and DNA.

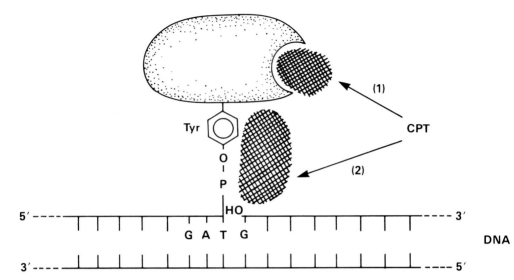

Figure 10.8. Hypothetical localization of the camptothecin binding site on the topoiso-merase I–DNA cleavage complex. A tyrosine residue (Tyr) of the enzyme (topo I) is covalently linked to the 3′ phosphoryl DNA terminus next to a thymine (T). The other DNA terminus is a 5′-OH next to a guanine (G). The shaded area represents the camp-tothecin molecule. Reversible binding can occur either on the protein only (1) or at the interface of the topoisomerase I–DNA complex (2). The latter possibility seems more likely because of the DNA sequence–selectivity of camptothecin action.

The exact structure of this complex remains to be determined. It is known that topoisomerase I is covalently linked by a tyrosine residue to the 3′ DNA ter-minus next to a thymine (Fig. 10.8) (11,31, and Jaxel et al. this volume). Since, for the camptothecin-induced DNA breaks, the 5′ hydroxyl terminus of the DNA break is next to a G, whereas for topoisomerase I–mediated DNA breaks detected in the absence of drug, it is more often an A (15), an attractive pos-sibility is that the G may be required for a camptothecin–topoisomerase I–DNA complex to form (Fig. 10.8).

In conclusion, analysis of the structure–activity relationship of campto-thecin analogs permits the modeling of a ternary drug–topoisomerase I–DNA complex. Moreover, the observation that the antitumor activity of the camp-tothecin derivatives against murine leukemia correlated well with their potency to inhibit purified mouse leukemia topoisomerase I (32) further supports evi-dence that topoisomerase I is the cellular target for camptothecins (33–35), and that in *in vitro* inhibition of mammalian topoisomerase I may be useful in eval-uating the potency of camptothecin derivatives.

REFERENCES

1. Wang, J. C. Recent studies of DNA to-poisomerases. Biochim. Biophys. Acta. **909:** 1–9, 1987.

2. Wang, J. C. DNA topoisomerases. Annu. Rev. Biochem. **54:** 665–697, 1985.
3. Liu, L. F. DNA topoisomerase poisons as

antitumor drugs. Annu. Rev. Biochem. **58**: 351–375, 1989.

4. Lynn, R. M., Bjornsti, M. A., Caron, P. R., and Wang, J. C. Pepide sequencing and site-directed mutagenesis identify tyrosine-727 as the active site tyrosine of Saccharomyces cerevisiae DNA topoisomerase I. Proc. Natl. Acad. Sci. USA. **86**: 3559–3563, 1989.

5. Hsiang, Y. H., Hertzberg, R., Hecht, S., and Liu, L. F. Camptothecin induces protein-linked DNA breaks via mammalian DNA topoisomerase I. J. Biol. Chem. **260**: 14873–14878, 1985.

6. Liu, L. F., Rowe, T. C., Yang, L., Tewey, K. M., and Chen, G. L. Cleavage of DNA by mammalian DNA topoisomerase II. J. Biol. Chem. **258**: 15365–15370, 1983.

7. Tewey, K. M., Rowe, T. C., Yang, L., Halligan, B. D., and Liu, L. F. Adriamycin-induced DNA damage mediated by mammalian DNA topoisomerase II. Science. **226**: 466–468, 1984.

8. Juan, C. C., Hwang, J. L., Liu, A. A., Whang-Peng, J., Knutsen, T., Huebner, K., Croce, C. M., Zhang, H., Wang, J. C., and Liu, L. F. Human DNA topoisomerase I is encoded by a single-copy gene that maps to chromosome region 20q12-13.2. Proc. Natl. Acad. Sci. USA. **85**: 8910–8913, 1988.

9. D'Arpa, P., Machlin, P. S., Ratrie, H., 3d., Rothfield, N. F., Cleveland, D. W., and Earnshaw, W. C. cDNA cloning of human DNA topoisomerase I: Catalytic activity of a 67.7-kDa carboxyl-terminal fragment. Proc. Natl. Acad. Sci. USA. **85**: 2543–2547, 1988.

10. Wall, M. E., Wani, M. C., Cooke, C. E., Palmer, K. H., McPhail, A. T., and Slim, G. A. The isolation and structure of camptothecin, a novel alkaloidal leukemia and tumor inhibitor from Camptotheca acuminata. J. Am. Chem. Soc. **88**: 3888–3890, 1966.

11. Thomsen, B., Mollerup, S., Bonven, B. J., Frank, R., Blocker, H., Nielsen, O. F., and Westergaard, O. Sequence specificity of DNA topoisomerase I in the presence and absence of camptothecin. EMBO J. **6**: 1817–1823, 1987.

12. Jaxel, C., Kohn, K. W., and Pommier, Y. Topoisomerase I interaction with SV40 DNA in the presence and absence of camptothecin. Nucleic Acids Res. **16**: 11157–11170, 1988.

13. Jaxel, C., Kohn, K. W., Wani, M. C., Wall, M. E., and Pommier, Y. Structure-activity study of the actions of camptothecin derivatives on mammalian topoisomerase I: Evidence for a specific receptor site and a relation to antitumor activity. Cancer Res. **49**: 1465–1469, 1989.

14. Kjeldsen, E., Mollerup, S., Thomsen, B., Bonven, B. J., Bolund, L., and Westergaard, O. Sequence-dependent effect of camptothecin on human topoisomerase I DNA cleavage. J. Mol. Biol. **202**: 333–342, 1988.

15. Porter, S. E. and Champoux, J. J. Mapping in vivo topoisomerase I sites on simian virus 40 DNA: Asymmetric distribution of sites on replicating molecules. Mol. Cell. Biol. **9**: 541–550, 1989.

16. Wall, M. E. A new look at older drugs in cancer treatment: Natural products. Biosci. Rep. **11**: 480A–489A, 1983.

17. Gottlieb, J. A., Guarino, A. M., Call, J. B., Olivero, V. T., and Block, J. B. Preliminary pharmacologic and clinical evaluation of camptothecin sodium (NSC-100880). Biochemistry. **56**: 461, 1970.

18. Muggia, F. M., Creaven, P. J., Hansen, H. H., Cohen, M. H., and Selawry, O. S. Phase I clinical trial of weekly and daily treatment with camptothecin (NSC-100800): Correlation with preclinical studies. Biochemistry. **56**: 515–521, 1972.

19. Johnson, R. K., McCabe, F. L., Faucette, L. F., Hertzberg, R. P., Kingsbury, W. D., Boehm, J. C.,Caranfa, M. J., and Holden, K. G. SK&F 10864, a water-soluble analog of camptothecin with broad-spectrum activity in preclinical tumor models. Proc. Am. Assoc. Cancer Res. **30**: 623, 1989.

20. Kunimoto, T., Nitta, K., Tanaka, T., Uebuara, N., Baba, H., Takeuchi, M., Yokokura, T., Sawada, S., Miyasaka, T., and Mutai, M. Antitumor activity of 7-ethyl-10-[4-(1-piperidino)-1-piperidino]carbonyloxy-camptothecin, a novel water-soluble derivative of camptothecin, against murine tumors. Cancer Res. **47**: 5944–5947, 1987.

21. Hsiang, Y. H. and Liu, L. F. Identification of mammalian DNA topoisomerase I as an intracellular target of the anticancer drug camptothecin. Cancer Res. **48**: 1722–1726, 1988.

22. Mattern, M. R., Mong, S. M., Bartus, H. F., Mirabelli, C. K., Crooke, S. T., and Johnson, R. K. Relationship between the intracellular effects of camptothecin and the inhibition of DNA topoisomerase I in cultured L1210 cells. Cancer Res. **47**: 1793–1798, 1987.

23. Covey, J. M., Jaxel, C., Kerrigan, D., Kohn, K. W., and Pommier, Y. Detergent and temperature sensitivity of protein-linked DNA single-strand breaks induced in mammalian cells by camptothecin, an inhibitor of topoisomerase I. Proc. Am. Assoc. Cancer Res. **29**: 272, 1989.

24. Gilmour, D. S. and Elgin, S. C. Localization of specific topoisomerase I interac-

tions within the transcribed region of active heat shock genes by using the inhibitor camptothecin. Mol. Cell. Biol. **7:** 141–148, 1987.

25. Stewart, A. F. and Schutz, G. Camptothecin-induced in vivo topoisomerase I cleavages in the transcriptionally active tyrosine aminotransferase gene. Cell. **50:** 1109–1117, 1987.

26. Culotta, V. and Sollner-Webb, B. Sites of topoisomerase I action on X. laevis ribosomal chromatin: Transcriptionally active rDNA has an approximately 200 bp repeating structure. Cell. **52:** 585–597, 1988.

27. Minford, J., Pommier, Y., Filipski, J., Kohn, K. W., Kerrigan, D., Mattern, M., Michaels, S., Schwartz, R., and Zwelling, L. A. Isolation of intercalator-dependent protein-linked DNA strand cleavage activity from cell nuclei and identification as topoisomerase II. Biochemistry. **25:** 9–16, 1986.

28. Hertzberg, R. P., Caranfa, M. J., Holden, K. G., Jakas, D. R., Gallagher, G., Mattern, M. R., Mong, S. M., Bartus, J. O., Johnson, R. K., and Kingsbury, W. D. Modification of the hydroxy lactone ring of camptothecin: Inhibition of mammalian topoisomerase I and biological activity. J. Med. Chem. **32:** 715–720, 1989.

29. Hertzberg, R. P., Caranfa, M. J., and Hecht, S. M. On the mechanism of topoisomerase I inhibition by camptothecin: Evidence for binding to an enzyme-DNA complex. Biochemistry. **28:** 4629–4638, 1989.

30. Fukada, M. Action of camptothecin and its derivatives on deoxyribonucleic acid. Biochem. Pharmacol. **34:** 1225–1230, 1985.

31. Been, M. D., Burgess, R. R., and Champoux, J. J. Nucleotide sequence preference at rat liver and wheat germ type I DNA topoisomerase breakage sites in duplex SV40 DNA. Nucleic Acids Res. **12:** 3097–3114, 1984.

32. Hsiang, Y.-H., Liu, L. F., Wall, M. E., Wani, M. C., Nicholas, A. W., Manikumar, G., Kirschenbaum, S., Silber, R., and Potmesil, M. DNA topoisomerase I-mediated DNA cleavage and cytotoxicity of camptothecin analogs. Cancer Res. **49:** 4385–4389, 1989.

33. Andoh, T., Ishii, K., Suzuki, Y., Ikegami, Y., Kusunki, Y., Takemoto, Y., and Okada, K. Characterization of a mammalian mutant with a camptothecin resistant DNA topoisomerase I. Proc. Natl. Acad. Sci. USA. **84:** 5565–5569, 1987.

34. Eng, W. K., Faucette, L., Johnson, R. K., and Sternglanz, R. Evidence that DNA topoisomerase I is necessary for the cytotoxic effects of camptothecin. Mol. Pharmacol. **34:** 755–760, 1988.

35. Nitiss, J. and Wang, J. C. DNA topoisomerase-targeting antitumor drugs can be studied in yeast. Proc. Natl. Acad. Sci. USA. **85:** 7501–7505, 1988.

Chapter 11
Topoisomerase Heterogeneity: Implications for the Discovery of Novel Antitumor Drugs

C. K. MIRABELLI, F. H. DRAKE, K. B. TAN,
S. R. PER, T. D. Y. CHUNG, R. D. WOESSNER, R. K. JOHNSON,
S. T. CROOKE, AND M. R. MATTERN

Of the relatively few cytotoxic compounds that have been found to possess significant antitumor activity, most have fallen into one of two categories. First are those compounds or treatments that compromise DNA metabolism in some way; for example, by interfering with the biosynthesis of DNA precursors (methotrexate) or by damaging the DNA directly (ionizing radiation, alkylating agents). Second are compounds, such as the vinca alkaloids, that disrupt critical cellular structures by interfering with tubulin formation. A novel group of antineoplastic compounds has recently been identified by similar mechanistic criteria. Several years ago, a group of clinically active antineoplastic agents— DNA intercalators and epipodophyllotoxins—were found to have as their intracellular target DNA topoisomerase II (1,2). More recently, the antineoplastic cytotoxic compound camptothecin was found to inhibit DNA topoisomerase I in cells (3). These nuclear enzymes were identified immunologically as relevant drug targets only after it was demonstrated that their inhibitors possessed antitumor activity. Clinically useful topoisomerase inhibitors kill tumor cells with some degree of selectivity. That this selectivity is modest is indicated by the toxicities sustained by patients during the course of their treatment regimes. A major goal of cancer chemotherapy is to increase the therapeutic index by increasing selective killing of malignant cells. That cell killing can be modulated by using topoisomerase enzymes as drug targets is suggested by the association of tumors that are hypersensitive or resistant to topoisomerase inhibitors with qualitative or quantitative alterations in topoisomerase I (4,5) or topoisomerase II (6,7).

One approach that we have taken toward this end is to test the hypothesis that malignant and nonmalignant cells differ in quantity, kind, or regulation of topoisomerases. In this chapter we present evidence that suggests that mammalian topoisomerases are heterogeneous owing to differences in primary structure as well as to posttranslational modification and regulation. The resulting alternate forms of the enzymes can differ in their biochemical and pharmacological properties. It is thus possible that malignant and nonmalignant cells differ in their spectra of topoisomerase targets.

TOPOISOMERASE I INTRACELLULAR ACTIVITY

DNA Single-Strand Breaks Induced in Cells by Camptothecin

U937 human monoblast cells were labeled overnight with .02 μCi/ml [^{14}C]methyl thymidine (New England Nuclear Corp: 50 mCi mmol^{-1}) and then subjected to various treatments whose effects on topoisomerase I were to be determined. These included overnight incubation at 37°C with 25 nM LTD$_4$ (kindly provided by Dr. J. Gleason, Dept. of Medicinal Chemistry, SmithKline Beecham Laboratories) in the presence or absence of 3 nM staurosporine; 0–6 h treatment with the differentiation inducer 12-0-tetradecanoylphorbol-13-acetate (TPA) (Sigma). After treatment, cells were incubated for 60 min at 37°C with indicated concentrations of camptothecin (obtained from the Drug Synthesis and Design Branch, NCI), after which DNA single-strand breakage was assayed by alkaline elution (in the presence of proteinase K) as described previously (8).

Topoisomerase I Catalytic Activity in Nuclear Extracts

In some experiments nuclei were prepared from cells treated as previously described according to published procedures (7). Topoisomerase I activity contained in these extracts was assayed using pBR322 supercoiled DNA as described previously (10). After the relaxation reaction and agarose gel electrophoresis, DNA was visualized by staining with ethidium bromide. Specific activity was estimated by dividing the topoisomerase I units/ml by the protein concentration, determined by the method of Bradford (11). One unit of topoisomerase I activity was defined as the minimum amount of enzyme capable of relaxing 100 ng of supercoiled DNA in the absence of ATP.

TOPOISOMERASE II INTRACELLULAR ACTIVITY

DNA Single-Strand Breaks Induced in Cells by Teniposide

CHO-Cd^r (cadmium-resistant) cells were prelabeled with [^{14}C]thymidine overnight and then for 60 min with or without CdCl$_2$ (to induce metallothionein gene expression). Induced and uninduced cultures were then incubated for 60 min at 37°C with 5 μM teniposide or 5 μM teniposide plus 50 μM merbarone. Topoisomerase II–induced lesions trapped by teniposide were assayed by alkaline elution as described for camptothecin-induced lesions.

SDS-POLYACRYLAMIDE GEL ELECTROPHORESIS
AND IMMUNOBLOTTING

SDS-Page was performed by the method of Laemmli (12). Immunoblotting with antibodies against topoisomerase I (scleroderma antiserum) or 170 kD or 180 kD topoisomerase II was as described previously (13).

cDNA CLONING

A cDNA library was prepared from human Raji-HN_2 cells by linker–ligation at the EcoRI site of bacteriophage λgt 11. The library was screened with a Drosophila topoisomerase II cDNA as described (14).

RESULTS

Topoisomerase I Heterogeneity

Discrete proteolysed forms. A single species of mammalian topoisomerase I has been reported to date. The intact polypeptide is believed to have a molecular weight of approximately 100 kD. In addition, a series of proteolysed forms having discrete molecular weights between 60 and 100 kDa is often present in cellular lysates (15). It is possible that the proteolysis of topoisomerase I has physiological significance and is a means of regulating the intracellular activity or location of the enzyme as well as contributing to the enzyme's heterogeneity.

Regulation of topoisomerase I activity by posttranslational modification. Purified topoisomerase I can be modified chemically in at least two ways: phosphorylation (16) and poly(ADP-ribosylation) (17) (Fig. 11-1). The former modification has been found capable of either increasing or decreasing activity, depending upon conditions, whereas the latter has been reported only to inhibit catalytic activity.

Whether posttranslational modification is an important cellular mechanism for regulating topoisomerase I activity is difficult to determine. Intracellular topoisomerase I activity can be estimated by assaying protein-concealed DNA single-strand breakage produced by camptothecin, a naturally occurring anti-tumor agent and highly selective inhibitor of topoisomerase I (3). Each protein-associated break induced by camptothecin is a site of cellular topoisomerase I activity, since the protein to which it is covalently linked has been identified immunologically as topoisomerase I (3). The yield of camptothecin-induced DNA strand breakage has been found to be modulated under a number of conditions. Because the cellular content of topoisomerase I appears to be invariant (18), changes in the numbers of DNA strand breaks induced by camptothecin are likely indicative of changes in the activity of the enzyme. Several studies that have employed this assay have provided evidence that topoisomerase I is

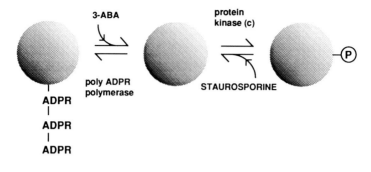

LEAST ACTIVE   **MOST ACTIVE**

Figure 11.1. Hypothetical mechanism for the regulation of topoisomerase I intracellular activity through posttranslational modification. Poly(ADP-ribosylation) is an inhibitory modification, indicated by the ability of 3-ABA to increase overall cellular activity of topoisomerase I. Under conditions of inositol phosphate-linked, induced gene expression, staurosporine, an inhibitor of protein kinase C, lowers cellular topoisomerase I activity, suggesting that phosphorylation of the enzyme (or of a regulatory protein) increases its activity.

modified by posttranslational regulation in cells. Treatment of cultured cells with 3-aminobenzamide (3-ABA), an inhibitor of poly(ADP-ribosylation) of proteins, increases the yield of camptothecin-induced DNA strand breakage (Fig. 11.2) (8). This result is circumstantial evidence that poly(ADP-ribosylation) of topoisomerase I attenuates its activity in cells, as it does that of the purified enzyme (17). At present it is not known whether or, if so, how topoisomerase I is phosphorylated in cells. Topoisomerase I activity has long been associated with active transcription (19). Recently, a number of physiologically important ligands have been found to activate the transcription of specific genes within minutes of binding to their receptors at the cell surface. These include c-fos, induced by vasopressin in rat smooth muscle cells (20); Il-6, induced by TNF, Il-1, or forskolin, in FS-4 human cells (21); and phospholipase A_2 activating protein (PLAP), induced by leukotriene D_4 (LTD_4) in human monoblast (U937) cells (22). In all of these cases, signals generated by ligand binding are transduced, via second messengers, to the nucleus, where enzymes necessary to transcription are activated. Second messengers implicated in the examples cited previously are either intermediates in inositol phosphate turnover, which leads to the activation of protein kinase C, or cyclic nucleotides, which activate protein kinases. Thus, the possibility exists that topoisomerase I is activated by a protein kinase when transcription is induced by a receptor agonist. Activation may be by direct phosphorylation of topoisomerase I or by phosphorylation of another protein, which then acts to increase topoisomerase I activity. Evidence consistent with these possibilities has recently been obtained using U937 cells treated with LTD_4. LTD_4 binding initiates phosphoinositol turnover, leading to the activation of protein kinase C and the rapid expression of PLAP (22). Topoisomerase I activity is very rapidly

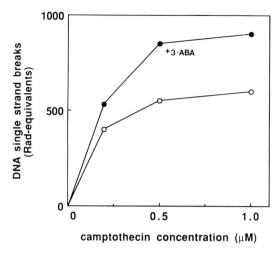

Figure 11.2. Increases in camptothecin-induced DNA strand breakage by 3-ABA treatment of L1210 cells. Cells were incubated overnight with 5 mM 3-ABA, an inhibitor of poly(ADP-ribose) modification of proteins, and then for 60 min with the topoisomerase I inhibitor camptothecin.

increased by LTD_4, as judged by camptothecin-induced DNA strand breakage (Fig. 11.3). This increase is blocked by low concentrations of staurosporine, a selective inhibitor of protein kinase C (23) (Fig. 11.3). Thus phosphorylation appears, either directly or indirectly, to activate topoisomerase I when tran-

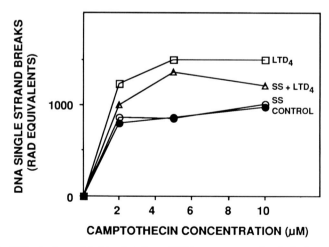

Figure 11.3. Effect of peptidyl leukotriene LTD_4 on camptothecin-induced, topoisomerase I–associated DNA strand breakage in human U937 cells; attenuation of this effect by the protein kinase C inhibitor staurosporine. LTD_4 concentration was 25 nM; staurosporine concentration was 3 nM. Cells treated with combinantions of LTD_4 and staurosporine were incubated with these drugs for 10 min before the addition of camptothecin. Camptothecin treatment was for 60 min.

scription is induced by cellular signaling. Similar activation of topoisomerases has been observed in A-10 rat aortic smooth muscle cells treated with vasopressin (which activates pKC) or forskolin (which increases cellular cAMP) (P. Nambi and M. Mattern, unpublished observation) and in U937 cells differentiated with phorbol esters (24). Thus, at least two cellular signaling pathways— inositol phosphate turnover and cyclic nucleotide activation of protein kinases—can regulate the activity of topoisomerase I.

Additional evidence that posttranslational modification of topoisomerase I may be important in regulating the enzyme's intracellular activity comes from studies of U937 human monoblast cells differentiated with DMSO or with the phorbol ester TPA (Fig. 11.4). Topoisomerase I activity in the differentiating cells increases with kinetics similar to that of the appearance of the differentiated phenotype and decreases thereafter (24), clearly indicating regulation. Concomitant with this regulation of topoisomerase I activity is the appearance of (or increase in prominence of) a protein that reacts with the scleroderma antibody for topoisomerase I (25) and migrates in a polyacrylamide gel somewhat less rapidly than does the 100 kD form of topoisomerase I (Fig. 11.5). The nature of this protein is not known, but one might speculate that it is a posttranslationally altered, inactivated topoisomerase I.

Topoisomerase II Heterogeneity

Multiple forms by proteolysis or posttranslational regulation. As in the case of type I topoisomerase, multiple forms of topoisomerase II may be generated through proteolysis and posttranslational modification. Published evidence

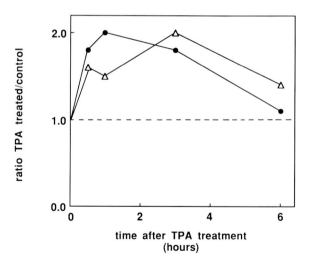

Figure 11.4. Camptothecin-induced DNA strand breakage and extractable topoisomerase I activity in U937 cells during the first 6 h after treatment with TPA. (Triangle) camptothecin-induced DNA strand breaks; (filled circle) specific activity of topoisomerase I extracted from nuclei in 0.35 *M* NaCl. Data are expressed as ratios of the same parameter measured with undifferentiated U937 cells seeded at the same time as the TPA-treated cells.

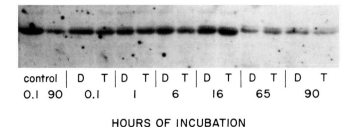

control	D	T	D	T	D	T	D	T	D	T	D	T
	0.1	90	0.1		1		6		16		65	90

HOURS OF INCUBATION

Figure 11.5. Topoisomerase I content of U937 cells differentiated with DMSO or TPA. Cells were differentiated for indicated times with either 1.3% DMSO or 30 nM TPA. Controls: untreated cells seeded at the same time as the differentiated cells. Cells were lysed at indicated times after seeding and topoisomerase I content was determined by immunoblotting, following SDS-PAGE.

suggests that topoisomerase II can be phosphorylated by protein kinase C in differentiating human HL-60 cells (26); more direct evidence suggests that this is the case in developing sponge cells (27). The production of protein-associated DNA strand breaks by topoisomerase II inhibitors such as amsacrine and teniposide (which, like camptothecin, trap a topoisomerase-strand-cleaved DNA reaction intermediate) is enhanced by prior treatment of cultured cells with 3-ABA. This result suggests that poly(ADP-ribosylation) is an inhibitory modification to topoisomerase II, as well as topoisomerase I, in cells (8).

Variants of topoisomerase II. It has recently been shown that topoisomerase II is present in cells as two forms, which likely differ in their primary sequence. Purification of topoisomerase II from mammalian cells typically yields two polypeptides, which migrate as about 170 and 180 kD molecules in SDS-polyacrylamide gels; the ratio of 170 to 180 kD enzyme differs among cell lines (Fig. 11.6) (13). The 170 kD form is not a proteolysis product of the 180 kD form, since peptide digestion products of the two proteins are quite different and antibodies raised against one form do not react with the other form. These variants of mammalian topoisomerase II have different biochemical properties, including ionic strength dependence, processivity of the catalytic reaction, and thermal stability (G. Hofmann and F. Drake, unpublished results). In addition, the two forms maybe regulated differently in cells. For example, in a number of cultured cell lines the 170 kD topoisomerase II is prominent during rapid growth, while the 180 kD form becomes dominant in cells whose growth is slowed.

A number of pharmacological experiments have further characterized and differentiated the 170 and 180 kD enzymes; these include sensitivity to merbarone (28) and cleavable complex–forming drugs such as amsacrine and teniposide. Novobiocin, a representative of a third class of inhibitor of topoisomerase II, does not discriminate between the two forms (G. Hofmann and F. Drake, unpublished observations). The 170 kD and the 180 kD enzymes cut DNA at preferred sites in the presence of teniposide. The two forms of topoisomerase II have some preferred cleavage sites in common but others that are peculiar to one or the other form (Fig. 11.7). In addition, the 170 kD form

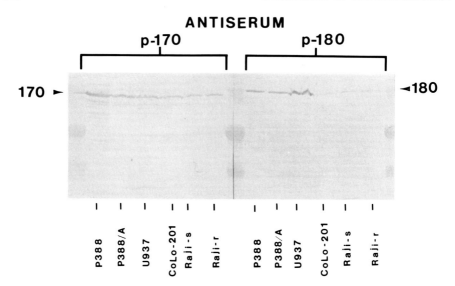

Figure 11.6. Mammalian topoisomerase II. Rodent (P388, P388/A) or human (U937, Colo 201, Raji-s [hypersensitive to nitrogen mustard], Raji-r [resistant to nitrogen mustard]) cells were lysed in SDS, and the lysates were electrophoresed on 15% polyacrylamide gels. Duplicate gels were transferred to nitrocellulose and reacted with antiserum specific for 170 kD (p170) or 180 kD (p180) topoisomerase II. Arrows indicate position of gel migration of the 170 kD or the 180 kD enzyme.

prefers AT-rich nucleotide sequences for binding, while the 180 kD form prefers GC-rich sequences (F. Drake, unpublished observation). These results provide very strong evidence that the 170 and 180 kD forms of topoisomerase II are biochemical variants.

At least three classes of inhibitors of eukaryotic topoisomerase II are known. Coumarin antibiotics such as novobiocin and coumerycin, which inhibit the ATPase activity of DNA gyrase, also inhibit the catalytic activity of mammalian topoisomerase II, likely through the same mechanism (29). A second class of inhibitor, consisting of epipodophyllotoxin derivatives (etoposide and teniposide) and certain intercalators such as amsacrine, the ellipticines, and Adriamycin, trap the topoisomerase II–DNA reacton intermediate in a DNA strand-cleaved state (1,2). In addition to blocking the catalytic activity of topoisomerase II, this class produces DNA lesions that are observable as cleavages upon treatment of cells or drug–topoisomerase II DNA mixtures with proteolysing enzymes and SDS (1,2). Recently, a third class of inhibitor, represented by the thiobarbituric acid derivative merbarone, has been identified. Merbarone is distinguishable from the coumarins in that it preferentially inhibits the 170 kD form of topoisomerase II and is not competitive with respect to ATP (G. Hofmann and F. Drake, unpublished results). Merbarone itself produces no cleavable complexes over a very broad range of concentrations, yet it inhibits the production of these lesions by amsacrine or teniposide (28). Thus, although merbarone and the cleavable complex inducers can have the same intracellular target, they inhibit it by different mechanisms.

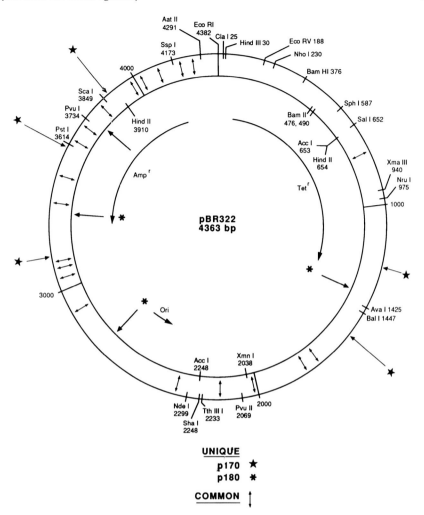

Figure 11.7. Cleavage sites induced in pBR322 DNA by teniposide plus 170 kD or 180 kD topoisomerase II. Teniposide-stimulated DNA cleavage sites of 170 kD and 180 kD topoisomerase II were determined by the method of Liu et al. (39), using [^{32}P]-labeled pBR322 DNA. (Star) sites unique to 170 kD topoisomerase II; (asterisk) sites unique to 180 kD topoisomerase II; (double-headed arrow) sites common to 170 kD and 180 kD topoisomerase II.

Topoisomerase II heterogeneity in induced gene expression. Topoisomerase II diversity and the possibility of selective intervention of malignancy are illustrated further in studies of induced gene expression. Chinese hamster ovary cells made resistant to cadmium (CHO-Cd^r) (30) contain amplified genes for the metallothioneins MT-II and express these genes in a coordinated fashion when treated for short periods of time with cadmium (31). The topoisomerase I inhibitor camptothecin produces DNA cleavage selectively near the induced genes and blocks induced transcription (32). This result is in agreement with those of others (33,34) and tends to support the notion that topoisomerase I participates in transcription. Recent studies suggest that (+) and (−) DNA supercoils are produced in actively transcribing cells, presumably at each RNA polymerase complex (35). Since topoisomerase I can relax both (+) and (−) supercoils, its inhibitor, camptothecin, could block all forms of RNA synthesis, whether induced or constitutive.

The role of topoisomerase II in transcription has not been clearly defined. Of the three known classes of topoisomerase II inhibitor, novobiocin and membarone inhibit induced MT expression, while amsacrine and teniposide do not, even at very high concentrations (32). Yet in CHO-Cd^r cells, as well as in others

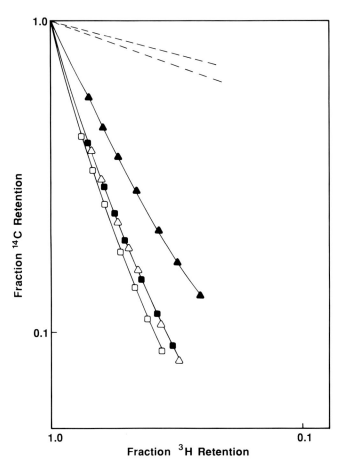

Figure 11.8. Topoisomerase II–associated DNA strand breakage produced by teniposide in CHO-Cd^r cells stimulated to express metallothionein genes; effects of merbarone. (Triangles) unstimulated cells; treated with 5 μM teniposide for 60 min; (squares) cells stimulated with 50 μM CdCl$_2$ for 30 min and then incubated for 60 min with 5 μM teniposide. (Open symbols) cells treated with 5 μM teniposide alone; (closed symbols) cells treated with 50 μM merbarone plus 5 μM teniposide. (Dashed lines) indicate control elution rates (untreated cells or cells treated with 50 μM CdCl$_2$ and/or 50 μM merbarone).

in which transcription of specific genes is activated, DNA is cleaved by amsacrine or teniposide preferentially at the site of the active genes (32,36). It is clear that at least one form of topoisomerase II—that involved in cleavable complex formation—is active during induced transcription. It is possible that a second form, inhibited by merbarone and novobiocin, is essential for RNA synthesis, while the form that is sensitive to amsacrine and teniposide may act subsequent to RNA synthesis to restore the template DNA to the pretranscription topological state. The latter would be consistent with published reports that locate intercalator- or epipodophyllotoxin-induced cleavages in the untranscribed regions of induced genes (36). It should be recalled that the only function of topoisomerase II in eukaryotes that has been confirmed by genetics experiments is the disentanglement of newly replicated daughter DNA molecules (36). In this case, the enzyme acts subsequent to DNA synthesis. An alternative explanation is that topoisomerase II–DNA complexes trapped by amsacrine or teniposide are not effective blockers of RNA polymerization. It is interesting to note, however, that in CHO Cd^r cells induced to express MT-I/MT-II, merbarone does not inhibit the formation of cleavable complexes by teniposide, as it does in uninduced cells (Fig. 11.8). Thus, in the case of induced gene expression, these two classes of inhibitor may not have a common target. It is possible that a novel form of topoisomerase II is activated when transcription is induced; this form may interact preferentially with merbarone.

The human gene(s) for topoisomerase II. The most definitive evidence for topoisomerase II heterogeneity will come from genetics experiments. We have cloned the topoisomerase II cDNA from human cells and found that the cDNA clones belong to two classes by restriction enzyme analysis (Fig. 11.9). Preliminary studies with members of these two cDNA classes showed that they hybridize to each other, to Drosophila genomic topoisomerase II sequences, to distinct restriction enzyme fragments of human DNA, and to a 6 kb mRNA (14 and K. B. Tan, unpublished data). Nucleotide sequence analysis of SP.1, a partial clone flanked by two natural Eco RI sites, showed that it is identical to nucleotides 1307 to 4338 of the human topoisomerase II sequence reported by Tsai-Pflugfelder et al. (38). SP.1 (Fig. 11.9) and SP.17 belong to the same class of cDNA. Antibodies raised against the protein expressed by this class of cDNA *in vitro* reacted principally with the 170 kD form of topoisomerase II (F. Drake, unpublished results). SP.3 (Fig. 11.9) and SP.12 (14) belong to the second class of cDNA. It is not known whether SP.1 and SP.3 result from differentially spliced mRNA or from different topoisomerase II genes.

CONCLUSION

The heterogeneity that characterizes topoisomerases in both form and function provides an opportunity for selective pharmacologic action against human tumors. Differences among cell types in the quantities of topoisomerases, in their regulation through posttranslational modification, or in their forms, can serve as bases for selective drug discovery. It is possible that functional heteroge-

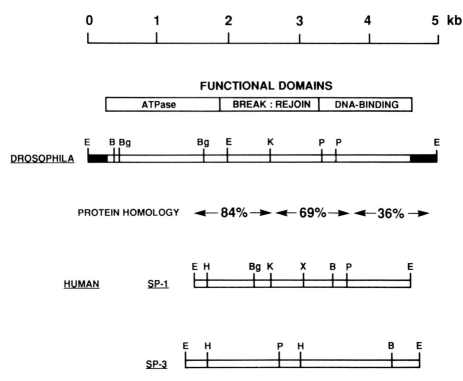

Figure 11.9. Human topoisomerase II cDNA. Clones were isolated from a cDNA library that was screened with a Drosophila topoisomerase II cDNA probe. Nucleotide sequence analysis suggests that SP .1 is 65% homologous to Drosophila topoisomerase II at the protein level. The homology between human and Drosophila topoisomerase II is greatest at the 5' portion and least at the 3' portion of the protein. The restriction map of SP .3 indicates that it belongs to a second class of cDNA. The restriction enzyme and suggested functional domain maps of the Drosophila cDNA were derived from data provided by Dr. T. Hsieh (personal communication). Solid black bar = noncoding sequences. B = Bam HI; Bg = Bgl II; E = Eco RI; H = Hind III; K = Kpn I; P = Pst I; x = Xba I

neity of topoisomerases in DNA replication, DNA damage repair, gene amplification, or recombination can be similarly exploited. A major goal of antineoplastic research remains to identify those forms and/or cellular functions of topoisomerase I and topoisomerase II that are peculiar to malignant cells. It may then be possible to design topoisomerase inhibitors having enhanced anticancer specificity.

Acknowledgments

This work was supported in part by grant #1-U01-C40884-01 from the National Cancer Institute. We thank Dr. Gerd Maul, Wistar Institute of Anatomy and Biology, for scleroderma antiserum and Dr. Leroy Liu, Johns Hopkins University, for antiserum reactive against a fragment of the expressed human topoisomerase II gene. We also thank Shau-Ming Mong, Joan O'Leary Bartus, Henry F. Bartus, Rebecca A. Boyce, Joseph P. Zimmerman, Francis L. McCabe, and Glenn A. Hofmann for invaluable assistance with the experiments, and Mrs. Susanne Young for expert editorial assistance.

REFERENCES

1. Rowe, T. C., Chen G. C., Hsiang, V., and Liu, L. F. DNA damage by antitumor acridines mediated by mammalian DNA topoisomerase II. Cancer Res. **46:** 2021–2026, 1986.

2. Yang, L., Rowe, T. C., and Liu, L. F. Identification of topoisomerase II as the intracellular target of antitumor epipodophyllotoxins in Simian virus 40 infected monkey cells. Cancer Res. **45:** 5872–5876, 1985.

3. Hsiang, Y. H. and Liu, L. F. Identification of mammalian DNA topoisomerase I as an intracellular target of the anticancer drug camptothecin. Cancer Res. **48:** 1722–1726, 1988.

4. Andoh, T., Ishii, K., Suzuki, Y., Ikegami, Y., Takemoto, Y., and Okada, K. Characterization of a mammalian mutant with camptothecin-resistant DNA topoisomerase I. Proc. Natl. Acad. Sci. USA. **84:** 5565–5569, 1987.

5. Gupta, R. S., Gupta, R., Eng, B., Lock, R. B., Ross, W. E., Hertzberg, R. P., Caranfa, M. J., and Johnson, R. K. Camptothecin-resistant mutant of Chinese hamster ovary cells containing a resistant form of topoisomerase I. Cancer Res. **48:** 6404–6410, 1988.

6. Per, S. R., Mattern, M. R., Mirabelli, C. K., Drake, F. H., Johnson, R. K., and Crooke, S. T. Characterization of a subline of P388 leukemia resistant to amsacrine: Evidence of altered topoisomerase II function. Mol. Pharmacol. **32:** 17–25, 1987.

7. Robson, C. N., Hoban, P. R., Harris, A. L., and Hickson, I. D. Cross-sensitivity to topoisomerase II inhibitors in cytotoxic drug-hypersensitive Chinese hamster ovary cell lines. Cancer Res. **47:** 1560–1565, 1987.

8. Mattern, M. R., Mong, S. M., Bartus, H. F., Mirabelli, C. K., Crooke, S. T., and Johnson, R. K. Relationship between the intracellular effects of camptothecin and the inhibition of DNA topoisomerase I in cultured L1210 cells. Cancer Res. **47:** 1793–1798, 1987.

9. Tan, K. B., Mattern, M. R., Boyce, R. A., and Schein, P. S. Elevated DNA topoisomerase II activity in nitrogen mustard-resistant human cells. Proc. Natl. Acad. Sci. USA. **84:** 7668–7771, 1987.

10. Hsiang, Y. H., Hertzberg, R., Hecht, S., and Liu, L. F. Camptothecin induces protein linked DNA breaks via mammalian DNA topoisomerase I. J. Biol. Chem. **27:** 14873–14878, 1986.

11. Bradford, M. A. A rapid and sensitive method for the quantitation of microgram quantities of protein utilizing principles of protein-dye binding. Anal. Biochem. **72:** 248–254, 1976.

12. Laemmli, U. K. Cleavage of structural proteins during the assembly of the head of bacteriophage T4. Nature. **227:** 680–685, 1970.

13. Drake, F. H., Zimmerman, J. P., McCabe, F. L., Bartus, H. F., Per, S. R., Sullivan, D. M., Ross, W. E., Mattern, M. R., Johnson, R. K., Crooke, S. T., and Mirabelli, C. K. Purification of topoisomerase II from amsacrine-resistant P388 leukemia cells: Evidence for two forms of the enzyme. J. Biol. Chem. **262:** 16739–16747, 1987.

14. Tan, K. B., Per, S. R., Boyce, R. A., Mirabelli, C. K., and Crooke, S. T. Altered expression and transcription of the topoisomerase II gene in nitrogen mustard-resistant human cells. Biochem. Pharmacol. **37:** 4413–4416, 1988.

15. Schmitt, B., Buhre, U., and Vosberg, H.-P. Characterization of size variants of type I DNA topoisomerase isolated from calf thymus. Eur. J. Biochem. **144:** 127–134, (1984).

16. Tse-Dinh, Y.-C., Wong, T. W., and Goldberg, A. R. Virus and cell encoded tyrosine protein kinase inactivates DNA topoisomerase *in vitro*. *Nature*. **312:** 785–786, 1984.

17. Ferro, A. M., Higgins, N. P., and Olivera, B. M. Poly (ADP-ribosylation) of a DNA topoisomerase. J. Biol. Chem. **258:** 6000–6003, 1983.

18. Champoux, J. J., Young, L. S., and Been, M. D. Studies on the regulation and specificity of the DNA-untwisting enzyme. Cold Spring Harbor Symp. Quant. Biol. **43:** 53–58, 1978.

19. Gilmour, D. S., Pflugfelder, G., Wang, J. C., and Lis, J. T. Topoisomerase I interacts with transcribed regions in *Drosophila* cells. Cell. **44:** 401–407, 1986.

20. Nambi, P., Watt, R., Whitman, M., Aiyar, N., Moore, J. P., Evan, G. I., and Crooke, S. T., Induction of c-fos protein by activation of vasopressin receptors in smooth muscle cells. FEBS Lett **245:** 61–64, 1989.

21. Zhang, Y., Lin, J-X., Yip Y. K., and Vilcek, J. Enhancement of cAMP levels and of protein kinase activity by tumor necrosis factor and interleukin 1 in human fibroblasts: Role of the induction of interleukin 6. Proc. Natl. Acad. Sci. USA. **85:** 6802–6805, 1988.

22. Clark, M. A., Littlejohn, T. M., Conway, S., Mong, S., Steiner, S., and Crooke, S. T. Leukotriene D₄ treatment of bovine aortic endothelial cells and murine smooth muscle cells in culture results in an increase in phospholipase A₂ activity. J. Biol. Chem. **261:** 10713–10718, 1985.

23. Tamaoki, T., Nomoto, I., Takahashi, Y., Kato, Y., Morimoto, M., and Tomita, I. Staurosporine, a potent inhibitor of phospholipid/Ca^{+2} dependent protein kinase. Biochem. Biophys. Res. Commun. **135:** 397–402, 1986.

24. Bartus, J. O., Mong, S-M., Zimmerman, J. P., Drake, F. H., Tan, K. B., Mirabelli, C. K., Mattern, M. R., and Crooke, S. T. Topoisomerases I and II: Increase in intracellular activity at the onset of differentiation of human U937 cells. Proc. Am. Assoc. Cancer Res. **29:** A121, 1988.

25. Maul, G. G., French, B. T., van Venrooij, W. J., and Jimenez, S. A. Topoisomerase I identified by Scleroderma 70 antisera: Enrichment of topoisomerase I at the centromere in mouse mitotic cells before anaphase. Proc. Natl. Acad. Sci. USA. **83:** 5145–5149, 1986.

26. Sahyoun, N., Wolf, M., Besterman, J., Hsieh, T., Sander, M., Levine, H., Chang, K-J., and Cuatrecasas, P. Protein kinase C phosphorylates topoisomerase II: Topoisomerase activation and its possible role in phorbol ester-induced differentiation of HL-60 cells. Proc. Natl. Acad. Sci. USA. **83:** 1603–1608, 1986.

27. Rottman, M., Schroder, H. C., Gramzow, M., Renneisen, K., Kurelec, B., Dorn, A., Friese, U., and Muller, W.E.G. Specific phosphorylation of proteins in pore complex laminae from the sponge *G. cydonium* by the homologous aggregation factor and phorbol ester. Role of protein kinase C in the phosphorylation of topoisomerase II. EMBO J. **6:** 3939–3944, 1987.

28. Drake, F. H., Hofmann, G. A., Mong, S-M., O'Leary Bartus, J., Hertzberg, R. P., Johnson, R. K., Mattern, M. R., and Mirabelli, C. K. *In vitro* and intracellular inhibition of topoisomerase II by the antitumor agent merbarone. Cancer Res. **49:** 2578–2583, 1989.

29. Vosberg, H-P. DNA topoisomerases: Enzymes that control DNA conformation. Curr. Top. Microbiol. Immunol. **114:** 19–102, 1985.

30. Enger, M. D., Rall, L. B., and Hildebrand, C. E. Thionein gene expression in Cd^{++}-resistant variants of the CHO cell: Correlation of thionein synthesis rates with translatable mRNA levels during induction, deinduction, and superinduction. Nucleic Acids Res. **7:** 271–288, 1979.

31. Crawford, B. D., Enger, M. D., Griffith, B. B., Griffith, J. K., Hammers, J. L., Longmire, J. L., Munk, A. C., Stallings, R. L., Tesmer, J. G., Walters, R. A., and Hildebrand, C. E. Coordinate amplification of metallothionein I and II genes in cadmium-resistant Chinese hamster cells: Implications for mechanisms regulating metallothionein gene expression. Mol. Cell. Biol. **5:** 320–329, 1985.

32. Zimmerman, J. P., Tan, K. B., Mong, S-M., Bartus, J. O., Mattern, M. R., Mirabelli, C. K., and Crooke, S. T. Topoisomerase I activation accompanies MT-II induction in Cd^{++}-resistant CHO cells. Proc. Am. Assoc. Cancer Res. **29:** A31, 1988.

33. Gilmour, D. S. and Elgin, S. C. R. Localization of specific topoisomerase I interactions within the transcribed region of active heat shock genes by using the inhibitor camptothecin. Mol. Cell. Biol. **7:** 141–148, 1987.

34. Stewart, A. F. and Schutz, G. Camptothecin-induced *in vivo* topoisomerase I cleavages in the transcriptionally active tyrosine aminotransferase gene. Cell. **50:** 1109–1117, 1987.

35. Wu, H-Y., Shyy, S., Wang, J. C., and Liu, L. F. Transcription generates positively and negatively supercoiled domains in the template. Cell. **53:** 433–440, 1988.

36. Yang, L., Rowe, T. C., Nelson, E. M., and Liu, L. F. *In vivo* mapping of topoisomerase II-specific cleavage sites on SV-40 chromatin. Cell. **41:** 127–132, 1985.

37. DiNardo, S., Voelkel, K., and Sternglanz, R. DNA topoisomerase II mutant of *S. cerevisiae:* Topoisomerase II is required for the segregation of daughter molecules at the termination of replication. Proc. Natl. Acad. Sci. USA. **81:** 2616–2620, 1984.

38. Tsai-Pflugfelder, M., Liu, L. F., Liu, A. A., Tewey, K. M., Whang-Peng, J., Knut-

sen, T., Huebner, K., Croce, C. M., and Wang, J. C. Cloning and sequencing of cDNA encoding human DNA topoisomerase II and localization of the gene to chromosome region 17q21-22. Proc. Natl. Acad. Sci. USA. **85:** 7177–7181, 1988.

39. Liu, L. F., Rowe, T. C., Yang, L., Tewey, K. M., and Chen, G. L. Cleavage of DNA by mammalian DNA topoisomerase II. J. Biol. Chem. **258:** 15365–15370, 1983.

Chapter 12
The Influence of Camptothecin on Topoisomerase I Interaction with Genomic Sequences

EIGIL KJELDSEN, CHRISTIAN BENDIXEN, BO THOMSEN,
KENT CHRISTIANSEN, BJARNE JUUL BONVEN,
OLE FREDERIK NIELSEN, AND OLE WESTERGAARD

Topoisomerase I has been shown to be the primary cellular target for the antitumor drug, camptothecin (2). The antitumor activity of this drug presumably results from its severe physiological effects, which include fragmentation of the genome and inhibition of RNA and DNA synthesis (3–5). These metabolic alterations are mediated solely by topoisomerase I, since a mutant cell line producing topoisomerase I, resistant to camptothecin, escapes the physiological effects of the drug (2,6). Several lines of evidence suggest that camptothecin inhibits the topoisomerase I–catalyzed DNA relaxation, by blocking the religation reaction of the normal catalytic cycle (1,6,7). To obtain a more detailed picture of the molecular mechanism, we have studied the interaction of topoisomerase I with DNA in the presence and absence of camptothecin. The studies take advantage of a strong recognition sequence at which the catalytic rate of relaxation is exceeded by three orders of magnitude relative to an average relaxation site (20). The information obtained on both the sequential and structural level is of potential interest for the design and evaluation of new drugs.

MATERIALS AND METHODS

Materials

Camptothecin (lactone form, no. 94600) was kindly provided by the National Cancer Institute (Bethesda, MD). Stock solutions of camptothecin, 10 mM in 100% DMSO were stored in −20°C. DMSO was from Merck. Radioactive nucleotides were obtained from ICN. DNA modifying enzymes were obtained from New England Biolabs, unless stated otherwise.

Purification of Eukaryotic Topoisomerase I

Cultures of *T. thermophila* and human Daudi cells were used for the purification as described (7,19).

Gel Electrophoresis and Autoradiography

Agarose gel electrophoresis and Southern blot hybridization were performed as described by Bonven et al. (17). Maxam-Gilbert sequencing reactions and topoisomerase I cleavage reactions were analyzed on denaturing polyacrylamide gels (7), unless otherwise mentioned.

Micrococcal Nuclease Digestion of Macronuclei

Macronuclei were prepared from early log-phase cells (5×10^4 cells/ml) of *Tetrahymena thermophila* strain B 1868-7 as previously described (17,38) except that 10 mM NaCl was not added to the solutions. Macronuclear DNA was immediately or after digestion with micrococcal nuclease (Worthington; 0,005 units/ml) extracted from macronuclei according to Bonven et al. (17).

Purification and Labeling of Restriction Fragments

Plasmid pTtrl, containing the central spacer of rDNA from *T. thermophila* cloned into the *Hind*III restriction site of pBr322 (36), was isolated and [^{32}P]labeled (17). Isolation and 3' end [^{32}P]labeling of the central *Hinf*I rDNA fragment from macronuclear DNA of *T. thermophila* was performed as described (27). The plasmid pNCl, containing the hexadecameric recognition sequence (AGACTTAGAAAAATTT) for topoisomerase I (19,20), was digested with *Hind*III and *Pvu*II. Isolation and 3' end [^{32}P]labeling was done as described previously (7).

Topoisomerase I Cleavage Induction

3'End-labeled restriction fragments (3 fmol) were incubated with 0 to 100 units of purified topoisomerase I with or without camptothecin (for details see 7). Induction of cleavage was accomplished by addition of SDS and EDTA to final concentrations of 1% and 10 mM, respectively. Quantification of cleavage was determined as described (7).

Prediction of Helical Parameters

The computer program AUGUR was used to predict helix twist angles and base pair roll angles of a given sequence. The program calculates minimum conformational energy suggested by Tung and Harvey for successive base pairs (21,22). This model distinguishes adenosines from guanosines and thymidine from cytidine unlike the Calladine-Dickerson model. The helix twist angle between two successive base pairs is defined as the angle between the projections of the base pair long axes on the xy-plane. The roll angle of a base pair is a measure of the rotation of the best fit base pair plane about the base pair long axis. By convention, the roll angle change of a base pair step is defined as positive if the angle between the best fit base pair planes opens toward the minor groove and negative if it opens toward the major groove (37).

RESULTS AND DISCUSSION

Topoisomerase I Has a High Affinity for a Hexadecameric Recognition Sequence Located within Hypersensitive Regions

The chromatin structure of eukaryotic genes undergoes profound alterations in connection with changes in gene expression. Current models depict series of sequential events resulting in transition from inactive to transcriptionally competent chromatin. A characteristic of transcriptionally competent chromatin is the presence of DNAase I hypersensitive sites (reviewed in 8,9). These constitute defined regions 200–400 bp in length where the underlying DNA is in a highly accessible, nonnucleosomal state (10–12). The hypersensitive regions often encompass regulatory sites at the 5' and/or 3' end of eukaryotic genes. Recent data have shed light on the molecular basis of hypersensitivity. The models suggested include both alternating DNA conformations (13,14) and specific protein–DNA interactions (15,16). Both mechanisms are likely to be involved in mediating a perturbation of histone–DNA interactions that lead to local nucleosome displacement. Such a localized opening of the chromatin structure provides a means to expose regulatory elements in DNA to specific effector molecules.

    As an example of a heavily transcribed gene we have studied the rRNA genes of Tetrahymena. The rDNA in this organism is organized as extrachromosomal, highly amplified giant palindromes, each containing two genes coding for 35S pre-RNA. The promoters are separated by a central spacer, while two distal spacers abut the coding regions at the transcription termination (Fig. 12.1A). Analysis of the chromatin structure of these minichromosomes has revealed the presence of three nucleosome-free, DNAase I hypersensitive sites upstream of the transcription initiation site (Fig. 12.1B, 1C). The nuclease hypersensitivity is due to nucleosome positioning, as digestion with naked rDNA does not reveal sequence selective cleavage (data not shown).

    Treatment of intact r-chromatin from Tetrahymena, in the absence of camptothecin, with a denaturing agent causes topoisomerase I–mediated single-strand cleavage of rDNA spacer sequences. Analysis of the cleaved products on a sequencing gel demonstrates that the endogenous topoisomerase I introduces site- and strand-specific single-strand cleavages (17). The cleavages occur base specifically within a hexadecameric sequence motif

$$\text{AGACTTAGA}^{\text{A}}_{\text{G}}\text{AAA}^{\text{AAA}}_{\text{TTT}}$$

present in two or three direct repeats located within each of the hypersensitive sites (Fig. 12.1D, lane 1). The same sequence specificity and strand selection is observed when topoisomerase I is reacted with naked rDNA, indicating that the repetitive element functions as a high affinity topoisomerase I attraction site in the r-chromatin (Fig. 12.1D, lane 2). Furthermore, the preference for the recognition sequence seems to be an intrinsic property of all type I topoisomerases (27).

It is interesting that we observe only a low level of topoisomerase I–mediated cleavage in the coding region of the Tetrahymena rRNA genes, suggesting that the enzyme was only weakly associated with this region. The data are in clear contrast to the results by Culotta and Sollner-Webb (18) on the mapping of topoisomerase I on ribosomal RNA genes of *Xenopus*. In these experiments extensive DNA cleavage was found in both the spacer and coding regions. The difference between the two observations might reflect the use of camptothecin in the Xenopus mapping experiments. Thus, we have recently mapped topoisomerase I on the Xenopus rDNA in the absence of camptothecin and have found strong cleavage sites at the promoter region only (K. Kristensen, et al., unpublished results). A similar observation has been done for the interaction of topoisomerase I with rDNA of *Dictyostelium* (35), and both sets of data support the idea of strong regulatory sites at the promoter region, originally observed for the Tetrahymena rDNA.

Camptothecin Alters the Cleavage Pattern of Topoisomerase I

To explain the discrepancies discussed before we have examined the effect of camptothecin on the topoisomerase I–mediated cleavage on naked DNA. For this purpose cleavage was investigated on a 3' end-labeled 1.6 kb *Hin*dIII-*Pvu*II-restriction-fragment of the plasmid pNCl (19,20), spanning the hexadecameric recognition sequence. As expected, cleavage in the absence of camptothecin was confined to the hexadecameric recognition sequence (Fig. 12.2, lane 1), while several additional cleavage sites were observed in the presence of low concentrations of camptothecin (0.5 μM, lane 2) (7). No further changes in the cleavage pattern resulted from increasing the concentration of camptothecin up to 125 μM (data not shown). The frequency of topoisomerase I–mediated DNA cleavage at the hexadecameric sequence was only slightly stimulated (< twofold) by camptothecin. Some of the camptothecin-induced cleavage sites can be provoked in the absence of drug by increasing the amount of topoisomerase I to an enzyme:DNA ratio of approximately 100. However, the cleavage efficiency at the additional sites obtained in the absence of camptothecin was very low (< 1%), relative to cleavage observed in the presence of drug.

It has been shown that camptothecin inhibits topoisomerase I catalysis and promotes cleavable complex formation (1). On this basis it was suggested that inhibition of relaxation occurred by a drug-mediated block of the religation reaction stabilizing cleavable enzyme–DNA complexes. According to this hypothesis it was of interest to examine the stability of complexes involving the hexadecameric sequence and the camptothecin-stimulated sequences. Dissociation kinetic studies were done in 0.6 M NaCl at 20°C and aliquots were removed at different times followed by treatment with SDS. The electrophoretic analysis of the resulting DNA fragments is shown in Figure 12.3. The enzyme–

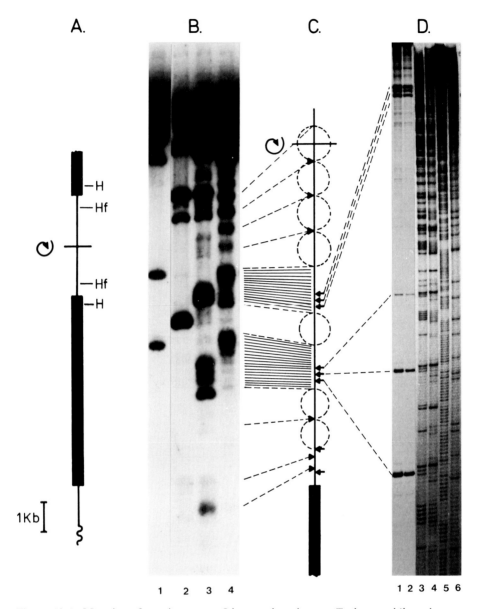

A.   B.   C.   D.

1   2   3   4

1 2 3 4 5 6

Figure 12.1. Mapping of topoisomerase I interaction sites on *T. thermophila* r-chromatin. **Panel A.** Schematic representation of an arm of the palindromic rDNA. The central
*Hin*d III fragment investigated for micrococcal nuclease cleavage sites in panel B and
the central *Hin*fI fragment investigated for topoisomerase I cleavage sites in panel D
are indicated. Thin lines: spacer regions. Filled bars: coding regions. Wavy line: telomere ends. Bent arrow: axis of symmetry. Hf: *Hin*fI, H: *Hind*III. **Panel B.** Micrococcal
nuclease cleavage sites in the central spacer. Macronuclei isolated from *T. thermophila*
log-phase cells were digested with micrococcal nuclease and the cleavage pattern in the
central spacer region was analyzed (lane 4). Partial digestions of macronuclear DNA
with *Dde*I (lane 3), *Sph*I (lane 2), and *Xba*I (lane 1) were used as markers. The micrococcal nuclease–treated macronuclear DNA sample (10 μg) and the macronuclear DNA
samples (10 μg) partially digested with appropriate restrictions enzymes were digested
to completion with *Hind*III, subjected to electrophoresis on a 1.5% agarose gel, transferred to nitrocellulose, and hybridized with [³²P]labeled *Hind*III-fragment of the plas-

152

Figure 12.2. Topoisomerase I cleavage in the presence and absence of camptothecin. 3 fmol of 3' end labeled 1.6 kb *Hind*III-*Pvu*II fragment of pNC1 was incubated with 30 units human topoisomerase I in the absence and presence of camptothecin for 30 min at 30° C. The reactions were terminated and processed for sequencing-gel analysis as described in Material and Methods. Lane 1, 0 μM camptothecin; lane 2, 0.5 μM camptothecin. Reaction mixture contained a final concentration of 6% DMSO. The arrow indicates the position of cleavage at the hexadecameric recognition sequence.

---

mid, pTtrI, containing the central spacer of *T. thermophila* rDNA (36). **Panel C.** Model for the chromatin structure and positions of topoisomerase I cleavage sites around the center of the rDNA. The location of micrococcal nuclease cleavage sites mapped in panel B and the location of topoisomerase I cleavage sites mapped in panel D are indicated. Thin lines: spacer regions. Filled bars: coding regions. Bent arrow: axis of symmetry. Dashed circles: nucleosomes. **Panel D.** Comparison of topoisomerase I cleavage sites *in situ* and *in vitro* by sequencing gel analysis. The 3' end-labeled 2.7 kb central fragment was subjected to Maxam-Gilbert chemical degradation reactions C + T (lane 3), C (lane 4), A > C (lane 5), G (lane 6). The 3' end-labeled 2.7 kb *Hin*fI fragment cleaved by topoisomerase I *in situ* was isolated directly from SDS-treated macronuclei according to Christiansen et al. (27) and run in parallel (lane 1). Purified *T. thermophila* topoisomerase I was reacted with the 3' end-labeled 2.7 kb *Hin*fI fragment and loaded on the gel (lane 2).

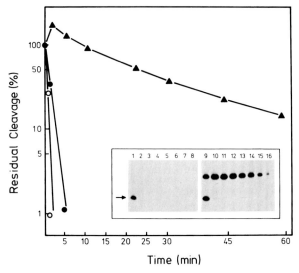

Figure 12.3. Dissociation kinetics of cleavable complexes. Two parallel 240-μl reactions, each containing 3' end labeled *Hin*dIII-*Pvu*III restriction fragment and topoisomerase I at an enzyme to DNA ratio of approximately 40, were preincubated at 30°C with or without 10 μM camptothecin (7). After 29.5 min a 30-μl sample of each series was taken to 1% SDS (final concentration). At 30 min the remainder of the reaction mixtures were quickly chilled at 20°C and adjusted to 0.6 M NaCl (final concentration). Samples (30 μl) were taken at different times after salt addition and rapidly mixed with 6 μl 6% SDS and processed for sequencing gels. The inserted box represents the cleavage products obtained at the hexadecameric sequence and a camptothecin-stimulated sequence. The arrow indicates the position of cleavage at the hexadecameric sequence. Lanes 1 to 8, no camptothecin; lanes 9 to 16, 10 μM camptothecin. Lanes 1 and 9, 29.5 min preincubation and 1% SDS. Lanes 2 to 8 and 10 to 16, time elapsed after adjusting to 0.6 M NaCl; lanes 2 and 10, 1 min; lanes 3 and 11, 5 min; lanes 4 and 12, 10 min; lanes 5 and 13, 20 min; lanes 6 and 14, 30 min; lanes 7 and 15, 45 min; lanes 8 and 16, 60 min. In each of the experimental series, the cleavage frequency at the hexadecameric sequence and at the camptothecin-stimulated site in any point were expressed as a percentage of the cleavage frequency in the sample taken after 29.5 min of preincubation. This percentage, the residual cleavage, was plotted against the time of sampling. The quantification are based on densitometric scanning of the whole autoradiogram shown in the box. (Open circle) residual cleavage frequency at the hexadecameric sequence in the absence of camptothecin; (filled circle) residual cleavage frequency at the hexadecameric sequence in the presence of camptothecin; (triangle) residual cleavage frequency at the camptothecin-stimulated site in the presence of camptothecin. The increased cleavage frequency at the camptothecin-stimulated site observed after 1 min is probably due to a decreased masking effect of cleavage at the hexadecameric sequence, supporting the idea that the residual cleavage at the hexadecameric sequence decreases much more rapidly than that at the camptothecin-stimulated site.

DNA complex formed at the hexadecameric recognition sequence dissociates rapidly in the presence of salt and was at the given temperature only marginally affected by camptothecin. The dissociation kinetics of the enzyme–DNA complex formed at a camptothecin-stimulated sequence (cf. Fig. 12.2, site b) decayed very slowly. Taken together, the data demonstrate a correlation between the degree of camptothecin stimulation and the salt stability of the enzyme–DNA complex in question. Thus, a high degree of stimulation of cleavage by camptothecin at a particular site is also reflected by a high stability in salt and vice versa (7).

Recent results from experiments with topoisomerase I, purified from a camptothecin-resistant human leukemia cell line, are consistent with the interpretation that camptothecin promotes cleavable complex formation (2,6). The drug inhibits relaxation catalyzed by wild-type topoisomerase I and stimulates cleavage at the additional sites on DNA. Drug-promoted stimulation of cleavage is not observed with topoisomerase I from resistant cells, and the catalytic activity of the enzyme is insensitive to camptothecin. When these data are considered together with the fact that camptothecin causes fragmentation of the cellular DNA in wild-type cells (2,4), but not in the resistant cell line, it seems reasonable to assume that topoisomerase I is the primary cellular target of the drug. It therefore seems plausible that it is the interaction of the drug with the enzyme that results in fragmentation of the genome.

Major DNA Determinants for Topoisomerase I Binding Site Selection

In general, eukaryotic topoisomerase I is highly promiscuous with respect to binding site selection. It has been shown that the enzyme cleaves duplex DNA as frequently as once per helical turn on the average (25,26). By comparative sequence analysis of such cleavage sites, a highly degenerate four (26) to five (25) base pair consensus sequence could be derived. Four of the consensus base pairs were located immediately 5′ to the cleavage site, i.e., to the side, where the enzyme attaches covalently. The fifth consensus base pair was located immediately 3′ to the cleavage site. These observations indicate that topoisomerase I primarily contacts DNA on the 5′ side of the cleavage position.

Our observations demonstrate, despite the loose sequence specificity indicated (25,26), that the hexadecameric motif from Tetrahymena rDNA is an unusually efficient substrate for topoisomerase I–mediated cleavage (17,19,27) and catalytic DNA relaxation (20). The hexadecamer consists of a core part surrounding the cleavage site, embedded between two homopolymeric AT runs. The core part obeys the five base pair minimal consensus, suggesting that the flanking AT runs play a role in conferring the high affinity.

As shown in Figure 12.2, addition of camptothecin causes topoisomerase I to cleave a great number of sequences with equally high cleavage efficiency. Determination of the underlying DNA sequences at the camptothecin-induced sites does not reveal any obvious homology (Table 12.1), except for a preference for the dinucleotide constellation TG at the position of the scissile bond and a G at position -3. These results are in agreement with results obtained by other groups (39,40).

Table 12.1. Determination of Potential Topoisomerase I–DNA Cleavage Sites

Hexadecameric recognition sequence

−10									−1									+10
A	A	A	A	A	G	A	C	T	T	A	G	A	A	A	A	A	T	T	T

Camptothecin-stimulated sequences

G	C	T	C	T	C	C	C	T	T	A	T	G	C	G	A	C	T	C	C
T	G	A	G	G	C	C	G	T	T	G	A	G	C	A	C	C	G	C	C
A	A	G	G	A	A	T	G	G	T	G	C	A	T	G	A	A	A	A	A
C	A	T	C	C	A	G	G	G	T	G	A	C	G	G	T	G	C	C	G
C	C	A	G	G	G	T	G	A	C	G	G	T	G	C	C	G	A	G	G
G	G	G	T	G	A	C	G	G	T	G	C	C	G	A	G	G	A	T	G
T	G	C	C	G	A	G	G	A	T	G	A	C	G	A	T	G	A	G	C
C	G	A	G	G	A	T	G	A	C	G	A	T	G	A	G	C	G	C	A
G	G	A	T	G	A	C	G	A	T	G	A	G	C	G	C	A	T	T	G
T	G	A	G	C	G	C	A	T	T	G	T	T	A	G	A	T	T	T	C

1.6 kb *Hind*III-*Pvu*II restriction fragments of pNC1, 3′ end [^{32}P]labeled, were subjected to Maxam-Gilbert chemical degradation reactions. For cleavage, 3′ end-labeled fragments were incubated with topoisomerase I (enzyme:DNA-ratio ≈80) in the presence and absence of camptothecin (10 μM, final concentration). The reactions were terminated with SDS and samples processed as described in Materials and Methods for co-electrophoresis with the Maxam-Gilbert reactions. The obtained sequences are listed. The positions of cleavage are indicated by −1.

The low sequence specificity in the presence of camptothecin suggests that other factors, such as local structures of the DNA helices, may play a central role in governing the recognition of the DNA by topoisomerase I. Studies of promoter sequences in *Escherichia coli* by Tung and Harvey have shown that sequences conferring very little sequence homology share a common DNA structure (23). To estimate the sequence-dependent variations in the helical parameters, twist angle, and base pair roll angle, we have used the computer program based on the conformational energy calculations by Tung and Harvey (21,22) to search for possible structural homologies of topoisomerase I binding sites.

Figure 12.4 shows the predicted helix geometry of the camptothecin-induced cleavage sequences, averaged over all the camptothecin-stimulated sequences listed in Table 12.1. All of the listed sequences, including the hexadecameric sequence, have a decreased helix twist angle spanning the dinucleotide step of the scissile bond (base pair step no. 10) and an overtwisting of the 5′ adjacent base pair step (Fig. 12.4A,4B). Outside this region the twist angles vary considerably. With respect to roll angles both the camptothecin-stimulated cleavage sequences and the hexadecameric sequence exhibit the highest positive value at the cleaved base pair step. Taken together, this might indicate that the camptothecin-stimulated sequences fulfill a minimal structural requirement that might be of functional significance in the enzyme–DNA interaction. However, investigation of a large number of camptothecin-stimulated sites reveals that approximately 20% of the sequences do not follow the structural motif, suggesting that the structural feature is not an absolute requirement and that other important parameters also are involved in the enzyme–DNA interaction.

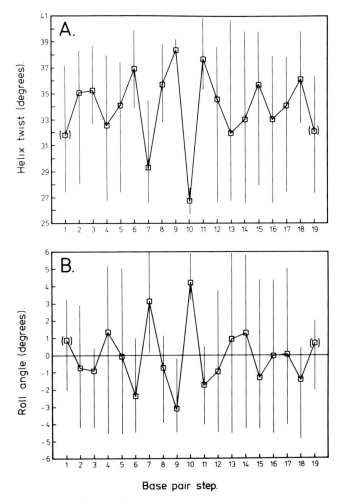

Figure 12.4. Prediction of the helix geometry of camptothecin-stimulated topoisomerase I cleavage sequences. **Panels A** and **B** display the expected local variations in helix twist angles and base pair roll angles, respectively, of sequences listed in Table 12.1. The curves connect the average values and the bars show the ranges of the estimated values.

To further characterize the interaction of topoisomerase I with DNA in the absence of camptothecin, the anatomy of the complex formed between topoisomerase I and the hexadecamer has been studied by footprinting and modification interference analysis (24). Assayed by nuclease footprinting, binding of topoisomerase I to the hexadecamer was tight and highly specific with $K_D \sim 10^{-10}$ M. The major contribution to the overall binding affinity was provided by the noncovalent association between the enzyme and the recognition site, while the transient formation of a cavalent enzyme–DNA intermediate contributed insignificantly (24).

The enzyme protects both strands over a ~20 base pair region in which the cleavage site is centrally located. However, only the nucleotides from -2 to -7 relative to the scissile bond were found to be essential for the binding of topoisomerase I. The essential region within the hexadecamer therefore extends beyond and only partially overlaps the four base pair minimal consensus. Furthermore, nucleotides from -8 to -11 relative to the site of the nick were found to modulate the efficiency of complex formation. At the present stage of analysis, there is no indication of essential contacts 3' to the cleavage site; however, nucleotides immediately 3' to the nick were found to influence the capability of the enzyme to perform a complete catalytic (i.e., nicking-closing) cycle.

CONCLUSION

Although, a complete understanding of the mechanisms of topoisomerase I–DNA interactions awaits further studies, some major DNA determinants have been described. Taken together, a simple interpretation of the data might be that the cleavage efficiency correlates with (1) the ease by which a given sequence can be deformed into the optimal conformation for topoisomerase I activity and (2) the location of essential bases in the enzyme–DNA complex.

Owing to their central role in macromolecular DNA metabolism (29–31), the topoisomerases are potentially interesting targets for chemotherapy. Topoisomerase II inhibitors, such as the epipodophyllotoxins, are well-known examples of clinically useful antitumor drugs (32,33). Topoisomerase I has been shown to be the primary cellular target for the antitumor drug camptothecin. However, the clinical use of this drug has been seriously hampered by its side effects (34). In an attempt to overcome this problem, a number of new derivatives of camptothecin have been developed. A detailed knowledge of the molecular interactions of these derivatives with topoisomerase I and DNA is therefore of potential interest.

Acknowledgments

This study was supported by the Commission of the European Communities (contract B-6-0170-DK), the Danish Medical Research Council (grant 5.1017.06), the Danish Cancer Society (grants 86-178, 87-025, and 87-088), the National Agency of Technology (contract 1985-133/001-85.521), and the Danish Programme of Biotechnology.

REFERENCES

1. Hsiang, Y.-H., Hertzberg, R., Hecht, S., and Liu, L. F. Camptothecin induces protein-linked DNA breaks via mammalian DNA topoisomerase I. J. Biol. Chem. **260:** 14873–14878, 1985.
2. Andoh, T., Ishii, K., Suzuki, Y., Ikegami, Y., Kusunoki, Y., Takamoto, H., and Okada, K. Characterization of a mammalian mutant with a camptothecin-resistant DNA topoisomerase I. Proc. Natl. Acad. Sci. USA. **84:** 5565–5569, 1987.
3. Horwitz, M. S. and Horwitz, S. B. Intracellular degradation of HeLa and adenovirus type 2 DNA induced by camptothe-

cin. Biochem. Biophys. Res. Commun. **45**: 723–727, 1971.

4. Sparato, A. and Kessel, D. Studies on camptothecin-induced degradation and apparent reaggregation of DNA from L1210 cells. Biochem. Biophys. Res. Commun. **48**: 643–648, 1972.

5. Abelson, H. T. and Penman, S. Selective interruption of high molecular weight RNA synthesis in HeLa cells by camptothecin. Nature [New Biol.]. **237**: 144–146, 1972.

6. Kjeldsen, E., Bonven, B. J., Andoh, T., Ishii, K., Okada, K., Bolund, L., and Westergaard, O. Characterization of a camptothecin-resistant human DNA topoisomerase I. J. Biol. Chem. **263**: 3912–3916, 1988.

7. Kjeldsen, E., Mollerup, S., Thomsen, B., Bonven, B. J., Bolund, L., and Westergaard, O. Sequence-dependent effect of camptothecin on human topoisomerase I DNA cleavage. J. Mol. Biol. **202**: 333–342, 1988.

8. Eissenberg, J. C., Cartwright, I. L., Thomas, G. H., and Elgin, S. C. R. Selected topics in chromatin structure. Annu. Rev. Genet. **19**: 485–536, 1985.

9. Igo-Kemenes, T., Hörz, W., and Zachau, H. G. Chromatin. Annu. Rev. Biochem. **51**: 89–121, 1982.

10. Saragosti, S., Moyne, G., and Yaniv, M. Absence of nucleosomes in a fraction of SV40 chromatin between the origin of replication and the coding region for the late leader RNA. Cell. **20**: 65–73, 1980.

11. McGhee, J. D., Wood, W. I., Dolan, M., Engel, J. D., and Felsenfeld, G. A 200 base pair region at the 5′-end of the chicken adult B-globin gene is accessible to nuclease digestion. Cell. **27**: 45–55, 1981.

12. Palen, T. E. and Cech, T. R. Chromatin structure at the replication origins and transcription-initiation regions of the ribosomal RNA genes of Tetrahymena. Cell. **36**: 933–942, 1984.

13. Weintraub, H. A dominant role for DNA secondary structure in forming hypersensitive structures in chromatin. Cell. **32**: 1191–1203, 1983.

14. Mace, H. A. F., Pelham, H. R. B., and Travers, A. A. Association of an S_1 nuclease-sensitive structure with short direct repeats 5′ of Drosophila heat shock genes. Nature. **304**: 555–557, 1983.

15. Emerson, B. M. and Felsenfeld, G. Specific factor conferring nuclease hypersensitivity of the 5′-end of the chicken adult B-globin gene. Proc. Natl. Acad. Sci. USA. **81**: 95–99, 1984.

16. Zareth, K. S., Yamamoto, K. R. Reversible and persistent changes in chromatin structure accompany activation of a glycocorticoid-dependent enhancer element. Cell. **38**: 29–38, 1984.

17. Bonven, B. J., Gocke, E., and Westergaard, O. A high affinity topoisomerase I binding sequence is clustered at DNAase I hypersensitive sites in Tetrahymena r-chromatin. Cell. **41**: 541–551, 1985.

18. Culotta, V. and Sollner-Webb, B. Sites of topoisomerase I action on X. laevis ribosomal chromatin: Transcriptionally active rDNA has an $\sqrt{200}$ bp repeating structure. Cell. **52**: 585–597, 1988.

19. Thomsen, B., Mollerup, S., Bonven, B. J., Frank, R., Blöcker, H., Nielsen, O. F., and Westergaard, O. Sequence specificity of DNA topoisomerase I in the presence and absence of camptothecin. EMBO J. **6**: 1817–1823, 1987.

20. Busk, H., Thomsen, B., Bonven, B. J., Kjeldsen, E., Nielsen, O. F., and Westergaard, O. Preferential relaxation of supercoiled DNA containing a hexadecameric recognition sequence for topoisomerase I. Nature. **327**: 638–640, 1987.

21. Tan, R.K.Z., Prabhakaran, M., Tung, C. S., and Harvey, S. C. AUGUR: A program to predict, display and analyze the tertiary structure of B-DNA. CABIOS. **4**: 147–151, 1988.

22. Tung, C.-S. and Harvey, S. C. Base sequence, local helix structure, and macroscopic curvature of A-DNA and B-DNA. J. Biol. Chem. **261**: 3700–3709, 1986.

23. Tung, C.-S. and Harvey, S. C. A common structural feature in promotor sequences of *E. coli*. Nucleic Acids Res. **15**: 4973–4985, 1987.

24. Stevsner, T., Mortensen, U. H., Westergaard, O., and Bonven, B. J. Interactions between eukaryotic DNA topoisomerase I and a specific binding sequence. J. Biol. Chem. **264**: 10110–10113, 1989.

25. Edwards, K. A., Halligan, B. D., Davis, J. L., Nivera, N. L., and Liu, L. F. Recognition sites sites of eukaryotic DNA topoisomerase I: DNA nucleotide sequence analysis of topoI cleavages sites on SV40 DNA. Nucleic Acids Res. **10**: 2565–2576, 1982.

26. Been, M. D., Burgess, R. R., and Champoux, J. J. Nucleotide sequence preference at rat liver and wheat germ type I DNA topoisomerase breakage sites in duplex SV40 DNA. Nucleic Acids Res. **12**: 3097–3114, 1984.

27. Christiansen, K., Bonven, B. J., and Westergaard, O. Mapping of sequence-specific chromatin proteins by a novel method: Topoisomerase I on Tetrahymena ribosomal chromatin. J. Mol. Biol. **193**: 517–525, 1987.

28. Brunelle, A. and Schleif, R. F. Missing

contact probing of DNA-protein interactions. Proc. Natl. Acad. Sci. USA. **84:** 6673–6676, 1987.

29. Wang, J. C. DNA topoisomerases. Annu. Rev. Biochem. **554:** 665–697, 1985.

30. Vosberg, H.-P. DNA topoisomerases: Enzymes that control DNA conformation. Curr. Topics Microbiol. Immunol. **114:** 19–102, 1985.

31. Maxwell, A. and Gellert, M. Mechanistic aspects of DNA topoisomerases. Adv. Protein Chem. **38:** 69–107, 1986.

32. Ross, W., Rowe, T., Glisson, B., Yalowich, J., and Liu, L. F. Role of topoisomerase II in mediating epipodophyllotoxin-induced DNA cleavage. Cancer Res. **44:** 5857–5860, 1984.

33. Tewey, K. M., Chen, G. L., Nelson, E. M., and Liu, L. F. Intercalative antitumor drugs interfere with the breakage-reunion reaction of mammalian DNA topoisomerase II. J. Biol. Chem. **259:** 9182–9187, 1984.

34. Nitta, K., Yokohura, T., Sadawa, S., Takeuchi, M., Tanaka, T., Uehara, N., Bab, H., Kunimoto, T., Miyasaka, T., and Mutai, M. In Ishigami, J., ed. *Recent Advances in Chemotherapy.* Tokyo: University of Tokyo Press, 1985, pp. 28–30.

35. Ness, P. J., Koller, T., and Thoma, F. Topoisomerase I cleavage sites identified and mapped in the chromatin of Dictyostelium ribosomal RNA genes. J. Mol. Biol. **200:** 127–139, 1988.

36. Challoner, P. B., Amin, A. A., Pearlman, R. E., and Blackburn, E. H. Conserved arrangements of repeated DNA sequences in nontranscribed spacers of ciliate ribosomal RNA genes: Evidence for molecular coevolution. Nucleic Acids Res. **13:** 2661–2680, 1985.

37. Fratini, A. V., Kopka, M. L., Drew, H. R., and Dickerson, R. E. Reversible bending and helix geometry in a B-DNA dodecamer: CGCGAATT^{Br}CGCG. J. Biol. Chem. **257:** 14686–14707, 1982.

38. Bonven, B. and Westergaard, O. DNase I hypersensitive regions correlate with a site-specific endogenous nuclease activity on the r-chromatin of *Tetrahymena.* Nucleic Acids Res. **10:** 7593–7608, 1982.

39. Jaxel, C., Kohn, K. W., and Pommier, Y. Topoisomerase I interaction with SV40 DNA in the presence and absence of camptothecin. Nucleic Acids Res. **16:** 11157–11170, 1988.

40. Porter, S. E. and Champoux, J. J. Mapping in vivo topoisomerase I sites on Simian virus 40 DNA: Asymmetric distribution of sites on replicating molecules. Mol. Cell. Biol. **9:** 541–550, 1989.

Chapter 13
Protection by DNA Synthesis Inhibition Against Cell Killing by Topoisomerase Blocking Drugs

CHRISTINE HOLM, JOSEPH M. COVEY,
DONNA KERRIGAN, KURT W. KOHN, AND YVES POMMIER

DNA topoisomerases I and II are found in the nuclei of all eukaryotic cells and play a major role in DNA replication and transcription (1,2). Topoisomerase I is specifically inhibited by camptothecin (3), while topoisomerase II is inhibited by demethylepipodophyllotoxins, such as etoposide (VP-16) and teniposide (VM-26) (4,5) and some DNA intercalators, such as adriamycin, amsacrine, or ellipticine (6–8). For both enzymes, drug-induced topoisomerase inhibition appears to result from the stabilization of covalent enzyme–DNA complexes. These complexes have been named "cleavable complexes" because they lead to DNA single-strand breaks upon protein and DNA denaturation (9). The cleavable complexes can be detected by alkaline elution as protein-associated DNA strand breaks (10,11).

Topoisomerase inhibitors are cytotoxic at concentrations that produce measurable protein-linked DNA strand breaks (cleavable complexes) (12,13). In addition, cells that are resistant to the cytotoxic effect of the drugs fail to produce cleavable complexes (14,15). These observations suggested that the cleavable complexes were the cytotoxic lesions produced by topoisomerase inhibitors. However, short exposures to cytotoxic concentrations of drugs produce only transient protein-associated DNA strand breaks, which reverse within minutes after drug removal (13,16). Therefore, if the stabilization of cleavable complexes is responsible for the cytotoxicity of topoisomerase inhibitors, it must represent only an initial event in the cytotoxic action of the drugs, and nonreversible lethal lesions have to occur secondary to the cleavable complexes. The cleavable complexes could lead to DNA recombination in the case of topoisomerase II (12,17), and form steric blocks for DNA replication, transcription, and repair for any of the two enzymes.

The present study was undertaken to test whether the conversion of cleavable complexes into lethal lesions could involve DNA replication. The effects of DNA replication inhibition by aphidicolin (18) and hydroxyurea upon the cytotoxicity and the formation of drug-induced topoisomerase-mediated DNA strand breaks were measured in order to monitor the relationship between these breaks and cytotoxicity.

MATERIALS AND METHODS

Drugs and Materials

Camptothecin (NSC 94600), amsacrine (*m*-AMSA) (NSC 249992), and VP-16 (NSC 122819) were obtained from the Drug Synthesis and Chemistry Branch, National Cancer Institute. Aphidicolin and hydroxyurea were purchased from Sigma Co. (St. Louis, MO). Hydroxyurea and VP-16 (10 mM) were dissolved immediately before use in culture medium and dimethylsulfoxide, respectively. VP-16 was further diluted in H_2O at 0.1 mM. Aphidicolin, camptothecin, and amsacrine stock solutions were made and kept frozen in dimethylsulfoxide at 10 mM. They were thawed and diluted in H_2O as needed. [^{14}C]thymidine and [^{3}H]thymidine were purchased from New England Nuclear (Boston, MA). Tissue culture medium and fetal calf serum were purchased from ABI (Columbia, MD) and GIBCO (Grand Island, NY), respectively.

Cell Culture and Drug Treatments

Chinese hamster lung fibroblasts DC3F cells were kindly provided by Dr. A. Jacquemin-Sablon (Institut Gustave Roussy, Villejuif, France) (19). Cells were grown in Eagles minimum essential medium supplemented with 10% fetal calf serum, 0.1 mM nonessential amino acids, 2 mM glutamine, 1 mM sodium pyruvate, 20 mM HEPES, and penicillin/streptomycin, at 37°C in the presence of 5% CO_2. DC3F cells had a doubling time of 12–18 h.

All experiments were performed with log phase DC3F cells that had been seeded 12–15 h before at approximately 3×10^5 cells per 25 cm^2 flask in 5 ml of medium. Camptothecin, VP-16, or amsacrine treatments were 30 min, unless otherwise indicated (see Fig. 13.2). Treatments with DNA synthesis inhibitors (aphidicolin and hydroxyurea) were started 5 min before camptothecin or VP-16 treatments, continued throughout the ensuing 30 min, and were ended at the same time as the camptothecin, VP-16, or amsacrine treatments (35 min total treatment time). Dimethylsulfoxide was added to control cell cultures at the concentration present in the treated flasks. The dimethylsulfoxide concentration never exceeded 1% and did not affect cell survival.

Clonogenic Assays

At the end of drug treatments, cells were washed 3 times with 10 ml warm medium, trypsinized, suspended in warm medium, and counted. 10^2, 10^3, and 10^4 cells were seeded in triplicate into 25 cm^2 flasks in 5 ml of medium for each treatment condition. Cell cultures were incubated for 5–7 days, after which they were washed twice with 10 ml phosphate-buffered saline. Colonies were fixed with 95% methanol (15 min), stained with methylene blue (20 min), and counted. The plating efficiency of drug-treated cells was divided by the plating efficiency of untreated cells, to yield a "survival fraction." The plating efficiency for untreated cells was 70–90%.

DNA Synthesis Inhibition

Cellular DNA was prelabeled by incubating the cell cultures with 0.005–0.01 μCi/ml [^{14}C]thymidine for approximately 18 h. The rate of DNA synthesis was measured by 5 min pulses with 1 μCi/ml [3H]thymidine. Thymidine incorporation was determined as follows: cells were washed twice with ice-cold Hanks' balanced salt solution (HBSS), and then scraped into 3 ml HBSS. One milliliter aliquots of this suspension were added to 100 μl 100% trichloroacetic acid (TCA) in duplicate, vortexed, and centrifuged for 6 min in an Eppendorf centrifuge, all at 0–4°C. The precipitates were dissolved with 1 ml 0.4 M NaOH, and counted by liquid scintillation spectrometry. DNA synthesis inhibition was determined as the ratio of [^{3}H]/[^{14}C] in the treated samples over the ratio of [^{3}H]/[^{14}C] in the untreated samples.

Measurement of DNA Single-Strand Breaks by Alkaline Elution

The alkaline elution methodology has been described in previous publications (16,11). Briefly, [^{14}C]thymidine labeled cells (0.02 μCi/ml for 18 h prior to drug treatments) were treated with camptothecin, amsacrine, or VP-16 for 30 min at 37°C. Cell cultures were then dispersed by scraping into 10 ml ice-cold HBSS. In the case of camptothecin the same drug concentration as for drug treatment was used in all the dilution tubes in order to avoid the reversal of the DNA breaks at 0°C (11). Cell suspensions were then loaded onto polycarbonate filters (2 μm pore diameter, Nucleopore Corp., Pleasanton, CA). When the HBSS containing the [^{14}C]labeled treatment cells had dripped through, approximately 0.5 ml ice-cold [^{3}H]thymidine labeled L1210 (internal standard) cells, which had been irradiated with 2000 rads, were loaded. Lysis was immediately performed with sodium dodecyl sulfate and proteinase K (SDS-ProK lysis solution). Elution was with tetrapropylammonium hydroxyl:EDTA, 0.1% SDS, pH 12.1. Fractions were collected every 5 min for 30 min (16). DNA single-strand breaks (SSB) were expressed in rad-equivalents.

RESULTS

Cytotoxicity of Camptothecin in DC3F Cells

Thirty minute exposures to various concentrations of camptothecin produced limited cytotoxicity with less than one log cell killing (Fig. 13.1). Drug concentration–dependence was clearest at low concentrations (0.1 and 0.25 μM). Increasing camptothecin concentrations above 0.25 μM did not increase cell killing significantly, even when the camptothecin concentration was 200-fold

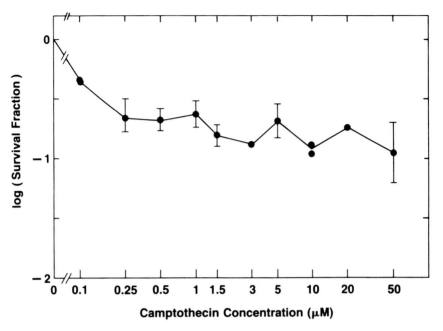

Figure 13.1. Concentration-dependence of camptothecin-induced cytotoxicity in DC3F cells.

higher (Fig. 13.1). Therefore 20–30% of the DC3F cells were naturally resistant to 30 min exposures to camptothecin.

This resistance was overcome by increasing the time of exposure to camptothecin (Fig. 13.2). An almost linear relationship was found between cytotox-

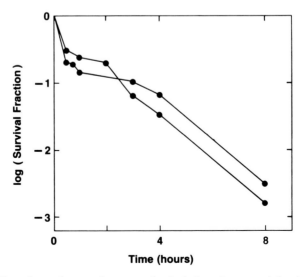

Figure 13.2. Time-dependence of camptothecin-induced cytotoxicity in DC3F cells. Cells were treated with 0.25 μM camptothecin for the indicated time periods. Two independent experiments are shown.

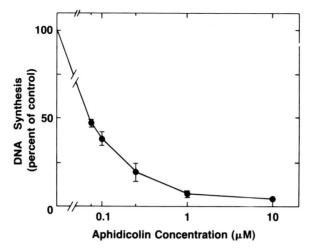

Figure 13.3. DNA synthesis inhibition by aphidicolin in DC3F cells. Aphidicolin treatments were for 35 min at 37°C.

icity and time of exposure. Approximately 3-logs of cell killing were observed after 8 h exposures. These results are in agreement with the previous finding that camptothecin is most cytotoxic in S-phase cells (20), since increasing the time of exposure to camptothecin would increase the fraction of S-phase cells exposed to the drug.

Protective Effect of DNA Synthesis Inhibition Against Camptothecin-Induced Cytotoxicity

First, the concentrations of aphidicolin that would inhibit DNA synthesis without killing a significant fraction of the cells were determined (Figs. 13.3–13.5). Ten micromolar aphidicolin blocked thymidine incorporation by more than 90%

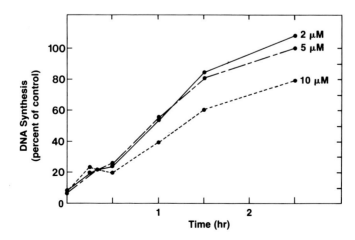

Figure 13.4. Kinetics of DNA synthesis recovery after 35 min treatments with aphidicolin.

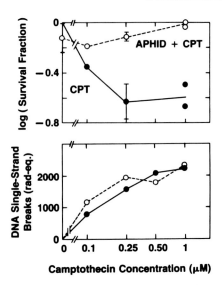

Figure 13.5. Effects of aphidicolin on camptothecin-induced cytotoxicity (**upper panel**) and DNA single-strand breaks (**lower panel**) in DC3F cells. Aphidicolin treatments were started 5 min before the addition of camptothecin and continued throughout the 30 min camptothecin treatments.

(Fig. 13.3). Kinetics experiments indicated that aphidicolin inhibited DNA synthesis within the first 5 min of exposure (data not shown). Following 35 min exposure to aphidicolin, DNA synthesis inhibition recovered slowly, and almost no reversal occurred during the first 30 min (Fig. 13.4). Under these conditions, aphidicolin produced minimal cell killing (10–20%) (Fig. 13.5, Table 13.1).

The protocol subsequently chosen to study the effect of DNA synthesis inhibition upon camptothecin-induced cytotoxicity and DNA breaks was the following: DC3F cells were treated with 10 μM aphidicolin; 5 min later, camptothecin was added while aphidicolin was kept in the culture medium; finally, both drugs were removed from the cell culture simultaneously after 30 min of co-incubation. Under these conditions, DNA synthesis was inhibited during

Table 13.1. DNA Synthesis Inhibitors Prevent Camptothecin Cytotoxicity

	Cell Survival (Percent of Control)	
	No Camptothecin	Camptothecin (0.25 μM)
No treatment[a]	100	28
Hydroxyurea (1 mM)	64	41
Aphidicolin (10 μM)	80	78

[a]DC3F cells were treated with hydroxyurea or aphidicolin for 5 min before the addition of camptothecin. Drugs were removed after 30 min and cells plated for colony formation assays.

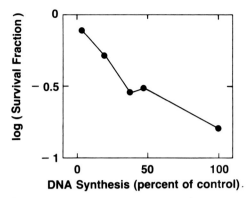

Figure 13.6. Relationship between camptothecin-induced cytotoxicity and DNA synthesis in DC3F cells. Different aphidicolin concentrations (0.075–10 μM; Fig. 13.3) were used to inhibit DNA synthesis and to determine the cytotoxicity of 0.25 μM camptothecin under these conditions.

the entire time that camptothecin-induced DNA breaks were present, since camptothecin-induced DNA breaks form within a few minutes after drug addition and reverse within 30 min after drug removal (13,11).

Ten micromolar aphidicolin protected from camptothecin cytotoxicity (Fig. 13.5). The protection was complete at camptothecin concentrations lower than 5 μM. It was partial at 5 and 10 μM and was not detectable at 20 and 50 μM camptothecin (not shown).

The same protocol was used to examine camptothecin-induced DNA single-strand breaks. Under these conditions, aphidicolin had no effect upon camptothecin-induced DNA break frequency (Fig. 13.5). Therefore, a dissociation between camptothecin-induced cytotoxicity and DNA breaks was produced by aphidicolin.

In order to confirm that the protective effect of aphidicolin was directly due to DNA synthesis inhibition, various aphidicolin concentrations producing different levels of DNA synthesis inhibition were used (Fig. 13.3). It was found that the greater the inhibition of DNA synthesis, the better the protection, and that an almost linear relationship existed between the rate of DNA synthesis and camptothecin-induced cytotoxicity (Fig. 13.6). An additional experiment using hydroxyurea showed also significant protection from camptothecin-induced cytotoxicity (Table 13.1). These results suggest that DNA synthesis inhibition is the mechanism of the protective effect of aphidicolin against the cytotoxicity of camptothecin.

Protective Effect of Aphidicolin Against VP-16– and Amsacrine–Induced Cytotoxicity

The same type of experiments were performed with the topoisomerase II inhibitors, VP-16 and amsacrine. As observed in the case of camptothecin, aphi-

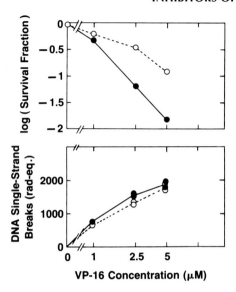

Figure 13.7. Effects of aphidicolin on VP-16–induced cytotoxicity (**upper pannel**) and DNA single-strand breaks (**lower panel**) in DC3F cells. Same protocol as in Fig. 13.5, except that VP-16 was used instead of camptothecin.

dicolin did not affect VP-16–induced DNA breaks (Fig. 13.7). However, in contrast to the case of camptothecin, aphidicolin protected only partially against VP-16–induced cytotoxicity (Fig. 13.7). Similar results were observed with amsacrine (Table 13.2). The frequency of amsacrine-induced DNA strand breaks was not significantly affected by aphidicolin and a partial protection against the cytotoxicity of amsacrine was produced by aphidicolin. Increasing aphidicolin concentration did not prevent the cytotoxicity of topoisomerase II inhibitors further but resulted in a significant cytotoxicity of aphidicolin (data not shown). These results indicate that the mechanism of the cytotoxicity of topoisomerase II inhibitors differs from that of camptothecin.

Table 13.2. Effects of Aphidicolin on the Cytotoxicity and the DNA Breaks Produced by Topoisomerase II Inhibitors

Aphidicolin Treatment[a]	Survival (Percent of Control)		DNA Single-Strand Breaks (Rad-Equivalents)	
	None	10 μM	None	10 μM
VP-16 (2.5 μM)	6.2	35.1	1548	1295
Amsacrine (0.5 μM)	3.0	23.9	1846	2013

[a]DC3F cells were treated with aphidicolin for 5 min before the addition of VP-16 or amsacrine. After 30 min drug treatments, DNA single-strand breaks were determined by alkaline elution and cell survival by colony formation assays.

DISCUSSION

Topoisomerase I inhibition by camptothecin appears to result from the stabilization of the enzyme within cleavable complexes (3), which can be detected as protein-associated DNA single-strand breaks by alkaline elution (11). Two types of studies strongly suggest that topoisomerase I inhibition is responsible for the cytotoxicity of camptothecin. First, cells that are resistant to camptothecin have a camptothecin-resistant topoisomerase I (15). Second, a good correlation is found between the antitumor activity of camptothecin analogs and their inhibitory activity against purified topoisomerase I (21). However, the camptothecin-induced DNA single-strand breaks reverse quickly after drug removal (20,13), which implies that their cytotoxicity results from a secondary interference with cellular processes. The present study showing that 5 min pretreatment with aphidicolin and hydroxyurea (which did not change the cell cycle distribution) did not affect the frequency of camptothecin-induced DNA breaks and yet protected against the cytotoxicity of camptothecin indicates that the topoisomerase I–induced DNA breaks are only a potentially lethal damage and that ongoing DNA replication is necessary for the induction of the lethal lesions responsible for camptothecin cytotoxicity. Therefore the cytotoxicity of camptothecin requires not only that the cells are in S-phase (20) but that DNA replication is active.

Topoisomerase I is likely to be present in close proximity to the DNA replication apparatus and to act as a swivel that relieves the torsional tension that accumulates near a moving replication fork (1,2,22). However, analysis of yeast topoisomerase mutants indicates that topoisomerase II can substitute for topoisomerase I during DNA replication, since topoisomerase I mutants replicate and are viable (23,24). Therefore, it seems unlikely that an accumulation of torsional tension within replicating DNA could explain the cytotoxicity of camptothecin. A more attractive possibility is that the covalent topoisomerase I–DNA complexes immobilized by camptothecin interact with moving DNA replication forks. Such a model is in agreement with the finding that camptothecin inhibits DNA synthesis by more than 60% under the conditions of the present study, and that this inhibition is almost immediate and not reversible after camptothecin removal (data not shown).

The mechanism of the cytotoxicity of topoisomerase II inhibitors appears to differ from that of camptothecin, since the protective effect of aphidicolin against VP-16–induced and amsacrine-induced cytotoxicity was only partial. These results are in agreement with those of other studies showing that aphidicolin and hydroxyurea protect only partially against the cytotoxicity of topoisomerase II inhibitors, while the protein synthesis inhibitor cycloheximide (25–27) and the RNA synthesis inhibitor cordycepin (27) give a more complete protection. The partial protective effect of DNA synthesis inhibition against VP-16–induced or amsacrine-induced cytotoxicity suggests that drug-induced topoisomerase II–mediated DNA breaks could exert their cytotoxic effect in the absence of ongoing DNA synthesis. DNA recombinations and mutations at the sites of drug-induced topoisomerase II–DNA complexes could be the lethal lesions induced by topoisomerase II inhibitors (12,14).

REFERENCES

1. Horwitz, S. B. and Horwitz, M. S. Effects of camptothecin on the breakage and repair of DNA during the cell cycle Cancer. Res. **33**: 2834–2836, 1973.
2. Huberman, J. A. New views of the biochemistry of eukaryotic DNA replication revealed by aphidicolin, an unusual inhibitor of DNA polymerase alpha. Cell. **23**: 647–648, 1981.
3. Zwelling, L. A., Michaels, S., Erickson, L. C., Ungerleider, R. S., Nichols, M., and Kohn, K. W. Protein-associated deoxyribonucleic acid strand breaks in L1210 cells treated with the deoxyribonucleic acid intercalating agents 4'-(9-acridinylamino) methanesulfon-m-anisidide and adriamycin. Biochemistry. **20**: 6553–6563, 1981.
4. Salles, B., Charcosset, J. Y., and Jacquemin-Sablon, A. Isolation and properties of Chinese hamster lung cells resistant to ellipticine derivatives. Cancer Treat. Rep. **66**: 327–338, 1982.
5. Liu, L. F., Rowe, T. C., Yang, L., Tewey, K. M., and Chen, G. L. Cleavage of DNA by mammalian DNA topoisomerase II. J. Biol. Chem. **258**: 15365–15370, 1983.
6. Chen, G. L., Yang, L., Rowe, T. C., Halligan, B. D., Tewey, K. M., and Liu, L. F. Nonintercalative antitumor drugs interfere with the breakage-reunion reaction of mammalian DNA topoisomerase II. J. Biol. Chem. **259**: 13560–13566, 1984.
7. DiNardo, S., Voelkel, K., and Sternglanz, R. DNA topoisomerase II mutant of Saccharomyces cerevisiae: Topoisomerase II is required for segregation of daughter molecules at the termination of DNA replication. Proc. Natl. Acad. Sci. USA. **81**: 2616–2620, 1984.
8. Ross, W., Rowe, T., Glisson, B., Yalowich, J., and Liu, L. Role of topoisomerase II in mediating epipodophyllotoxin-induced DNA cleavage. Cancer Res. **44**: 5857–5860, 1984.
9. Tewey, K. M., Rowe, T. C., Yang, L., Halligan, B. D., and Liu, L. F. Adriamycin-induced DNA damage mediated by mammalian DNA topoisomerase II. Science. **226**: 466–468, 1984.
10. Charcosset, J. Y., Bendirdjian, J. P., Lantieri, M. F., and Jacquemin-Sablon, A. Effects of 9-OH-ellipticine on cell survival, macromolecular syntheses, and cell cycle progression in sensitive and resistant Chinese hamster lung cells. Cancer Res. **45**: 4229–4236, 1985.
11. Holm, C., Goto, T., Wang, J. C., and Bolstein, D. DNA topoisomerase II is required at the time of mitosis in yeast. Cell. **41**: 553–563, 1985.
12. Hsiang, Y. H., Hertzberg, R., Hecht, S., and Liu, L. F. Camptothecin induces protein-linked DNA breaks via mammalian DNA topoisomerase I. J. Biol. Chem. **260**: 14873–14878, 1985.
13. Pommier, Y., Minford, J. K., Schwartz, R. E., Zwelling, L. A., and Kohn, K. W. Effects of the DNA intercalators 4'-(9-acridinylamino)methanesulfon-m-anisidide and 2-methyl-9-hydroxyellipticinium on topoisomerase II mediated DNA strand cleavage and strand passage. Biochemistry. **24**: 6410–6416, 1985.
14. Pommier, Y., Zwelling, L. A., Kao-Shan, C. S., Whang-Peng, J., and Bradley, M. O. Correlations between intercalator-induced DNA strand breaks and sister chromatid exchanges, mutations, and cytotoxicity in Chinese hamster cells. Cancer Res. **45**: 3143–3149, 1985.
15. Wang, J. C. DNA topoisomerases. Annu. Rev. Biochem. **54**: 665–697, 1985.
16. Minford, J., Pommier, Y., Filipski, J., Kohn, K. W., Kerrigan, D., Mattern, M., Michaels, S., Schwartz, R., and Zwelling, L. A. Isolation of intercalator-dependent protein-linked DNA strand cleavage activity from cell nuclei and identification as topoisomerase II. Biochemistry. **25**: 9–16, 1986.
17. Pommier, Y., Schwartz, R. E., Zwelling, L. A., Kerrigan, D., Mattern, M. R., Charcosset, J. Y., Jacquemin-Sablon, A., and Kohn, K. W. Reduced formation of protein-associated DNA strand breaks in Chinese hamster cells resistant to topoisomerase II inhibitors. Cancer Res. **46**: 611–616, 1986.
18. Andoh, T., Ishii, K., Suzuki, Y., Ikegami, Y., Kusunki, Y., Takemoto, Y., and Okada, K. Characterization of a mammalian mutant with a camptothecin resistant DNA topoisomerase I. Proc. Natl. Acad. Sci. USA. **84**: 5565–5569, 1987.
19. Chow, K. C. and Ross, W. E. Topoisomerase-specific drug sensitivity in relation to cell cycle progression. Mol. Cell. Biol. **7**: 3119–3123, 1987
20. Kohn, K. W., Pommier, Y., Kerrigan, D., Markovits, J., and Covey, J. M. Topoisomerase II as a target of anticancer drug action in mammalian cells. NCI Monogr. **4**: 61–71, 1987.
21. Mattern, M. R., Mong, S. M., Bartus, H. F., Mirabelli, C. K., Crooke, S. T., and Johnson, R. K. Relationship between the intracellular effects of camptothecin and the inhibition of DNA topoisomerase I in cultured L1210 cells. Cancer Res. **47**: 1793–1798, 1987.
22. Wang, J. C. Recent studies of DNA to-

poisomerases. Biochim. Biophys. Acta. **909:** 1–9, 1987.

23. Avemann, K., Knippers, R., Koller, T., and Sogo, J. M. Camptothecin, a specific inhibitor of type I DNA topoisomerase, induces DNA breakage at replication forks. Mol. Cell. Biol. **8:** 3026–3034, 1988.

24. Pommier, Y., Kerrigan, D., Covey, J. M., Kao-Shan, C. S., and Whang-Peng, J. Sister chromatid exchanges, chromosomal aberrations, and cytotoxicity produced by antitumor topoisomerase II inhibitors in sensitive (DC3F) and resistant (DC3F/ 9-OHE) Chinese hamster cells. Cancer Res. **48:** 512–516, 1988.

25. Covey, J. M., Jaxel, C., Kohn, K. W., and Pommier, Y. Protein-linked DNA strand breaks induced in mammalian cells by camptothecin, an inhibitor of topoisomerase I. Cancer Res. **49:** 5016–5022, 1989.

26. Jaxel, C., Kohn, K. W., Wani, M. C., Wall, M. E., and Pommier, Y. Structure-activity study of the actions of camptothecin derivatives on mammalian topoisomerase I: Evidence for a specific receptor site and a relation to antitumor activity. Cancer Res. **49:** 1465–1469, 1989.

27. Schneider, E., Lawson, P. A., and Ralph, R. K. Inhibition of protein synthesis reduces the cytotoxicity of 4'-(9-acridinylamino)methanesulfon-m-anisidide without affecting DNA breakage and DNA topoisomerase II in a murine mastocytoma cell line. Biochem. Pharmacol. **38:** 263–269, 1989.

Chapter 14

Modulation of Topoisomerase-Targeted Drugs by DNA Minor-Groove Binding Agents

TERRY A. BEERMAN, JAN M. WOYNAROWSKI,

AND MARY M. McHUGH

Topological enzymes that are essential for replication and transcription (1,2) are the primary targets of several clinically significant antitumor drugs (for review see 1,3,4). Both epipodophyllotoxins (such as VM-26) and anilinoacridines (e.g., *m*-AMSA) convert topoisomerase II to a cellular poison by stabilizing a reaction intermediate ("cleavable complex") in which the enzyme is bound covalently to DNA (3,4). The plant alkaloid camptothecin stabilizes an analogous complex between DNA and topoisomerase I (3,4). The formation of DNA lesions related to stabilization of cleavable complexes correlates with the antiproliferative effects of topoisomerase-targeted antitumor drugs (1,3–5).

The action of topoisomerases can also be affected by DNA intercalators that are unable to stabilize the cleavable complexes. Intercalators, such as ethidium bromide or *o*-AMSA, have been shown to inhibit catalytic activity of topoisomerases and also DNA lesions induced by topoisomerase-targeted drugs (6). However, intercalator-induced unwinding of DNA leads to significant changes in the DNA structure apart from the drug binding site (7). Consequently, the contribution of DNA intercalation to the interference with enzyme action is difficult to assess (8).

An alternative approach was to determine whether nonintercalative binding to DNA could modulate the action of topoisomerases. Unlike intercalators, agents that bind to the minor groove of DNA associate tightly with the DNA surface while producing little or no distortion of the helix (7). Minor-groove binders are known to affect the activities of enzymes that use DNA as a substrate. For example, the minor-groove binder distamycin inhibits the reaction between *Escherichia coli* RNA polymerase and the *lac* promoter sequence (9). A related drug, netropsin, causes an enhancement of S1 nuclease digestion of DNA (10).

Distamycin, Hoechst 33258, and DAPI (Fig. 14.1) are agents whose interaction with the minor groove is well characterized (11–16). While all three compounds show preference for AT sequences in the DNA, the size of their binding site varies. Distamycin occupies a 5 base pair region (13), while Hoechst and

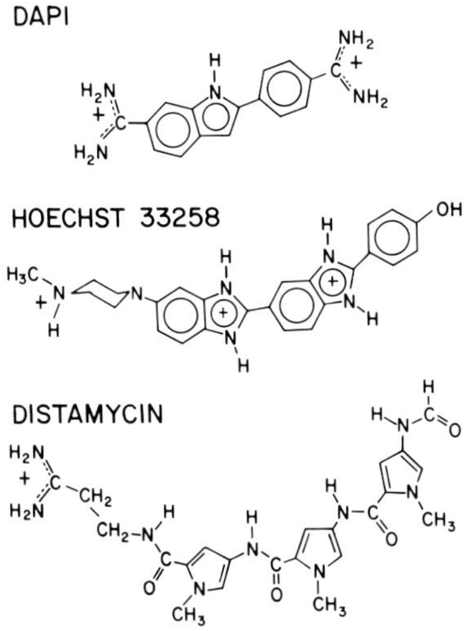

Figure 14.1. Structures of minor-groove binders.

DAPI bind to 4 and 3 base pair sites, respectively (15,16). Our studies evaluated these three model minor-groove binders for their ability to modulate topoisomerase-related effects. This report summarizes the results of these studies and shows that minor-groove binders can (1) influence the catalytic function of topoisomerase I and II (17,18), and (2) alter the formation of cleavable complex induced by various antitopoisomerase agents (19,20). These results point to a new approach to the modulation of topoisomerase-targeted drugs.

CATALYTIC ACTIVITY OF TOPOISOMERASE I AND II

The initial studies determined the effects of distamycin, Hoechst 33258, and DAPI on topoisomerase-mediated relaxation of supercoiled DNA. Figure 14.2A, 2B show the effect of distamycin on topoisomerase I and II, respectively. At low levels of distamycin ($<5.0 \mu M$), increased production of relaxed form I was observed. This stimulatory effect was more pronounced for topoisomerase II yielding two- to threefold enhancement at 1.0 μM distamycin. Above 5.0 μM distamycin, the relaxation activity of both enzymes was reduced, and by 10 μM the reaction was almost completely suppressed; 90% inhibition of topoisomerase I and II catalysis was observed at 9 and 12 μM distamycin, respectively. Incubation with distamycin in the absence of enzyme had no effect on DNA migration (data not shown).

Analogous experiments using two other minor-groove binding agents, Hoechst 33258 and DAPI, demonstrated that the ability to modulate the activity of topological enzymes was not limited to distamycin. Both enzymes were affected similarly by each of the drugs. However, DAPI, which occupies the fewest number of DNA base pairs, was clearly less inhibitory than distamycin and Hoechst (data not shown). Additionally, neither Hoechst nor DAPI produced pronounced stimulation of catalytic activity (data not shown).

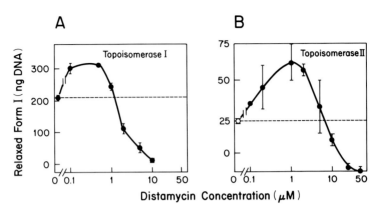

Figure 14.2. Effects of distamycin on the catalytic activity (relaxation of supercoiled DNA) of topoisomerase I (**A**) and II (**B**). Partially purified topoisomerases I and II were isolated from L1210 cells using a modification of a previously published procedure (21) as described elsewhere (18). Topoisomerase II relaxation assays (21,22) contained (in 25 μl): 0.15 μg pBR322 DNA, 50 mM Tris-HCl (pH 7.5), 0.4 mM ATP, 50 mM KCl, 5 mM MgCl₂, 0.1 mM EDTA, 0.5 mM dithiothreitol, and 30 μg/ml bovine serum albumin. After addition of drugs and topoisomerase II (0.5 unit) samples were incubated at 37°C (for 10 min). One unit of topoisomerase II was defined as the quantity that fully relaxed 0.15 μg of pBR322 DNA in 15 min. Conditions for topoisomerase I reaction were identical except that samples containing 0.35 μg of pLTL-1 DNA were incubated with 3 units enzyme for 7.5 min in the absence of ATP. One unit of topoisomerase I effected complete relaxation of 0.5 μg supercoiled pLTL-1 DNA in 30 min at 37°C. All reactions were terminated with 0.5% sodium dodecyl sulfate and 50 μg/ml proteinase K followed by addition of EDTA (10 mM) and incubation for 30 minn at 37°C. The samples were electrophoresed on 1% agarose gels, stained with ethidium bromide, and photographed as described previously (23). The amount of DNA in individual bands was determined by densitometry of photographic negatives. The results are expressed as the amounts of fully relaxed form I DNA generated by topoisomerase I and II in the absence and presence of distamycin. Error bars correspond to SEM.

INHIBITION OF CLEAVABLE COMPLEX STABILIZATION IN NUCLEI

Binding of a ligand to the minor groove could influence stabilization of cleavable complex by a topoisomerase-targeted drug in addition to altering the catalytic activities of topological enzymes. Three representative drugs capable of trapping cleavable complexes were examined: (1) VM-26, a non-DNA binder that acts via topoisomerase II, (2) *m*-AMSA, a DNA intercalator also targeted toward topoisomerase II, and (3) camptothecin, targeted toward topoisomerase I. The study was conducted in isolated nuclei and determined the effects of minor-groove binders on DNA lesions that reflect stabilization of cleavable complexes (DNA–protein crosslinks and DNA breaks).

DNA–Protein Crosslinks

Distamycin, Hoechst 33258, and DAPI failed to induce any DNA–protein crosslinks in L1210 nuclei (data not shown). Thus these agents were unable to stabilize cleavable complexes. This observation facilitated the studies in which minor-groove binders were used in combination with drugs that stabilized cleavable complexes.

Addition of distamycin (10–50 μM) to the nuclear reaction decreased in a concentration-dependent manner the crosslinks induced by camptothecin, VM-26, and m-AMSA (Fig. 14.3). The inhibitory effects were also produced by Hoechst 33258 and DAPI. While Hoechst 33258 was less effective than distamycin, DAPI was the least active of all three agents (Fig. 14.3). In addition, 5 μM distamycin produced a small enhancement of VM-26–induced crosslinks. Such enhancement may reflect the previously observed stimulation of topoisomerase activity by low concentrations (1–5 μM) of distamycin (Fig. 14.2). However, Figure 14.3 shows also that camptothecin and m-AMSA–induced DNA–protein crosslinks were inhibited at 5 μM distamycin. While the difference between VM-26 and m-AMSA and camptothecin is consistent, it is unclear whether this result reflects distinct aspects of the action of these drugs.

Further experiments examined the time dependence of distamycin's inhibitory effect on DNA lesions induced by camptothecin and VM-26. The results (Table 14.1) indicated that preformed lesions were unaffected by the addition of distamycin and that formation of new lesions was reduced. Moreover, reversal of camptothecin and VM-26–induced DNA–protein crosslinks in nuclei resuspended in fresh buffer was not inhibited by distamycin (data not shown).

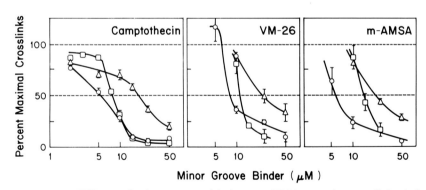

Figure 14.3. Effects of minor-groove binders on DNA–protein crosslinks induced in L1210 nuclei by camptothecin (5 μM), VM-26 (10 μM), or m-AMSA (20 μM): distamycin (open circle); Hoechst 33258 (open box); or DAPI (open triangle). Nuclei were isolated from [2-^{14}C]thymidine labeled leukemia L1210 cells as described elsewhere (19) and suspended in 2 mM KH$_2$PO$_4$, 5 mM MgCl$_2$, 150 mM NaCl, 1 mM EGTA (pH 6.9). In the case of VM-26 and m-AMSA treatments, aliquots of nuclei also contained 0.4 mM ATP. Antitopoisomerase drugs were added to nuclei immediately before the addition of minor-groove binding agents. After incubation at 37°C for 30 min (VM-26 or mAMSA) or for 5 min (camptothecin), the samples were analyzed for DNA–protein crosslinks by coprecipitation with potassium dodecyl sulfate as described previously (19). Maximal crosslinking (100%) corresponded to the effect of camptothecin, VM-26, or m-AMSA in the absence of minor-groove binder and amounted to 40%, 32%, and 39% total DNA, respectively,. Error bars correspond to SEM.

Table 14.1. Effect of Distamycin on Preformed DNA–Protein Crosslinks Induced by Camptothecin or VM-26

Distamycin Added at[a]: (min)	Percent Maximal Crosslinks[b]	
	Camptothecin (5 μM)	VM-26 (10 μM)
0	19	3
1	30	N.D.
4	64	N.D.
5	100	41
10		75
25		91
30		100

[a]Distamycin concentration was 10 μM in camptothecin reactions and 25 μM in VM-26 reactions. Camptothecin or VM-26 were always added at 0 min. Total incubation time with camptothecin or VM-26 was 5 or 30 min, respectively.
[b]Maximal crosslinks corresponded to the effect of camptothecin alone after 5 min incubation or VM-26 alone after 30 min incubation.
N.D.—not determined.

DNA–Strand Breaks

The interference of the minor-groove binders with the stabilization of the cleavable complexes was also evaluated by determining the effects on DNA strand breaks. While distamycin, Hoechst 33258, and DAPI were unable to cleave DNA themselves (data not shown), they inhibited the induction of DNA breaks by camptothecin and VM-26 (Fig. 14.4). Comparable inhibitory effects were seen for topoisomerase I–mediated lesions induced by camptothecin and for topoisomerase II–related cleavage by VM-26. The drug concentration-dependence of DNA breaks inhibition (Fig. 14.4) paralleled the data on inhibition of DNA–protein crosslinks (cf. Fig. 14.3). Again, distamycin was the most potent inhibitor, followed by Hoechst 33258, then DAPI. A similar inhibitory effect was produced by distamycin on DNA breaks induced by another topoisomerase II–targeted drug, *m*-AMSA (data not shown).

Comparison of Minor-Groove Binders' Effects on DNA–Protein Crosslinks and DNA Breaks

To compare the effects of all three minor-groove binders on both types of DNA lesions, the results were expressed as the concentrations of minor-groove binders causing 50% inhibition of topoisomerase I and II–mediated DNA–protein crosslinks and DNA breaks (C_{50}, Table 14.2). DNA lesions induced by different antitopoisomerase drugs were similarly affected by the minor-groove binders. The C_{50} values for DNA–protein crosslinks also showed that distamycin was more potent than Hoechst 33258, while DAPI was the least active. The same order of activity was seen for DNA breaks.

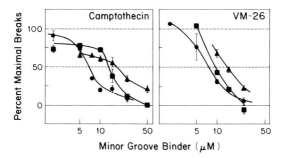

Figure 14.4. Effects of minor-groove binders on DNA single-strand breaks induced in L1210 nuclei by camptothecin (5 µM) and on DNA double-strand breaks induced by VM-26 (10 µM) as determined by the filter elution technique: distamycin (solid circle); Hoechst 33258 (solid square); or DAPI (solid triangle). Nuclei were treated with drugs as described in the legend to Figure 14.1. DNA double-strand breaks were monitored by filter elution under nondenaturing conditions (24). Single-strand breaks were determined similarly except that filter elution was performed at pH 12. Maximal elution (100%) corresponded to DNA cleavage by camptothecin or VM-26 in the absence of minor-groove binder and amounted to 46% and 63% total DNA, respectively. Error bars correspond to SEM. For other details see Figure 14.3.

INHIBITION OF CLEAVABLE COMPLEX STABILIZATION IN INTACT L1210 CELLS

The effects of a minor-groove binder on topoisomerase-mediated DNA lesions in intact cells resemble those in nuclei. Hoechst 33258 significantly inhibited ($p<0.01$) VM-26–induced DNA–protein crosslinks in intact L1210 cells (Table 14.3). This groove binder also inhibited DNA double-strand breaks by VM-26 (Table 14.3).

Table 14.2. Comparison of the Ability of Distamycin, Hoechst 33258, and DAPI to inhibit DNA Lesions Induced in L1210 Cell Nuclei by Camptothecin, VM-26, or *m*-AMSA[a]

	Camptothecin (5 µM)	VM-26 (10 µM)	*m*-AMSA (20 µM)
DNA–protein crosslinks			
Distamycin	5	8	6
Hoechst 33258	8	12	15
DAPI	18	25	22
DNA double-strand breaks			
Distamycin	6	6	3
Hoechst 33258	12	9	N.D.[b]
DAPI	17	13	<<25[c]

[a]The values represent concentrations of minor-groove binders inhibiting formation of DNA–protein crosslinks or DNA double-strand breaks by 50% (C_{50} [µM]).
[b]Not determined.
[c]100% inhibition at 25 µM DAPI.

Table 14.3. Effects of Hoechst 33258 on DNA–Protein Crosslinks and DNA Double-Strand Breaks Induced in Intact L1210 Cells by VM-26[a]

Treatment	DNA–Protein Crosslinks (Fraction Crosslinked[b])	DNA Double-Strand Breaks (Fraction Eluted[c])
No drugs (control)	0.070 ± 0.012	0.058
VM-26 alone	0.618 ± 0.027	0.939
VM-26 and Hoechst 33258	0.420 ± 0.027	0.647

[a]Cells were incubated without or with Hoechst 33258 (50 µM) for 60 min at 37°C followed by addition of VM-26 (10 µM) and further incubation for 30 min.
[b]The cells were analyzed for DNA–protein crosslinks as described for nuclei (cf Figs. 14.1 and 14.2). Hoechst 33258 alone did not induce any DNA–protein crosslinks or DNA breaks (data not shown). The reduction of VM-26–induced crosslinks by Hoechst 33258 was highly significant (p<0.01) as found by paired t-test.
[c]The cells were analyzed for DNA double-strand breaks as described for nuclei by filter elution under nondenaturing conditions. The results represent the fraction of DNA eluted after 60 min.

Our recent study indicated that an analog of Hoechst 33258 modified in one benzimidazole moiety (substitution of pyridine for the benzene ring, obtained from Professor W. Lown, University of Alberta) is an even more potent inhibitor of topoisomerase-mediated lesions in whole cells. On the other hand, distamycin, DAPI, and netropsin failed to produce inhibition in intact cells (unpublished data).

DISCUSSION

Compounds interacting with the minor groove in DNA, such as distamycin, Hoechst 33258, and DAPI, represent a new class of agents interfering with the action of DNA topoisomerases. Our studies demonstrated that the minor-groove binders inhibit (1) the catalytic activity of isolated mammalian topoisomerase I and II, and (2) lesions in nuclear DNA that are mediated by these enzymes. Additionally, distamycin at low concentrations stimulated both enzymes. The effects of all three minor-groove binders on both topoisomerases were similar. Likewise, in nuclei these minor-groove binders did not differentiate between DNA lesions induced by camptothecin (and mediated by topoisomerase I) and the lesions caused by VM-26 and *m*-AMSA, which exemplify two types of topoisomerase II–targeted drugs.

The inhibition of enzyme activities and interference with drug-induced lesions in nuclei are produced by similar drug concentrations in the micromolar range. These low concentrations suggest that the observed effects are not due to a simple saltlike effect of cationic molecules of the minor-groove binders. Also, a series of Hoechst 33258 analogs that exhibit similar ionization states showed profound differences in their abilities to interfere with topoisomerase action. On the other hand, it is likely that the effects of distamycin, Hoechst 33258, and DAPI originate from specific ligand binding in the minor groove, which alters the interaction between topoisomerases and DNA. Such interference has been proposed as an explanation for the inhibitory or stimulatory effects of minor-groove binders on other DNA processive enzymes (10,25–27). For topoisomerases, the stimulation of catalytic activity might reflect enhanced enzyme binding resulting from local alterations in DNA structure. Possibly, the stimulation could be due to DNA bending induced by low levels of distamycin (11). Higher levels of drug bound to DNA would be likely to diminish the accessibility of reaction sites to the enzymes yielding inhibition of topoisomerization. Consistent with this interpretation is the fact that the inhibitory effects of minor-groove binders in nuclei result from the prevention of formation of new lesions. Interestingly, the interference of distamycin, for example, with the action of m-AMSA did not seem to reflect simply prevention of m-AMSA binding to DNA; the level of inhibition (in nuclei) was essentially unchanged when the groove binder was added as the last component of the reaction mixture after allowing m-AMSA to interact with the DNA. While the exact molecular nature of the inhibitory and stimulatory effects of minor-groove binders remains to be determined, some light is shed by a recent independent study by Fesen and Pommier (28). These authors found that distamycin potentiated topoisomerase II cleavage in the proximity of distamycin binding sites while suppressing the cleavage directly at the binding sites (28).

Camptothecin, VM-26, and m-AMSA differ in their target (topoisomerase I or II) as well as in their ability to interact with DNA (only m-AMSA binds to DNA). Conceivably, these drugs may trap cleavable complexes by different mechanisms. In spite of these differences, the response of these drugs to modulation by distamycin, Hoechst 33258, and DAPI was strikingly similar. Thus, minor-groove binders may affect a stage in the formation of DNA lesions that is common to both types of topoisomerases and to each of the topoisomerase-targeted drugs. Possibly, the minor groove is involved in the action of both topoisomerase I and II and, consequently, in the action of drugs that stabilize cleavable complexes.

Interestingly, a recent study of m-AMSA–DNA complexes proposed that the drug's aniline side chain is located in the minor groove at AT sequences while its chromophore intercalates into DNA (29). It has been suggested that this side chain is responsible for the interaction with topoisomerase II, leading to stabilization of the cleavable complex (29). This suggestion is consistent with our findings implying a role for the minor groove in the action of topoisomerases.

The ability of the minor-groove binders to inhibit topoisomerase-mediated DNA–protein crosslinks and DNA breaks correlates with the size of their DNA binding sites: distamycin [5 base pairs (13)] > Hoechst 33258 [4 base pairs (14,15)] > DAPI [3 base pairs (16)]. These correlations again suggest that the observed effects are due to specific, localized interactions with the minor groove.

Distamycin, Hoechst 33258, and DAPI are not the only minor-groove binders with the ability to disturb topoisomerase action. Recently, we observed similar effects for netropsin and two series of novel minor-groove binders obtained from Professor W. Lown (unpublished data). The first series included analogs of Hoechst 33258. Some of these agents were found active not only with isolated enzyme and in nuclei but also in intact cells. The second group comprised netropsin dimers linked with varying numbers of methylene groups. Interestingly, dimeric analogs were typically 5–6 times more potent than monomeric netropsin.

Each of the studied compounds binds preferentially to AT regions (11–16). Binding of topoisomerase I to DNA occurs also at a specific sequence that consists predominantly of A and T (30,31). Possibly, the inhibitory effects of AT-specific ligands are due to blocking such distinct sequences. It remains to be determined if ligands interacting with GC regions would cause effects corresponding to those of AT-specific minor-groove binders.

In conclusion, DNA minor-groove binders appear to be useful as modulators of the action of topoisomerases and topoisomerase-targeted drugs. Additional studies on the relevance of such modulation to cytotoxicity of topoisomerase-targeted drugs might be helpful in providing leads for the mechanism-based development of promising new drug combinations.

Acknowledgments

This work was supported by American Cancer Society Grant CH-293 and National Cancer Institute Grant CA-24538. The authors thank Rita D. Sigmund and Loretta S. Gawron for excellent technical assistance.

REFERENCES

1. Wang, J. C. Recent studies of DNA topoisomerases. Biochim. Biophys. Acta. **909:** 1–9, 1987.
2. Liu, L. F. and Wang, J. C. Supercoiling of the DNA template during transcription. Proc. Natl. Acad. Sci. USA. **84:** 7024–7027, 1987.
3. Drlica, K. and Franco, R. J. Inhibitors of DNA topoisomerases. Biochemistry. **27:** 2253–2259, 1988.
4. Glisson, B. S. and Ross, W. A. DNA topoisomerase II: A primer on the enzyme and its unique role as a multidrug target in cancer chemotherapy. Pharmacol. Ther. **32:** 89–106, 1987.
5. Mattern, M. R., Mong, S.-M., Bartus, H. F., Mirabelli, C. K., Crooke, S. T., and Johnson, R. K. Relationship between the intracellular effects of camptothecin and the inhibition of DNA topoisomerase I in cultured L1210 cells. Cancer Res. **47:** 1793–1798, 1987.
6. Rowe, T., Kupfer, G., and Ross, W. Inhibition of epipodophyllotoxin cytotoxicity by interference with topoisomerase-mediated DNA cleavage. Biochem. Pharmacol. **34:** 2483–2487, 1987.
7. Neidle, S., Pearl, L. H., and Skelly, J. V. DNA structure and perturbation by drug binding. Biochem. J. **243:** 1–13, 1987.
8. Pommier, Y., Covey, J., Kerrigan, D., Mattes, W., Markovits, J., and Kohn, K. W. Role of DNA intercalation in the inhibition of purified mouse leukemia (L1210)

DNA topoisomerase II by 9-aminoacridines. Biochem. Pharmacol. **36:** 3477–3486, 1987.
9. Straney, D. C. and Crothers, D. M. Effect of drug-DNA interactions upon transcription initiation at the *lac* promoter. Biochemistry. **26:** 1987–1995, 1987.
10. Shishido, K., Sakaguchi, R., and Nosoh, Y. Enhancement of S1 nuclease-susceptibility of negatively superhelical DNA by netropsin. Biochem. Biophys. Res. Commun. **124:** 388–392, 1984.
11. Kopka, M. L., Yoon, C., Goodsell, D., Pjura, P., and Dickerson, R. E. The molecular origin of DNA-drug specificity in netropsin and distamycin. Proc. Natl. Acad. Sci. USA. **82:** 1376–1380, 1985.
12. Dattagupta, N., Hogan, M., and Crothers, D. M. Interaction of netropsin and distamycin with deoxyribonucleic acid: Electric dichroic study. Biochemistry. **19:** 5998–6005, 1980.
13. Coll, M., Frederick, C. A., Wang, A. H-J., and Rich, A. A bifurcated hydrogen-bonded conformation in the d(AT) base pairs of the DNA dodecamer d(cgcaaatttgcg) and its complex with distamycin. Proc. Natl. Acad. Sci. USA. **84:** 8385–8389, 1987.
14. Pjura, P. E., Grzeskowiak, K., and Dickerson, R. E. Binding of Hoechst 33258 to the minor groove of B-DNA. J. Mol. Biol. **197:** 257–271, 1987.
15. Teng, M-K., Usman, N., Frederick, C.

A., and Wang, A. H-J. The molecular structure of the complexes of Hoechst 33258 and the DNA dodecamer d(CGGAATTCGCG). Nucleic Acids Res. **16:** 2671–2690, 1988.

16. Manzini, G., Barcellona, M. L., Avitabile, M., and Quadrifoglio, F. Interaction of diamidino-2-phenylindole (DAPI) with natural and synthetic nucleic acids. Nucleic Acids Res. **11:** 8861–8876, 1983.

17. McHugh, M. M., Woynarowski, J. M., Sigmund, R. D., and Beerman, T. A. The effect of minor groove binding drugs on mammalian topoisomerase I activity. Biochem. Pharmacol. **38:** 2323–2328, 1989.

18. Woynarowski, J. M., McHugh, M. M., Sigmund, R. D., and Beerman, T. A. Modulation of topoisomerase II catalytic activity by DNA minor groove binding agents distamycin, Hoechst 33258, and 4′,6-diamidine-2-phenylindole. Mol. Pharmacol. **35:** 177–182, 1989.

19. Woynarowski, J. M., Sigmund, R. D., and Beerman, T. A. DNA minor-groove binding agents interfere with topoisomerase II-mediated lesions induced by epipodophyllotoxin derivative VM-26 and acridine derivative m-AMSA in nuclei from L1210 cells. Biochemistry. **28:** 3850–3855, 1989.

20. McHugh, M. M., Sigmund, R. D., and Beerman, T. A. The effect of minor groove binding drugs on camptothecin induced DNA lesions in L1210 nuclei. Biochem. Pharmacol. **39:** 707–714, 1990.

21. Miller, K. G., Liu, L. F., and Englund, P. T. A homogeneous type II DNA topoisomerase from HeLa cell nuclei. J. Biol. Chem. **256:** 9334–9339, 1981.

22. Osheroff, N., Shelton, E. R., and Brutlag, D. L. DNA topoisomerase II from Drosophila melanogaster: Relaxation of supercoiled DNA. J. Biol. Chem. **258:** 9356–9543, 1983.

23. Grimwade, J. E., and Beerman, T. A.

Measurement of bleomycin, neocarzinostatin, and auromomycin cleavage of cell-free and intracellular Simian Virus 40 DNA and chromatin. Mol. Pharmacol. **30:** 358–363, 1986.

24. Bradley, M. O. and Kohn, K. W. X-ray induced DNA double strand breaks production and repair in mammalian cells as measured by neutral filter elution. Nucleic Acids Res. **7:** 793–804, 1979.

25. Zimmer, C. Effects of the antibiotics netropsin and distamycin A on the structure and function of nucleic acids. Progress Nucl. Acid. Mol. Biol. **15:** 285–318, 1975.

26. Bruzik, J. P., Auble, D. T., and deHaseth, P. L. Specific activation of transcription initiation by the sequence-specific DNA-binding agents distamycin A and netropsin. Biochemistry. **26:** 950–956, 1987.

27. Fox, K. R. and Waring, M. J. DNA structural variations produced by actinomycin and distamycin as revealed by DNAase footprinting. Nucleic Acids Res. **12:** 9271–9285, 1984.

28. Fesen, M. and Pommier, Y. Mammalian topoisomerase II activity is modulated by the DNA minor groove binder distamycin in Simian Virus 40 DNA. J. Biol. Chem. **264:** 11354–11359, 1989.

29. Chen, K-X., Gresh, N., and Pullman, B. Energetics and stereochemistry of DNA complexation with the antitumor AT specific intercalators tilorone and m-AMSA. Nucleic Acids Res. **16:** 3061–3073, 1988.

30. Thomsen, B., Mollerup, S., Bonven, B. J., Frank, R., Blocker, H., Nielsen, O. F., and Westergaard, O. Sequence specificity of DNA topoisomerase I in the presence and absence of camptothecin. EMBO J. **6:** 1817–1823, 1987.

31. Busk, H., Thomsen, B., Bonven, B. J., Kjeldsen, E., Nielson, O. F., and Westergaard, O. Preferential relaxation of supercoiled DNA containing a hexadecameric recognition sequence for topoisomerase I. Nature. **327:** 638–640, 1987.

Chapter 15

DNA Sequence at Sites of Topoisomerase I Cleavage Induced by Camptothecin in SV40 DNA

CHRISTINE JAXEL, GIOVANNI CAPRANICO,
KARSTEN WASSERMANN,
DONNA KERRIGAN,
KURT W. KOHN, AND YVES POMMIER

Two types of eukaryotic DNA topoisomerases have been identified (for review, see 1,2): type I DNA topoisomerases, which break transiently duplex DNA one strand at a time; and type II DNA topoisomerases, which break both strands in concert. Cellular content of topoisomerase II increases during cell proliferation and during the S-phase of the cell cycle (3–5). Topoisomerase II is essential for DNA replication (6), for condensation–decondensation of chromosomal DNA during the cell cycle (7), and for chromosome segregation during mitosis (8,9). This could be related to the observation that topoisomerase II is a major structural protein of the nuclear matrix for interphase nuclei and of the scaffold of mitotic chromosomes (10).

In contrast, cellular content of topoisomerase I is less variable during cell cycle (11), and topoisomerase I activity is required for DNA replication elongation (6,12) and transcription (13,14).

At the present time, camptothecin is the only antitumor drug known to inhibit topoisomerase I specifically. Camptothecin is a plant alkaloid (15,16) that has a strong antitumor activity against a wide range of experimental tumors (16). It produces reversible topoisomerase I–mediated single-strand breakage in cellular DNA (17) followed by RNA and DNA syntheses inhibition (18) and subsequently by an irreversible DNA fragmentation (19). The antitumor activity of camptothecin is related to topoisomerase I inhibition (20,21). Camptothecin inhibits purified topoisomerase I by stimulating the formation of topoisomerase I–DNA cleavable complexes and inhibiting the enzyme catalytic activity (20,22). Camptothecin has been used to show the involvement of topoisomerase I in SV40 DNA replication (11,23) and transcription and to map topoisomerase I cleavage sites in active genes from different cellular systems (24–26).

In order to investigate the interaction of camptothecin with topoisomerase I, we have sequenced the cleavage sites of purified mouse leukemia topoisomerase I in SV40 DNA. We have used SV40 DNA for three main reasons. First, the SV40 genome is well known in terms of structural and functional characteristics. Second, it forms minichromosomes that are replicated as the cellular DNA by using cellular enzymes including topoisomerases. And third, the cleavage pattern induced by topoisomerases and drugs in this small viral DNA can be easily compared in a purified system *in vitro* and in the cell *in vivo*.

MATERIALS AND METHODS

Materials, Enzymes, and Drug

SV40 DNA, Ban I and Hpa II restriction enzymes, and agarose were purchased from Bethesda Research Laboratories (Gaithersburg, MD). Fok I restriction enzyme and Klenow polymerase were purchased from Biolabs and Pharmacia, respectively. Polyacrylamide and [^{32}P]-alpha-dGTP were purchased from Bio-Rad, Inc. (Richmond, CA) and New England Research Products (Boston, MA), respectively. Autoradiographies were performed with XAR-5 films (Eastman Kodak Company, Rochester, NY).

Type I and type II DNA topoisomerases were purified from mouse leukemia (L1210) cells, as described previously (27). One unit of topoisomerase I was defined as the amount of enzyme yielding 70% of closed circular-relaxed SV40 DNA (0.14 μg) in 10 min at 37°C (20). One unit of topoisomerase II was the amount of enzyme yielding 90% DNA relaxation in 30 min at 37°C.

Camptothecin was provided by Drs. Wani and Wall (Research Triangle Institute, Research Triangle Park, NC).

Labeling Procedures of SV40 DNA

[^{32}P]-end-labeled SV40 DNA was prepared as follows: first, the DNA was linearized with Ban I restriction endonuclease at position 295 of the genome and its termini were labeled with [^{32}P]-alpha-dGTP and Klenow polymerase; then, [^{32}P]-end-labeled DNA was cut with Hpa II restriction endonuclease at position 347. Such a procedure generates two [^{32}P]-3'-end-labeled fragments, one of 5191 base pairs and the other of 52 base pairs. Therefore, any DNA fragment longer than 53 base pairs could be localized unequivocally in the SV40 genome, as only one strand remains [^{32}P]-labeled.

In order to prepare the smaller DNA fragment (137 bp) containing the major topoisomerase I cleavage site, SV40 DNA was cut with Fok I restriction endonuclease, 3'-end labeled with [^{32}P]-alpha-dGTP and the 4912-5049 fragment was separated by electroelution after electrophoresis on a 6% polyacrylamide gel. This fragment will be referred as Fok I DNA. Since only one of the DNA termini (nucleotide 5049) of the 4912-5049 fragment was labeled, the isolated 4912-5049 fragment could be used directly for DNA sequencing.

DNA Cleavage Assays

Reactions were performed in 30 μl reaction buffer (0.01 M Tris-HCl, pH 7.5, 0.15 M KCl, 5 mM $MgCl_2$, 0.1 mM EDTA, 15 μg/ml bovine serum albumin). Approximately 0.04 μg and 0.002 μg of [^{32}P]-3′-end-labeled Ban I-Hpa II fragment and Fok I fragment, respectively, were incubated with 220 units of topoisomerase I, or 10 units of topoisomerase II for 30 min at 37°C. Reactions were stopped by adding sodium dodecyl sulfate ($NaDodSO_4$), EDTA, and proteinase K (1%, 20 mM, and 0.5 mg/ml, respectively) and incubated for an additional 60 min at 37°C. After extraction with phenol-chloroform, samples were submitted to either agarose or DNA sequencing gel electrophoresis as described previously (28).

RESULTS

Topoisomerase-Mediated DNA Breaks Induced by Anticancer Drugs in SV40 DNA

Figure 15.1A shows the DNA single-strand breakage produced by topoisomerases I and II in the absence or presence of different antitumor drugs. Topoisomerase I in the absence of drug produced very few breaks (lane 3). In the presence of camptothecin (lane 4), however, the enzyme cleaved the DNA at discrete sites, including a single major site (arrow). The SV40 fragment used covered nearly the entire SV40 genome (5191 bp, nucleotides 295-347 deleted). Camptothecin had no effect upon topoisomerase II (compare lanes 5 and 6). The topoisomerase II inhibitors, m-AMSA, VM-26, and 2-methyl-9-hydroxyellipticinium, stimulated topoisomerase II–mediated DNA cleavage (lanes 7–9) but did not stimulate cleavage in the case of topoisomerase I (data not shown). The topoisomerase II inhibitors did not stimulate a predominant cleavage site such as was induced by topoisomerase I plus camptothecin.

Figure 15.1B examines DNA double-strand cleavage produced by topoisomerases I and II. Topoisomerase I by itself produced little or no double-strand cleavage (lane 3) and camptothecin produced only slight cleavage (lane 4). Thus camptothecin induces predominantly single-strand breaks in this system. By contrast, topoisomerase II produced double-strand cleavage that was markedly increased by m-AMSA, VM-26, and 2-methyl-9-hydroxyellipticinium (lanes 7–9) and was not affected by camptothecin (lane 6).

The genomic localization of the DNA cleavage sites observed in Figure 15.1 was determined after densitometer scanning of the autoradiographies and computer analysis. The major sites induced by camptothecin was estimated to be localized at position 4928 ($\pm$ 30 base pairs) under DNA denaturing conditions, and 4985 under neutral conditions (28). The comparison of the DNA cleavage profiles under DNA denaturing conditions showed that camptothecin increased DNA cleavage at preexisting topoisomerase I sites. However, this increase was much stronger at some sites than at others. Camptothecin thus alters the distribution pattern of topoisomerase I–mediated DNA breaks.

DNA Sequence Selectivity of Topoisomerase I–Mediated DNA Cleavage Induced by Camptothecin in Purified DNA

In order to sequence the preferential topoisomerase I cleavage sites induced by camptothecin in SV40 DNA, the Ban I-Hpa II fragment (3′-end-labeled at the Ban I site) was first used (Fig. 15.2A). This fragment enabled us to study the location of topoisomerase I–mediated DNA breaks in the region spanning the SV40 origin of replication and transcription (see Fig. 15.4).

Three main DNA cleavage sites were induced by camptothecin (arrows). Two of them were easily localized at positions 127 and 199 of the genome. These two sites have the same DNA sequence: 5′-AGAT/GCATGCTTTGC-3′

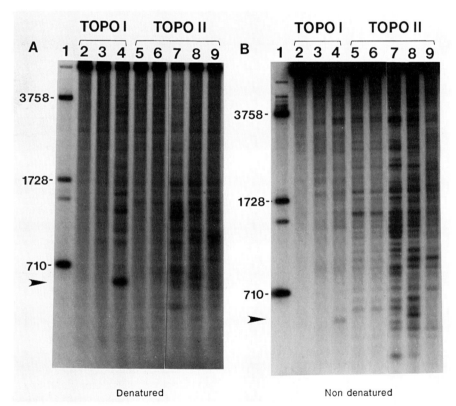

Figure 15.1. Cleavage sites induced by topoisomerase I or II in the presence of antitumor drugs in a fragment of SV40 DNA. **Panel A.** Single-strand cleavage sites (DNA denatured in 145 mM NaOH). **Panel B.** Double-strand cleavage sites (samples as in panel A, but not denatured). Lanes 2, DNA alone. Lanes 3, DNA plus topoisomerase I; lanes 4, same with 10 μM camptothecin added. Lanes 5, DNA plus topoisomerase II; lanes 6–9, same with 10 μM camptothecin (lanes 6), 10 μM m-AMSA (lanes 7), 10 μM VM-26 (lanes 8), or 1 μM 2-methyl-9-hydroxyellipticinium (lanes 9). Incubation times with topoisomerase with or without drugs were 30 min at 37°C. The DNA fragment (5191 bp, Ban I-Hpa II) was 3′-[^{32}P]-end labeled at the Ban I site. Electrophoresis in 1% agarose gels. Lanes 1, size markers as indicated. Arrowhead, major camptothecin-induced cleavage site.

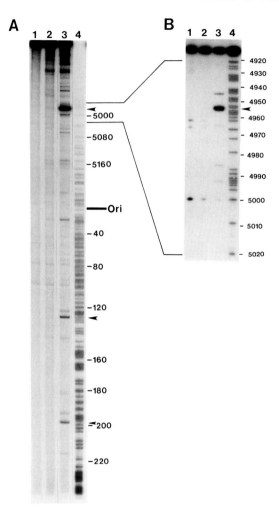

Figure 15.2. DNA sequence locations of camptothecin-induced topoisomerase I–mediated cleavage sites. In **panel A,** reactions were performed with the Ban I-Hpa II SV40 DNA fragment (5191 bp, genomic positions 295-347), and in **panel B** with the Fok I fragment (137 bp, genomic positions 4912-5049). In both cases, DNA fragments (lanes 1) were reacted with topoisomerase I in the absence (lanes 2) or in the presence of 10 μM camptothecin (lanes 3). Lanes 4 are purine sequencing lanes (formic acid treatment). Ori is the position of SV40 replication origin. Arrows indicate the most intense sites of camptothecin-induced cleavage.

(the slash indicates the location of the break), and are at corresponding positions in the two 72 bp repeats (Fig. 15.4).

The third site of cleavage, which was more intense and is the predominant site, was localized around position 4955. This site was sequenced precisely by using a 137 bp fragment 3′-end-labeled at position 5049 (Fok I DNA) (see Materials and Methods). This major site of cleavage was localized at position 4955 of SV40 genome (Fig. 15.2B, arrow) in the sequence: 5′-TGAT/GAGCATATTTT-3′.

Table 15.1 shows the available sequence data for known camptothecin-

Table 15.1. DNA Consensus Sequence of Topoisomerase I Cleavage Sites

−5	−4	−3	−2	−1	+1	+2	+3	+4	+5	+6	+7	+8	+9	+10	DNA (position)	CPT[a]	Ref
G	T	A	A	T	G	A	C	T	A	A	C	A	T	T	SV40 (4955)	+	(28)
T	G	C	G	T	G	C	T	G	G	T	G	T	T	G	SV40 (127,199)	+	(28)
G	A	G	C	T	G	G	G	A	A	A	C	A	G	C	pBR (113)[b]	+	(29)
C	A	G	A	T	G	A	G	C	G	G	C	C	C	G	pBR (128)[b]	+	(29)
A	A	T	C	T	G	A	A	A	A	A	A	A	A	A	pNCI (187)	+	(29)
G	C	C	G	T	G	G	C	C	C	C	C	G	C	C	pNCI (208)	+	(29)
A	A	A	A	T	G	A	G	T	C	C	G	T	C	A	rDNA (847)[b]	+	(31)
G	T	T	G	A	A	G	T	A	T	A	A	C	C		rDNA (1041)[b]	+	(31)
C	T	T	C	T	T	G	C	A	C	C	T	A	T	C	rDNA (840)	+	(31)
		$\frac{A}{T}$	$\frac{G}{C}$	T				$\frac{A}{T}$							SV40 consensus	−	(32)
		$\frac{A}{T}$	$\frac{G}{A}$	T	G		$\frac{A}{T}$	T	A						SV40 consensus	+	(34)
A	A	C	T	T	A	G	A	A	A	A	A	T	T	T	rDNA	−	(30)

[a]CPT: camptothecin was either present (+) or absent (−) in the topoisomerase I cleavage reactions.
[b]Indicates the lower DNA strand.

induced topoisomerase I cleavage sites (28–34). In seven of nine camptothecin-induced sites, including the two independent sites that we have sequenced in SV40, the break is between T and G in the sequence 5'-TG-3'. In at least eight of the nine reported instances, the 3' terminal nucleotide to which the topoisomerase I molecule becomes covalently attached when the break is formed is a T. This suggests that a 3' terminal T is a specific structural requirement in the stabilized ternary cleavage complex, DNA–camptothecin–topoisomerase I. In addition, at least eight of the nine sites have a G at position -3, and this may also be an invariant. Seven of the nine sites have G at $+1$, and eight sites have a purine at -2. Hence the current evidence suggests a consensus sequence for camptothecin-induced topoisomerase I cleavage sites of 5'-GRTG-3' (R = purine), the cleavage being between the TG dinucleotide and the topoisomerase being covalently linked to the T.

Camptothecin Enhances DNA Cleavage Mediated by Topoisomerase I at Specific Sites

In order to determine whether camptothecin induces topoisomerase I to create new DNA cleavage sites or enhances DNA cleavage sites of the enzyme alone, we attempted to optimize the conditions of DNA cleavage by the enzyme alone. First, we showed that in the presence of low salt (50 mM Na/KCl), the main camptothecin-induced DNA cleavage site (4955) was produced to a small extent, even in the absence of camptothecin (28). Under these conditions, topoisomerase I produced a discernible cleavage pattern of Fok I DNA in the absence of camptothecin (Fig. 15.3, lane 1). Camptothecin affected topoisomerase I–induced DNA cleavage in three ways (Fig. 15.3, lane 2): (1) it increased some of the cleavage sites (4955, 4965, 4985); (2) it did not change the 4976 site; and finally, (3) it decreased two sites (4997, 5006). This observation is in agreement with the results of Kjeldsen et al. (29).

Even if all these sites do not correspond to the consensus sequence (Fig. 15.3, Table 15.1), these results indicate that camptothecin does not induce new topoisomerase I cleavage sites but rather increases markedly DNA cleavage at some of the sites generated by topoisomerase I alone.

The finding that the sites of topoisomerase I cleavage induced by camptothecin correspond to cleavage sites detected in the absence of drug is consistent with the hypothesis that camptothecin inhibits topoisomerase I by stabilizing the cleavage intermediates of topoisomerase I reactions. The stabilization of the enzyme presumably results in the inhibition of its catalytic reaction of DNA relaxation by an inhibition of its turnover (20,22).

It is important to note that the presence of a GATG sequence is not sufficient for topoisomerase I trapping by camptothecin, since some GATG sequences of SV40 DNA were not cleaved by topoisomerase I and camptothecin (Table 15.2). This suggests that other DNA sequences are required for topoisomerase I recognition.

Further consideration of the DNA region between positions 4912 and 243 (Fig. 15.4) yielded another interesting finding. Figure 15.4 shows the principal characteristics of the studied SV40 DNA region; particularly, the alternating

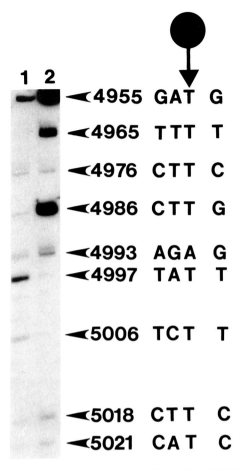

Figure 15.3. Comparison between topoisomerase I–mediated DNA cleavage induced in the absence and presence of camptothecin. The SV40 DNA Fok I fragment (137 bp, genomic positions 4912-5049) was reacted with 145 units topoisomerase I in the absence (lane 1) and in the presence of 10 μM camptothecin (lane 2).

Table 15.2. DNA Sequence Determinants of Camptothecin-Induced DNA Cleavage

SV40 Sites[a]	GAT G[b]	A/T,G/A,T/A,T G[c]	Purine/Pyrimidine[d]
4955	+	+	[4958–4963]
4965	−	−	[4958–4963]
4985	−	−	[4986–4991]
20	−	−	[12–17]
122	−	+	[126–133]
127	+	+	[126–133]
144	−	−	[136–142]
194	−	+	[198–205]
199	+	+	[198–205]
216	−	−	[208–214]

[a]Nucleotide covalently linked to topoisomerase I.
[b]Consensus DNA sequence of cleavage determined in the presence of camptothecin in the present study (28).
[c]Consensus DNA sequence of cleavage determined in the presence of camptothecin in SV40 by Porter and Champoux (34).
[d]First and last nucleotides of alternating purine/pyrimidines sequences of at least six nucleotides.
In the studied SV40 sequence [4912–243], 2 GATG sequences (positions 5039 and 83) and 1 A/T,G/A,T/A,T G sequence (position 4924) were uncut.

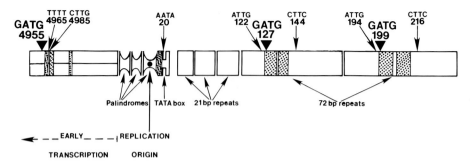

Figure 15.4. Cleavage sites induced by topoisomerase I with camptothecin within the regulatory region of SV40 DNA (between positions 4912 and 243). The structural and functional characteristics of this region are indicated. Dashed boxes represent the alternating purine-pyrimidine sequences (> six nucleotides).

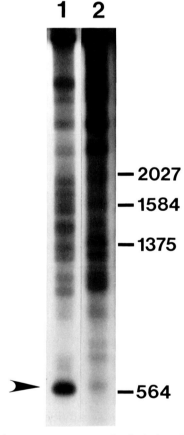

Figure 15.5. Effect of nucleosomes on camptothecin-induced topoisomerase I cleavage sites. The Ban I-Hpa II SV40 DNA fragment (5191 bp, genomic positons 295–347, 3'-[^{32}P]-end label) was reconstituted with purified mononucleosomes. The free (lane 1) or nucleosome-reconstituted (lane 2) DNA was reacted with topoisomerase I in the presence of 10 μM camptothecin. Samples were denatured prior to electrophoresis.

purine-pyrimidine ($>$ 6 nucleotides; dashed boxes). Less than 4 nucleotides away from each of these alternating purine-pyrimidines was a topoisomerase I cleavage site induced by camptothecin (Fig. 15.4, Table 15.2). These particular sequences may interact with camptothecin, topoisomerase I, or both. Fukada has reported that camptothecin by itself is able to bind to Z-DNA structures under particular conditions (35). Such structures are often found within the regulatory regions of active genes and have been implicated in controlling transcription. However, it is unlikely that the alternating purine-pyrimidines sequences shown in Figure 15.4 were in a Z configuration under our experimental conditions (reactions in low salt and in the absence of DNA supercoiling). Nevertheless, the location of potentially Z-DNA forming sequences near topoisomerase I sites could have a functional significance.

Influence of Nucleosomes Upon Camptothecin-Induced DNA Cleavage

In order to study the influence of chromatin structure on camptothecin-induced DNA cleavage, we reconstituted SV40 nucleosomal DNA by using the Ban I-Hpa II labeled DNA fragment and mononucleosomes from HeLa cells (36). In the nucleosome-reconstituted fragment, the major camptothecin site (4955) was completely suppressed (Fig. 15.5, compare lanes 2 and 1). Mapping of the nucleosomes positions by micrococcal nuclease digestion (not shown) indicated that this region formed a nucleosome between positions 4814 and 5042 (37). The suppression of camptothecin cleavage probably results from the presence of this nucleosome, which does not permit the binding of topoisomerase I at its preferential site and its trapping by camptothecin. It may be that the binding of topoisomerase I to its preferential site involves a dynamic state of chromatin, such as may occur during replication or transcription.

DISCUSSION

DNA topoisomerase I may release torsional stress in chromatin by relaxing DNA through transient single-strand breaks at specific DNA sequences (present study, 28–34). Since the frequency of occurrence of these sequences is high, it is likely that topoisomerase I can act in most regions of the genome. DNA torsional stress has been shown to accumulate as a result of transcription and replication (38). During replication, topoisomerase I probably acts as a swivel and seems to be located in the near proximity of replication forks (23,39,40). In addition, the finding of a high density of camptothecin-induced cleavage sites at the replication termination region of SV40 suggests that topoisomerase I might be involved in the separation of daughter molecules at the end of replication (34,41). Kerrigan et al. have isolated an unusual topoisomerase I from cells resistant to topoisomerase II inhibitors; the topoisomerase II being apparently unmodified (42). This topoisomerase I was able to decatenate kDNA, a function similar to the decatenation of daughter DNA molecules at the end of the replication, a role usually attributed to the topoisomerase II.

It has also been shown that topoisomerase I is involved in transcription (24–26,30,31,43), that the amount of cellular enzyme is related to the genetic expression (24), and that the camptothecin-induced DNA breaks are concentrated in transcribed region (24). In addition, Garg et al. have shown that camptothecin inhibits supercoiled rDNA transcription but not that of linear rDNA (26). Nevertheless, similar patterns of DNA cleavage were obtained in supercoiled and linear SV40 DNA (28). These two results together suggest that this is not only the blockage of RNA polymerase by camptothecin-trapped topoisomerase I–DNA abortive complex but also the absence of a "swivel" in the DNA, which blocks transcription.

The *in vivo* experiments of Porter and Champoux have studied the SV40 DNA cleavage produced by camptothecin in infected cells (34). Two main regions of the SV40 genome were analyzed: the origin (nucleotides 4745 to 500) and the termination of replication (nucleotides 2025 to 3020). In each one, strong cleavage sites were induced by camptothecin. Our major cleavage site localized at position 4955 was also observed in this study, suggesting that this site may, at least part of the time, be free of nucleosomes *in vivo*.

In addition, Porter and Champoux have observed a DNA strand preference of camptothecin-induced cleavage sites both in the origin and termination regions of SV40 genome. Cleavage sites were found almost exclusively on the template strand for discontinuous DNA synthesis (34). In fact, by analyzing

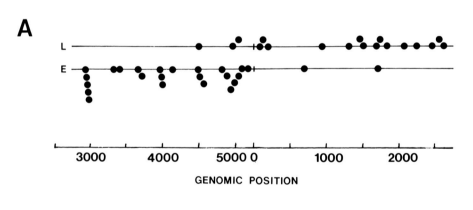

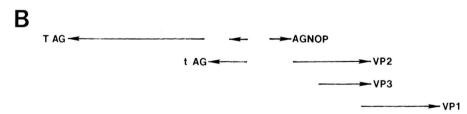

Figure 15.6. A. Distribution of topoisomerase I recognition sequence (GATG) in SV40 DNA (L: late strand; E: early strand) (see text). **B.** Relation to transcripts. Abbreviations: T AG, large t antigen; t AG, small t antigen; AGNOP, agnoprotein; VP, viral capsid protein. Arrows to the left indicate early transcripts and to the right late transcripts.

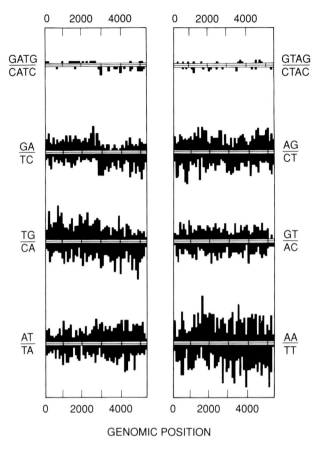

Figure 15.7. Asymmetry of the distribution of GATG sequences (**upper panels**), and comparison of the dinucleotide frequency in SV40 DNA. Each strand is represented above and under a line indicating the genomic positions.

the primary DNA sequence of SV40, it appears that the distribution of GATG sequences corresponds to that of the topoisomerase I cleavage sites observed by Porter and Champoux (34): on the late strand (same sense as the late mRNA), there are 14 GATG sites between nucleotides 0 and 2620 versus 3 between nucleotides 2621 and 5243, but on the early strand (complementary strand), there are 2 GATG sequences between nucleotides 0 and 2620 versus 21 between nucleotides 2621 and 5243 (Fig. 15.6A). This asymmetry coincides with the late and early transcription regions of SV40 DNA; late transcription proceeds from left to right in the first half of the genome, and early transcription proceeds from right to left in the second half of the genome (Fig. 15.6B). The asymmetry of GATG sequences in SV40 is at least in part attributable to asymmetries in dinucleotide frequencies (GA and TG, Fig. 15.7). These sequence asymmetries are not evident in the genomes of polyoma virus or lymphotrophic papovavirus. The dinucleotide asymmetries in SV40 appear to be dependent upon the reading frame (data not shown). Although the origin of the sequence asymmetries in SV40 is not clear, the asymmetries may affect the distribution of topoisomerase sites.

Acknowledgments

This work was supported by awards from the Associazione Italiana per la Ricerca sul Cancro and from the EORTC-NCI Research Training Program.

REFERENCES

1. Wang, J. C. DNA topoisomerases. Annu. Rev. Biochem. **54**: 665–697, 1985.
2. Osheroff, N. Biochemical basis for the interactions of type I and type II topoisomerases with DNA. Pharmacol. Ther. **41**: 223–241, 1989.
3. Duguet, M., Lavenot, C., Harper, F., Mirambeau, G., and De Recondo, A. M. DNA topoisomerases from rat liver: Physiological variations. Nucleic Acids Res. **11**: 1059–1075, 1983.
4. Taudou, G., Mirambeau, G., Lavenot, C., Der Garabedian, A., Vermeersch, J., and Duguet, M. DNA topoisomerase activities in convanavalin A-stimulated lymphocytes. FEBS Lett. **176**: 431–435, 1984.
5. Markovits, J., Pommier, Y., Kerrigan, D., Covey, J. M., Tilchen, E. J., and Kohn, K. W. Topoisomerase II-mediated DNA breaks and cytotoxicity in relation to cell proliferation and the cell cycle in NIH 3T3 fibroblasts and L1210 leukemia cells. Cancer Res. **47**: 2050–2055, 1987
6. Yang, L., Wold, M. S., Li, J. J., Kelly, T. J., and Liu, L. F. Roles of DNA topoisomerases in simian virus 40 DNA replication *in vitro*. Proc. Natl. Acad. Sci. USA. **84**: 950–954, 1987.
7. Newport, J. Nuclear reconstitution *in vitro*: Stages of assembly around protein-free DNA. Cell. **48**: 205–217, 1987.
8. Holm, C., Goto, T., Wang, J. C., and Boldstein, D. DNA topoisomerase II is required at the time of mitosis in yeast. Cell. **41**: 553–563, 1985.
9. Uemura, T., Ohkura, H., Adachi, Y., Morino, K., Shiozaki, K., and Yanagida, M. DNA topoisomerase II is required for condensation and separation of mitotic chromosomes in *S. pombe*. Cell. **50**: 917–925, 1987.
10. Heck, M.M.S. and Earnshaw, W. C. Topoisomerase II: A specific marker for cell proliferation. J. Cell. Biol. **103**: 2569–2581, 1986.
11. Hsiang, Y-H. and Liu, L. F. Identification of mammalian DNA topoisomerase I as an intracellular target of the anticancer drug camptothecin. Cancer Res. **48**: 1722–1726, 1988.
12. Kim, R.A., and Wang, J.C. Function of DNA topoisomerases as replication swivels in *Saccharomyces cerevisiae*. J. Mol. Biol. **208**: 257–267, 1989.
13. Weisbrod, S. Properties of active nucleosomes as revealed by HMG 14 and 17 chromatography. Nucleic Acids Res. **10**: 2017–2042, 1982.
14. Fleischmann, G., Pflugfelder, G., Steiner, E. K., Javaherian, K., Howard, G. C., Wang, J. C., and Elgin, S.C.R. Drosophila DNA topoisomerase I is associated with transcriptionally active regions of the genome. Proc. Natl. Acad. Sci. USA. **81**: 6958–6962, 1984.
15. Wall, M. E., Wani, M. C., Cooke, C. E., Palmer, K. H., Mc Phail, A. T., and Sim, G. A. Plant antitumor agents. I. The isolation and structure of camptothecin, a novel alkaloidal leukemia and tumor inhibitor from *Camptotheca acuminata*. J. Am. Chem. Soc. **88**: 3888–3890, 1966.
16. Wall, M. E. A new look at older drug in cancer treatment: Natural products. Med. Pediatr. Oncol. **11**: 480A–489A, 1983.
17. Covey, J. M., Jaxel, C., Kohn, K. W., and Pommier, Y. Protein-linked DNA strand breaks induced in mammalian cells by camptothecin, an inhibitor of topoisomerase I. Cancer Res., **49**: 5016–5022, 1989.
18. Horwitz, M. S. and Horwitz, S. B. Intracellular degradation of HeLa and adenovirus type 2 DNA induced by camptothecin. Biochem. Biophys. Res. Commun. **45**: 723–727, 1971.
19. Jaxel, C., Taudou, G., Portemer, C., Mirambeau, G., Panijel, J., and Duguet, M. Topoisomerase inhibitors induce irreversible fragmentation of replicated DNA in concanavalin A stimulated splenocytes. Biochemistry. **27**: 95–99, 1988.
20. Jaxel, C., Kohn, K. W., Wani, M. C., Wall, M. E., and Pommier, Y. Structure-activity study of the actions of campto-

thecin derivatives on mammalian topoisomerase I: Evidence for a specific receptor site and a relation to antitumor activity. Cancer Res. **49:** 1465–1469, 1989.

21. Andoh, T., Ishii, K., Suzuki, Y., Ikegami, Y., Kusunoki, Y., Takemoto, Y., and Okada, K. Characterization of a mammalian mutant with a camptothecin resistant DNA topoisomerase I. Proc. Natl. Acad. Sci. USA. **84:** 5565–5569, 1987.

22. Hsiang, Y-H., Hertzberg, R., Hecht, S., and Liu, L. F. Camptothecin induces protein-linked DNA breaks via mammalian DNA topoisomerase I. J. Biol. Chem. **260:** 14873–14878, 1985.

23. Snapka, R. M. Topoisomerase inhibitors can selectively interfere with different stages of simian virus 40 DNA replication. Mol. Cell. Biol. **6:** 4221–4227, 1986.

24. Gilmour, D. S. and Elgin, S.C.R. Localization of specific topoisomerase I interactions within the transcribed region of active heat shock genes by using the inhibitor camptothecin. Mol. Cell. Biol. **7:** 141–148, 1987.

25. Stewart, A. F. and Schutz, G. Camptothecin-induced *in vivo* topoisomerase I cleavages in the transcriptionally active tyrosine aminotransferase gene. Cell. **50:** 1109–1117, 1987.

26. Garg, L. C., DiAngelo, S., and Jacob, S. T. Role of DNA topoisomerase I in the transcription of supercoiled rRNA gene. Proc. Natl. Acad. Sci. USA. **84:** 3185–3188, 1987.

27. Minford, J., Pommier, Y., Filipski, J., Kohn, K. W., Kerrigan, D., Mattern, M., Michaels, S., Schwartz, R., and Zwelling, L. A. Isolation of intercalator-dependent protein-linked DNA strand cleavage activity from cell nuclei and identification as topoisomerase II. Biochemistry. **25:** 9–16, 1986.

28. Jaxel, C., Kohn, K. W., and Pommier, Y. Topoisomerase I interaction with SV40 DNA in the presence and absence of camptothecin. Nucleic Acids Res. **16:** 11157–11170, 1988.

29. Kjeldsen, E., Mollerup, S., Thomsen, B., Bonven, B. J., Bolund, L., and Westergaard, O. Sequence-dependent effect of camptothecin on human topoisomerase I DNA cleavage. J. Mol. Biol. **202:** 333–342, 1988.

30. Busk, H., Thomsen, B., Bonven, B. J., Kjeldsen, E., Nielsen, O. F., and Westergaard, O. Preferential relaxation of supercoiled DNA containing a hexadecameric recognition sequence for topoisomerase I. Nature. **327:** 638–640, 1987.

31. Culotta, V. and Sollner-Webb, B. Sites of topoisomerase I action on *X. laevis* ribosomal chromatin: Transcriptionally active rDNA has an 200 bp repeating structure. Cell. **52:** 585–597, 1988.

32. Been, M. D., Burgess, R. R., and Champoux, J. J. Nucleotide sequence preference at rat liver and wheat germ type I DNA topoisomerase breakage sites in duplex SV40 DNA. Nucleic Acids Res. **12:** 3097–3114, 1984.

33. Bonven, B. J., Gocke, E., and Westergaard, O. A high affinity topoisomerase I binding sequence is clustered at DNAase I hypersensitive sites in *Tetrahymena* R-chromatin. Cell. **41:** 541–555, 1985.

34. Porter, S. E. and Champoux, J. J. Mapping *in vivo* topoisomerase I sites on simian virus 40 DNA: Asymmetric distribution of sites on replicating molecules. Mol. Cell. Biol. **9:** 541–550, 1989.

35. Fukada, M. Action of camptothecin and its derivatives on deoxyribonucleic acid. Biochem. Pharmacol. **34:** 5944–5947, 1985.

36. Drew, H. R. and Mc Call, M. J. Structural analysis of a reconstituted DNA containing three histone octamers and histone H5. J. Mol. Biol. **197:** 485–511, 1987.

37. Capranico, G., Jaxel, C., Roberge, M., Kohn, K.W., and Pommier, Y. Nucleosome positioning as a critical determinant for the DNA cleavage sites of mammalian DNA topoisomerase II in reconstituted simian virus 40 chromatin. Nucleic Acids Res., **18:** 4553–4558, 1990.

38. Wu, H-W., Shyy, S., Wang, J. C., and Liu, L. F. Transcription generates positively and negatively supercoiled domains in the template. Cell. **53:** 433–440, 1988.

39. Snapka, R. M., Powelson, M. A., and Strayer, J. M. Swiveling and decatenation of replicating simian virus 40 genomes *in vivo*. Mol. Cell. Biol. **8:** 515–521, 1988.

40. Avemann, K., Knippers, R., Koller, T., and Sogo, J.M. Camptothecin, a specific inhibitor of type I DNA topoisomerase, induces DNA breakage at replication forks. Mol. Cell. Biol. **8:** 3026–3034, 1988.

41. Champoux, J. J. Topoisomerase I is preferentially associated with isolated replicating simian virus 40 molecules after treatment of infected cells with camptothecin. J. Virol. **62:** 3675–3683, 1988.

42. Kerrigan, D., Pommier, Y., Jaxel, C., Covey, J. M., and Kohn, K. W. A new DNA topoisomerase isolated from drug resistant Chinese hamster cells. Proc. Am. Assoc. Cancer Res. **29:** 1191, 1988.

43. Zhang, H., Wang, J. C., and Liu, L. F. Involvement of DNA topoisomerase I in transcription of human ribosomal RNA genes. Proc. Natl. Acad. Sci. USA, **85:** 1060–1064, 1988.

PART III

INHIBITORS OF TOPOISOMERASE II

Chapter 16

On the Mechanism of Interaction of DNA Topoisomerase II with Chemotherapeutic Agents

TIMOTHY L. MACDONALD, ERICH K. LEHNERT,
JOHN T. LOPER, K.-C. CHOW, AND WARREN E. ROSS

DNA topoisomerase II has emerged as the chemotherapeutic target for a diverse group of antitumor agents (1–4). Through mechanisms that are at present unclear, these drugs can induce topoisomerase II to produce "cleavable complexes," in which the enzyme has cleaved DNA and formed a concomitant covalent association with the broken strand(s) of duplex DNA (5–8). These ternary complexes of drug, DNA, and enzyme appear to be closely related to intermediates formed during the course of the catalytic cycle of the enzyme. In fact, the formation of drug-induced cleavable complexes of DNA topoisomerase II has been attributed to the stabilization by the drug of a covalent, DNA-bound catalytic intermediate in the cleavage–resealing sequence of the enzyme (1–8). The cleavable complex apparently represents a significant cellular lesion, perhaps a unique type of DNA damage, and the level of formation in experiments in cell culture has been demonstrated to correlate directly with the expression of cytotoxicity (1–4). We have been attempting to elucidate the mechanisms of cleavable complex formation with DNA topoisomerase II by five distinct classes of agents—the anthracyclines, epipodophyllotoxins, ellipticines, aminoacridines, and anthracenediones (Fig. 16.1). This report will outline the present status of our efforts.

The focus of our studies has been the resolution of two mechanistic questions. The first and primary issue has been the nature of the binding site(s) for these agents in the ternary complex. The second question has been the sequence of "events" through which the ternary complex is formed. These questions, despite common mechanistic underpinnings, are not interdependent. Thus, it is possible that each class of agents binds at a distinct site in the drug–DNA–enzyme complex, but the order of addition for ternary complex is the same; alternatively, it is possible that each class of agents binds at a common site in the ternary complex, but a different sequence of events occurs in the formation of the complex for each drug class. Currently, limited data are available that address either question.

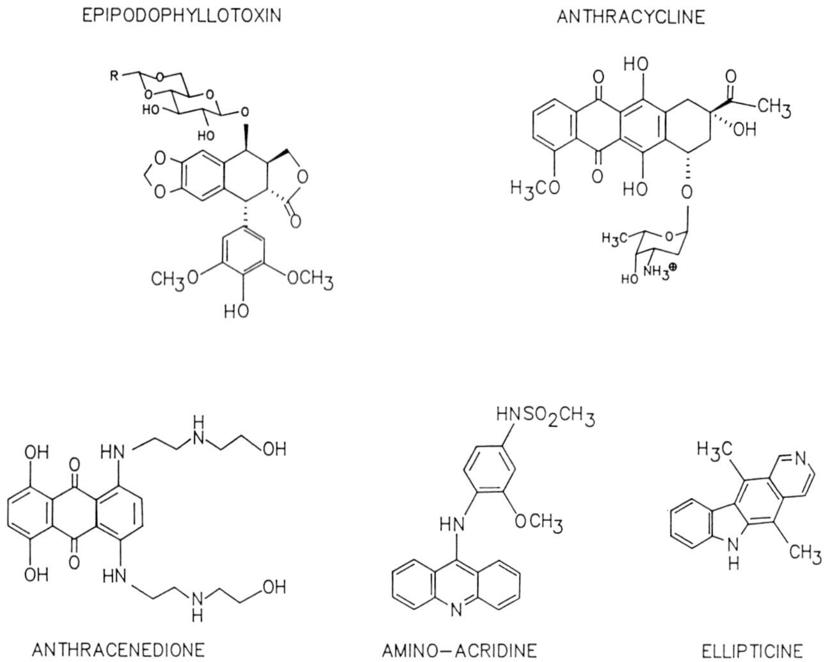

EPIPODOPHYLLOTOXIN   ANTHRACYCLINE

ANTHRACENEDIONE   AMINO–ACRIDINE   ELLIPTICINE

Figure 16.1. Representatives of the classes of DNA topoisomerase II–active agents.

THE NATURE OF THE BINDING SITE FOR TOPOISOMERASE II–ACTIVE AGENTS

In a ternary drug–DNA–topoisomerase II complex, the drug association site could reside *a priori* on either the enzyme or DNA exclusively or could be at a DNA–enzyme interface in which the drug exhibits close contact with both components. Investigating the nature of the drug association site in such complexes typically involves studying the binding of the drug to DNA and enzyme independently and, when feasible, elucidating the effects on ternary complex formation of agents proposed to associate at identical sites through competitive binding studies. When structurally distinct drug classes are active in complex formation, as is the case with topoisomerase II (Fig. 16.1), studies directed at identification of common and unique structural parameters of each drug class can assist in the "mapping" of the binding site(s) for the individual classes of agents and provide support for the postulation of similar or distinct ligand association sites. With regard to the classes of topoisomerase II–active drugs under our investigation, four classes of agents were established to interact with DNA via intercalation—the anthracyclines, ellipticines, aminoacridines, and anthracenediones (5–7, 9–11). Such data are compatible with the association of these agents in the ternary complex with either DNA exclusively or with both DNA and the enzyme. Alternatively, it is possible that DNA could act as a "reservoir" for these classes of agents, which are released as the enzyme approaches the intercalation site to provide locally high, but kinetically unstable, concentrations of the agent for subsequent interaction at the target site. At the outset of our investigations, existing evidence and prevailing attitudes suggested that the epipodophyllotoxin class did not associate with DNA via intercalation or through alternate modes of interaction (8,12). In addition, evidence regarding the direct interaction of these classes of agents with the enzyme was not available.

Our approach to investigating the nature of the drug association site on the drug–DNA–enzyme ternary complex centered on developing a fundamental understanding of the structural features of the ligands and on identifying the potential interactions of these ligands with DNA and protein. As our understanding of the structural features of these classes of topoisomerase active agents evolved, a unique composite pharmacophore became apparent through molecular modeling studies. This putative pharmacophore was produced by the superimposition of the five classes of topoisomerase-active agents so as to "carve out" the mutual space that the composite "super-structure" occupied (Fig. 16.2). All of the existing topoisomerase-active agents could be accommodated within this composite structure, by virtue of the method through which it was developed, although not each class of agents satisfied each of its structural domains.

Three domains of this composite structure (Fig. 16.3) could be identified: a planar, polycyclic molecular surface, which overlaps with the portion of these molecules postulated to intercalate with DNA; a pendant, *para*-hydroxy- or sulfonylamino-phenyl ring; and a molecular region, in which considerable structural diversity can be accommodated, as illustrated by the glycosyl residues of the anthracyclines and the epipodophyllotoxins. In each of the pendant substituent domains—those domains represented by the *para*-substituted phenyl region and the variable substituent region—a rigid stereochemical chirality is required (13,14). The model enabled a prediction regarding the "active" conformations of the conformationally mobile aminoacridine and anthracenedione systems. The model additionally enabled the assignment of substructures of each class to domains of the pharmacophore, and, through molecular modeling studies, we have been able to assign specific interactions for these domains with a putative target site in the ternary complex.

The unique character of this proposed composite pharmacophore stems from the laxity in adherence to a requisite occupancy of each of these domains by these families of agents. Thus, only the epipodophyllotoxins possess substructures that occupy each of the pharmacophore domains, although this class exhibits a "truncated" intercalation domain. The anthracyclines define the limit of the "intercalation domain" and possess a substituent in the variable domain; the aminoacridines exhibit substituents in both the planar, intercalation domains and the pendant, *para*-substituted phenyl domain. The anthracenediones have substituents in the planar and variable domains and a substituent that occupies the domain represented by the *para*-phenyl substituent and possibly accommodates the structural requirements of this domain. The ellipticines exhibit overlap only with the planar, intercalation domain. Strict occupancy of all of the domains in a composite pharmacophore over a series of molecular classes is generally observed in the medicinal chemical probing of

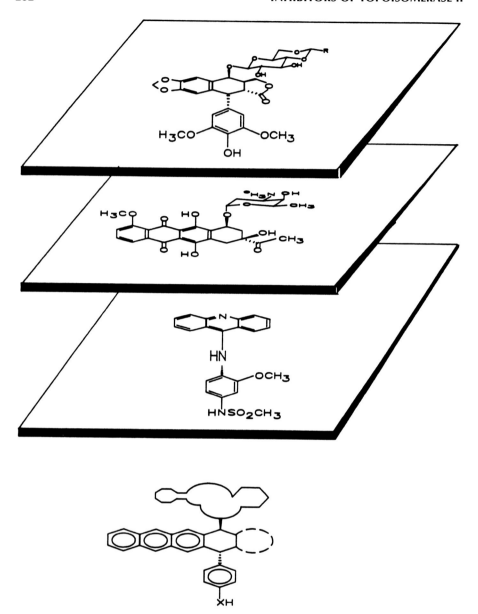

Figure 16.2. Superimposition of structural subunits of topoisomerase II inhibitors of the epipodophyllotoxin, anthracycline, and aminoacridine classes.

drug target or receptor sites, particularly sites on proteins. The composite pharmacophore that we have identified demands a binding site that paradoxically exhibits a fascinating lack of restriction for ligands that associate with it and yet, upon occupancy, exhibit considerable specificity in producing ternary drug–DNA–topoisomerase complexes.

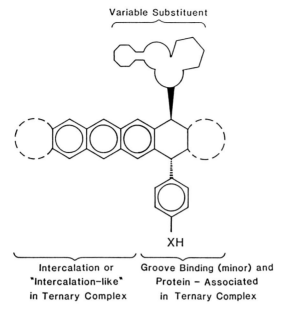

Variable Substituent

XH

Intercalation or
"Intercalation–like"
in Ternary Complex

Groove Binding (minor) and
Protein – Associated
in Ternary Complex

Figure 16.3. A composite pharmacophore for expression of topoisomerase activity.

Our hypothetical pharmacophore has defined three structural domains and assigned substructures within each class of agents to these domains. Thus, we have been able to evaluate and are proceeding to refine our pharmacophore hypothesis through the definition of a family of hybrid structures that incorporate substructural elements of each of these classes of agents.

The first hybrid class of topoisomerase II–active molecules that we synthesized incorporated subunits from the aminoacridine and epipodophyllotoxin families. Our selection of initial target molecules was dictated by synthetic access and was guided by the observation that the aminoacridine and epipodophyllotoxin classes exhibit strict structural requirements for the pendant *para*-substituted phenyl substituent. In both classes, methylation of either the phenol or methanesulfonanilide nitrogen moieties results in a significant depression of activity (-10^3-fold) (13–16). In the aminoacridine class, methoxylation *meta* to the methanesulfonanilide substituent (termed *m*-AMSA **1**) has a small effect, whereas methoxylation *ortho* to the methanesulfonanilide substituent (a structure termed *o*-AMSA **2**) significantly depresses activity ($>10^2$-fold) (1–5,16,17). These observations may appear to conflict with our postulated "laxity" of occupation of the proposed domains of our composite pharmacophore. However, strict structural requirements for the domains of a molecular class that are occupied are not only compatible with our model, such precise structural limitations and requirements for each domain are expected. We anticipated that data on the topoisomerase activity of our target molecules would provide preliminary confirmation or rejection for the concept of a unified pharmacophore for topoisomerase-active agents. If support for the model was forthcoming, the interdigitation of structure–activity data for the domains of these families of agents would enable a significant refinement of the domains of our model pharmacophore. Moreover, the strict structural requirements of the pendant phenyl ring of both the epipodophyllotoxin and aminoacridine classes, although at present unexplained, would have to be accommodated in any putative binding site model.

Structure–activity data on hybrid molecules with a planar acridine nucleus appended to a pendant podophyllotoxinlike, substituted phenol substituent in an *in vitro* assay are compiled in Figure 16.4. As is apparent from the data, these aminoacridine–epipodophyllotoxin analogs exhibit an SAR profile analogous to the epipodophyllotoxins with regard to phenol methylation. Thus, phenol 3 is more active than anisole 5, and dimethoxyphenol 5 is more active than trimethoxyphenol 7. Interestingly, the activity order for the aminoacridine phenols (3, 4, and 6) in this *in vitro* assay follows the sequence: phenol 3 (the most active aminoacridine) > methoxyphenol 4 > dimethoxylphenol 6. This SAR sequence for the substituted phenol series parallels that observed in the methanesulfonanilide aminoacridine series—*ortho*-methoxylation of either the methoxyphenol 4 (to provide 6) or the methanesulfonanilide aminoacridine (to provide *o*-AMSA 2) results in a substantial diminution of activity. The parallel SAR profiles suggest that the o-methoxyphenol and methanesulfonanilide groups, due to their steric similarities (Fig. 16.5) and their similar pKa values (pKa = -10), display a common mechanistic process at the binding site. The nature of that process must underlie the difference in activities between *m*-AMSA and *o*-AMSA, which has been considered a "Gordian knot" for topoisomerase II structure–activity relationships. We hypothesize that the protons of the oxygen and nitrogen functionalities of the *para*-substituted aminoacridine and epipodophyllotoxin series are engaged in a critical hydrogen bonding interaction in the binding site and that methylation of these proton-donating moieties or steric encumbrance surrounding these sites abolishes or inhibits this interaction. We have also shown that *m*-AMSA 1, phenol 3, and dimethoxyphenol 5 exhibit indistinguishable patterns of topoisomerase II–induced DNA cleavage. Although the molecular basis for distinct cleavage patterns by drugs is not understood, each drug class possesses a differential and characteristic DNA "fingerprint" of enzyme-induced cleavage (1–8); the structural determinants for the aminoacridine class must reside in the acridine nucleus. In addition, we are currently refining our composite pharmacophore model through the synthesis of additional hybrid molecules, which integrate the postulated domain subunits of established classes of topoisomerase-active into composite structures.

Implicit in our postulate of a unified pharmacophore for topoisomerase II activity is a common target site for these agents. However, a unified pharmacophore does not suggest the nature of this putative common target site—even at the level of DNA, enzyme, or DNA–enzyme complex. Nonetheless, our pharmacophore model and a *single* assumption has allowed the elaboration of a unified picture of the target site for all topoisomerase-active species. Certainly, this initial target site model will be refined as additional data become available. However, the present hypothesis has considerable power in rationalizing in mechanistic terms a body of extant data and in predicting future avenues for topoisomerase drug development.

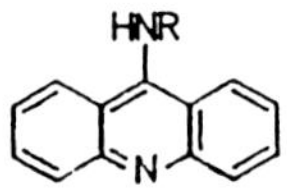

HNR

Concentration (in uM) for DNA strand breaks

R	(at 500 Rad eq.)	(at 1000 Rad eq.)
3 — OH	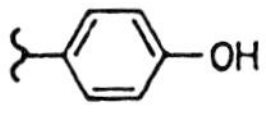 0.87	1.75
1 H₃CO — NHSO₂CH₃	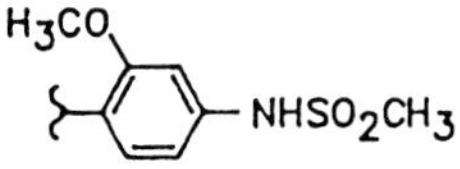 1.27	2.54
4 OCH₃ — OH	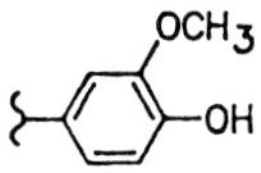 3.0	6.5
5 — OCH₃	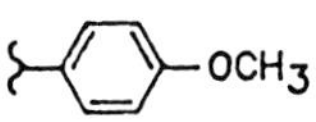 12.3	40.0
6 OCH₃ — OH OCH₃	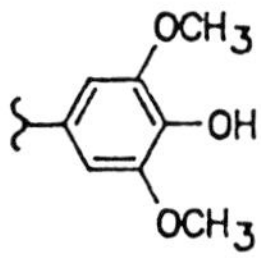 22.2	50.6
7	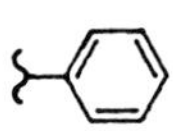 60.7	Inactive
2 OCH₃ — NHSO₂CH₃ 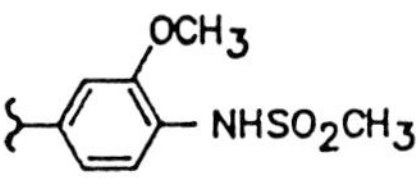	Inactive	
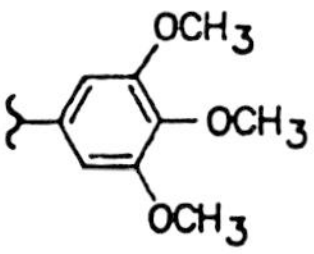 8 OCH₃ — OCH₃ OCH₃	Inactive	

Figure 16.4. Structure–activity data for the cleavage of DNA by aminoacridine analogs that possess the methanesulfonanilide and phenolic (epipodophyllotoxin) pendant aryl ring systems.

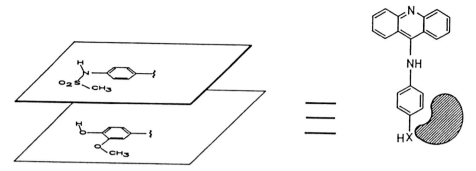

Figure 16.5. The superimposition of the aminoacridine methanesulfonanilide and epipodophyllotoxin methoxyphenol pendant rings. The hatched region indicated in the aminoacridine composite represents the region of space occupied by both the methanesulfonanilide and methoxyphenol moieties.

The assumption that we have adopted in developing our target site model is that the anthracyclines, perhaps the best understood class of topoisomerase-active drugs, associate with DNA via their thermodynamically favored mode of interaction in the ternary complex. Our assumption does not specify whether the drug association site on DNA is in contact with the enzyme or whether this site acts at distance from the enzyme in the ternary complex; we assume simply that a critical parameter in the ternary complex is anthracycline–DNA thermodynamic association. We have produced data that indicate that anthracycline intercalation is essential for topoisomerase activity—a finding consistent with our assumption (18). The observation of intercalation for N-acylanthracyclines resolves an apparent contradiction in the activities of this class of anthracycline derivatives.

This assumption expresses its full potential when the excellent resolution (1.2Å) of the Rich group's X-ray crystal structure of daunomycin associated with a duplex DNA hexamer (10) (Fig. 16.6) is combined with molecular modeling. Although the crystal structure provides extraordinary insight into the structural factors that dictate association of this drug–DNA complex, two features should be highlighted as background for our discussion. Foremost, the interaction of the aromatic region of daunomycin with DNA, which occurs with the long axis of the π-framework of the drug perpendicular to the H-bonding network of the nucleotide bases, illustrates a "perpendicular" mode of intercalation. Second, the energetic factors that assist DNA association of the aminoglycoside moiety, which resides in the minor groove of the DNA helix, are primarily derived from hydrophobic forces and a nonspecific electrostatic interaction of the protonated amine with the phosphate backbone (rather than "specific" H-bonding interactions). Importantly, the drug–DNA complex results in a net $-9°$ helix unwinding in the region of the intercalation site. Through the overlap of analogous pharmacophore domains of topoisomerase active agents with the anthracycline system in the daunomycin–DNA crystal structure, hypothetical depictions of DNA complexes with these classes of

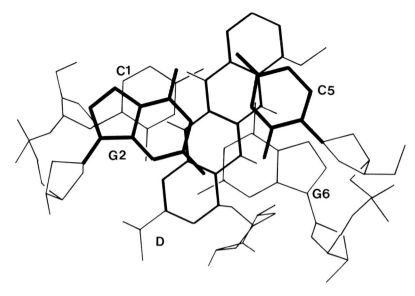

Figure 16.6. A view of the daunomycin–DNA duplex hexamer. (Reproduced from the structure determined by X-ray crystallography [Wang et al. (10)] through computer graphics.)

agents can be derived. A representative epipodophyllotoxin complex is illustrated in Figure 16.7. This hypothetical complex illustrates the excellent fit afforded the DNA–drug complex by the complementary chirality of the drug and the DNA. Furthermore, this hypothetical complex "hints" at the postulated critical interaction for the pendant phenol ring hydroxylic proton through a bifurcated hydrogen bond to a proximate (2.6 Å) guanine–cytosine base pair.

To summarize a considerable series of studies of this type, we now believe that an essential criterion for expression of topoisomerase II activity by these classes of drugs is their ability to distort DNA in a specific manner upon association. The precise nature of this structural alteration cannot be defined at present, although we believe it to be embodied in a local unwinding angle of approximately 10° in the DNA double helix induced by the drugs that we have investigated. Such a limited DNA distortion is a typical consequence of perpendicular intercalation, which is less sterically demanding to the DNA duplex than "parallel intercalation" (19) (Fig. 16.8). A common signature of "parallel intercalation," in which the long axis of the drug and base pair π-systems are aligned, is a considerably larger unwinding angle, illustrated by the 26° unwinding angle of ethidium bromide (20). We believe that the pendant substituents of topoisomerase-active agents (bound in their "active" intercalation modes) serve to "enforce" perpendicular association of the intercalation functionality, while providing additional and often critical stabilization energy through their (generally "nonspecific") interaction with the minor groove of DNA. Although perpendicular intercalation appears to be a predominant means for the production of a small unwinding angle and it has been the focus of our discussion, it is presumably not the only interaction by which a drug

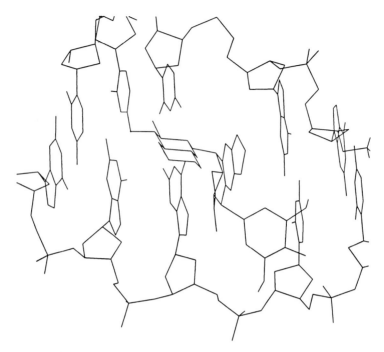

Figure 16.7. A simulated etoposide–DNA intercalated structure produced by pharma-cophore domain-dictated superimmposition of etoposide with daunomycin in the DNA complex (Fig. 16.5) and subsequent removal of daunomycin.

may induce the postulated DNA distortion. Moreover, it is unlikely that an unwinding angle of $-10°$ will be sufficient for activity or that an unwinding angle in this range will necessarily be the optimum for expression of cytotox-icity.

Consistent with the postulation of some DNA distortion represented by a $-10°$ unwinding angle as critical to the expression of topoisomerase activity are the unwinding angles of the anthracycline and ellipticine families of agents, all of which exhibit small ($<12°$) unwinding angles (21). In addition, this hy-pothesis is consistent with the inactivity of many intercalators that exhibit large unwinding angles and cannot produce a perpendicular intercalated species, such as ethidium bromide. However, the unwinding angle of the aminoacridine ($-20°$) (22) and anthracenedione ($-26°$) (22–24) classes are much larger than the unwinding angle postulated, and, although the epipodophyllotoxin class has been recently demonstrated to associate with DNA (18), there is no indication that these agents intercalate (as is suggested in Figure 16.7). With regard to the intercalative classes, the model of drug–DNA association obtained from our modeling studies proposes that the "active" mode of DNA association is *not* the primary mode of DNA association for the anthracenedione (23–25) and aminoacridine (26,27) classes. We do not believe that this inconsistency is a weakness in the hypothesis; on the contrary, we believe that the "active" in-tercalation species for both of these classes is either induced upon association of DNA by enzyme or is a minor contributor to the overall profile of DNA-associated complexes. Since the unwinding angle does not represent the DNA alteration caused by a single molecular interaction, but instead the average unwinding angle per ligand of a presumed statistical mix of DNA-associated species, the second possibility would imply that these classes of agents are relatively "inefficient" in inducing cleavable complex per intercalation event. We postulate that the hypothetical model resulting from the superimposition of these classes with daunomycin and exhibiting a perpendicular mode of acridine intercalation would exhibit the requisite unwinding angle. In addition, we believe that the *o*-AMSA–*m*-AMSA activity difference resides in the comparative inability of *o*-AMSA to accommodate this "essential" perpendicular orientation adopted by *m*-AMSA, as a consequence of the steric inhibition to the critical hydrogen bond formed by the sulfonanilide proton (see Fig. 16.8).

A more difficult issue is the inability to observe any degree of unwinding for the epipodophyllotoxins. This observation is most likely a reflection of the lack of sensitivity in determining unwinding angles for low levels of DNA association or of the ability of the large regions of uncomplexed DNA to "dampen" the unwinding associated with the limited number of complexed drug sites. It is also possible that the epipodophyllotoxins achieve the putative, requisite DNA alteration via different structural adjustments, which are not revealed as DNA unwinding. Alternatively, the epipodophyllotoxins could associate with the DNA double helix subsequent to, rather than prior to, enzyme association. Nonetheless, the predicted unwinding angle for this class would be similar to the anthracyclines, as a consequence of the excellent "fit" of epipodophyllotoxins with DNA in the perpendicular intercalation mode (Fig. 16.7). However, more extensive energy minimization protocols will be needed to refine our present picture of the perpendicular intercalation of the aminoacridine, anthracenedione, and epipodophyllotixin classes with DNA.

Thus, we postulate that the target site for the topoisomerase-active agents under our investigation is the DNA double helix. Association of the drug with DNA causes a local distortion in the duplex, which is the factor we propose to be essential for formation of the cleavable complex and expression of topo-

Models Of Drug – DNA Intercalation

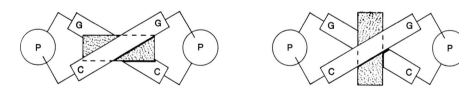

Parallel Intercalation   Perpendicular Intercalation

Figure 16.8. Depictions of parallel and perpendicular intercalation. For purposes of clarity, a DNA duplex dimer is illustrated with the drug (the darkened rectangle) intercalated between the base pairs with the long axis of the π-framework of the drug parallel or perpendicular to the long axis of the DNA base pairs.

isomerase activity. We next address the mechanistic order of formation of the cleavable complex and the issue of whether the postulated drug–DNA complex resides proximate or distant to the enzyme in the ternary complex.

THE SEQUENCE OF FORMATION OF THE CLEAVABLE COMPLEX

A second issue that we have addressed is the mechanism through which the cleavable complex, a ternary species composed of drug, DNA, and enzyme, is formed. The three potential sequences for the formation of the ternary complex, omitting the entropically implausible simultaneous "three body collision," are presented in Figure 16.9. This simplified scheme does not illustrate the complexity of this issue, because of its lack of the variety of binary or ternary complexes that may serve as intermediates preceding the cytotoxic species (the cleavable complex). It should also be recalled that although we believe that DNA is the target for these agents, their order of ternary complex formation is not required to be identical. An *a priori* mechanistic sequence for cleavable complex formation with any class of agents cannot be assumed, as can be, for example, in gene activation by steroid hormones, which presumably involves the initial complexation of steroid and receptor and subsequent DNA association of the steroid hormone–receptor complex (28,29). Consequently, to rigorously define an exclusive pathway of cleavable complex formation for a single drug, *all* of the *kinetic* parameters for the sequences illustrated in Figure 16.9 would have to be elucidated—an effort of considerable magnitude. This conclusion is inescapable because of the thermodynamic nature of the ternary complex.

A less rigorous means to approach the issue of sequence is through "order of addition" experiments. In such experiments, the different pairwise combinations (cf. Fig. 16.9) are preincubated and the relative proportions of ternary complex and normal catalytic complex (binary complex) are assessed upon addition of the third component after a single enzymic event. We have performed such experiments with the epipodophyllotoxin, etoposide. Although the rapid

Mechanisms of Ligand Association in Ternary Complex

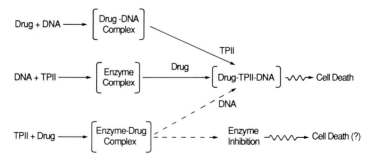

Figure 16.9. Potential sequences for the formation of the cleavable complex.

rate of binary complex formation between enzyme and DNA renders unambiguous evaluation difficult, our data are most consistent with the order of addition proceeding via the formation of an initial drug–DNA complex, which subsequently associates with the enzyme.

We selected the epipodophyllotoxin class for examination because of its low relative association with DNA, as compared with the other classes under investigation (18). The indication of initial drug–DNA association preceding the ternary complex is therefore consistent with the behavior of these families of drugs. Alternative hypotheses for the sequence of cleavable complex formation can be envisioned, such as the proposal outlined by Shen et al. for quinolone antibiotic–DNA gyrase–DNA complex formation (30–32). Clearly, considerable work lies before us, if the sequences of ternary complex formation for these drugs are to be determined.

The postulation of an initial drug–DNA association is consistent with the observation of distinct cleavage sites on DNA for each drug class, presumably reflecting the formation of a family of cleavable complexes at specific sites on DNA. The drug-induced cleavage sites appear to represent an enhancement of native, but minor, cleavage sites that occur in the normal catalytic process (33). Thus, the characteristic cleavage pattern of each drug class, its cleavage "fingerprint," would be a consequence of the selectivity in drug binding sites on DNA, which are known to differ from one class to another. In order to so profoundly influence the endogenous cleavage pattern of the enzyme, the site of drug–DNA distortion might be expected to be in close proximity to or in contact with the enzyme in the cleavable complex.

What are the benefits of knowing the sequence of ternary complex formation? Fundamental knowledge concerning the molecular recognition of the species in the ternary complex and the mechanistic details of the catalytic sequence may accrue. Obviously, a knowledge of the sequence improves our ability to design more specific agents and, assuming the principle of microscopic reversibility holds, less reversible therapeutic agents. This knowledge will unravel at the molecular level *the* fundamental process of an important class of chemotherapeutic agents.

A HYPOTHETICAL UNIFIED MECHANISM FOR DNA TOPOISOMERASE ACTIVITY

We have begun to develop a rudimentary knowledge of the mechanism by which a small group of molecules interact with DNA and DNA topoisomerase II to produce a ternary complex. To translate this knowledge into a coherent picture, we will conclude with speculations about the process of cleavable complex formation—a hypothetical "unified mechanism" for topoisomerase activity. Based on our current level of knowledge, we anticipate that the initial step in the sequence to cleavable complex is association of the drug with DNA. The drug–DNA complex must meet two essential criteria in order to initiate enzyme recognition and cleavable complex formation. The first condition is that the drug must distort the DNA duplex in a specific manner, which we speculate is embodied in the DNA alteration witnessed upon $-10°$ unwinding. The second condition is that DNA association must occur within a specific "window" of nucleotides that have a defined relationship with the consensus cleavage sequence for the enzyme (33–35). When these two criteria are met, a "hot spot" in the DNA is produced, which subsequent catalytic processing by enzyme results in the formation of a cleavable complex. We envision that the resealing process of the cleavable complex is inhibited as a consequence of the stabilization of this catalytic intermediate by the drug. It is also possible that the initial drug–DNA "hot spot" promotes enzyme association by distorting the DNA in a specific fashion resulting in a noncovalent stabilized "recognition complex."

What are the mechanisms by which the drug–DNA complex could stabilize a DNA–enzyme covalent intermediate in the catalytic cycle or enhance enzyme recognition? We believe that the answer to this question emanates from the foundations of mechanistic enzymology: enzymes bind transition states—high energy intermediates in the reaction pathway—with greater affinity than ground states. Since the energies of enzyme intermediates are related to the transition states leading to them, stabilization of transition states results in stabilization of transient intermediates. This concept underlies the process of transition state inhibition of enzymes. We believe that the structural distortion induced in DNA upon drug association simulates an altered DNA structure that is an intermediate in the cleavage–resealing sequence—that the drug–DNA complex is a "transition state analog" of DNA at some point in the catalytic cycle.

Clearly, there are alternatives to this hypothesis. We offer it not as an absolute but as a point of departure for the imagination, as the intimate details of this fundamental process begin to be understood at the molecular level. At its present level of refinement, this unified mechanism for topoisomerase activity has consolidated a body of fragmented observations into a simple mechanistic fabric and has suggested a range of experiments as "litmus tests." Most importantly, this hypothesis has allowed us to identify critical structural elements in molecules for the expression of topoisomerase activity, as we search for more specific and potent inhibitors of this important chemotherapeutic target.

Acknowledgments

We wish to acknowledge support for this research from the National Institutes of Health through CA 40884.

REFERENCES

1. Ross, W. E. DNA topoisomerases as targets in cancer chemotherapy. Biochem. Pharmacol. **34**: 4191–5, 1985.
2. Ross, W. E., Sullivan, D. M., and Chow, K-C. Altered function of DNA topoisomerases as a basis for antineoplastic drug action. In V. DeVita, S. Hellman, and S. Rosenberg, eds. *Important Advances in Oncology 1988*. Philadelphia: J. B. Lippincott Company, 1988, pp. 65–81.
3. Drlica, K. and Franco, R. J. Inhibitors of DNA topoisomerases. Biochemistry. **27**: 2253–9, 1988.
4. Lock, R. B. and Ross, W. E. DNA topo-

isomerases in cancer therapy. Anticancer Drug Design. **2**: 151–64, 1987.

5. Nelson, E. M., Tewey, K. M., and Liu, L. F. Mechanism of antitumor drug action poisoning of mammalian DNA-topoisomerase II on DNA by 4'-(9-acridinylamino)-methanesulfon-m-anisidide. Proc. Natl. Acad. Sci. USA. **81**: 1361–5, 1984.

6. Tewey, K. M., Chen, G. L., Nelson, E. M., and Liu, L. F. Intercalative antitumor drugs interfere with the breakage-reunion reaction of mammalian DNA-topoisomerase II. J. Biol. Chem. **259**: 9182–7, 1984.

7. Tewey, K. M., Rowe, T. C., Yang, L., Halligan, B. D., and Liu, L. F. Adriamycin-induced DNA damage mediated by mammalian DNA-topoisomerase II. Science. **226**: 466–8, 1984.

8. Chen, G. L., Yang, L., Rowe, T. C., Halligan, B. D., Tewey, K. M., and Liu, L. F. Non-intercalative antitumor drugs interfere with the breakage-reunion reaction of mammalian DNA topoisomerase II. J. Biol. Chem. **259**: 13560–6, 1984.

9. Waring, M. J. DNA modification and cancer. Annu. Rev. Biochem. **50**: 159–92, 1981.

10. Wang, A. H-J., Ughetto, G., Quigley, G. J., and Rich, A. Interaction between an anthracycline antibiotic and DNA: Molecular structure of daunomycin complexed to d(CpGpTpApCpG) at 1.2 Å resolution. Biochemistry. **26**: 1152–63, 1987.

11. Lown, J. W., Morgan, A. R., Yen, S-F., Wang, Y-H., and Wilson, W. D. Characteristics of the binding of the anticancer agent mitoxantrone, ametantrone and related structures to DNA. Biochemistry. **24**: 4028–35, 1985.

12. Wozniak, A. J., Glisson, B. S., Hande, K. R., and Ross, W. E. Inhibition of etoposide-induced DNA damage and cytotoxicity in L1210 cells by dehydrogenase inhibitors and other agents. Cancer Res. **44**: 626–32, 1984.

13. Issell, B. F., Rudolph, A. R., and Louie, A. C. Etoposide (VP-16-213): An overview. In B. F. Issell, F. M. Muggia, and S. K. Carter, eds. *Etoposide (VP-16), Current Status and New Developments*. Orlando, FL: Academic Press, 1984, pp. 1–13.

14. Doyle, T. W. The chemistry of etoposide. In B. F. Issell, F. M. Muggia, and S. K. Carter, eds. *Etoposide (VP-16), Current Status and New Developments*. Orlando, FL: Academic Press, 1984, pp. 15–32.

15. Long, B. H., Musial, S. T., and Brattian, M. G. Comparison of cytotoxicity and DNA breakage activity of cogeners of podophyllotoxin including VP-16-213 and VM-26: A quantitive structure activity relationship. Biochemistry. **23**: 1183–8, 1984.

16. Denny, W. A. and Wakelin-Lawrence, P. G. Kinetic and equilibrium studies of the interaction of amsacrine and aniline ring-substituted analogs with DNA. Cancer Res. **46**: 1717–21, 1986.

17. Baugley, B. C. and Nash, R. Antitumor activity of substituted 9-anilinoacridines: Comparison of in vivo and in vitro testing systems. Eur. J. Cancer. **17**: 671–79, 1981.

18. Chow, K-C., Macdonald, T. L., and Ross, W. E. DNA binding by epipodophyllotoxins and N-acyl anthracyclines: Implications for mechanism of topoisomerase II inhibition. Mol. Pharmacol. **34**: 467–73, 1988.

19. Wang, J. C. The degree of unwinding of the DNA helix by ethidium I. Titration of twisted PM2 DNA molecules in alkaline cesium chloride density gradients. J. Mol. Biol. **89**: 783–801, 1974.

20. Sobell, H. M., Tsal, C. C., Gilbert, S. G., Jain, S. C., and Sakore, T. D. Organization of DNA in chromatin. Proc. Natl. Acad. Sci. USA. **73**: 3068–72, 1976.

21. Auclair, C. Multimodal action of antitumor agents on DNA: The ellipticine series. Arch. Biochem. Biophys. **259**: 1–14, 1987.

22. Waring, M. DNA binding characteristics of acridinylmethanesulphon-anilide. Eur. J. Cancer. **12**: 995–1001, 1976.

23. Kapuscinski, J., Darzyrinkewicz, Z., Traganos, F., and Melamed, M. R. Interactions of a new antitumor agent, 1,4-dihydroxy-5,8-bis{[2-[(2-hydroxyethl)amino]-ethyl]amino}-9,10-anthracenedione, with nucleic acids. Biochem. Pharmacol. **30**: 231–40, 1981.

24. Collier, D. A. and Neidel, S. Synthesis, molecular modeling, DNA binding, and antitumor properties of some substituted amido-anthraquinones. J. Med. Chem. **31**: 847–57, 1988.

25. Fox, K. R., Waring, M. J., Brown, J. R., and Neidel S. DNA sequence preferences for the anti-cancer drug mitoxanthrone and related anthraquinones revealed by DNase I footprinting. FEBS Lett. **202**: 289–94, 1986.

26. Waring, M. Variations of the supercoils in closed circular DNA by binding antibiotics and drugs: Evidence for molecular models involving intercalation. J. Mol. Biol. **54**: 247–79, 1970.

27. Neidle, S., Webster, G. D., Baguley, B. C., and Denny, W. A. The crystal structure of 1-methyl amsacrine hydrochloride: Relationships to DNA binding ability and antitumor activity. Biochem. Pharmacol. **35**: 3915–21, 1986.

28. Green, S. and Chambon, P. A superfamily of potentially oncogenic hormone receptors. Nature. **324**: 615–17, 1986.

29. Yamamoto, K. R. Steroid receptor regulated transcription of specific genes and gene networks. Annu. Rev. Genet. **19:** 209–52, 1985.

30. Shen, L. L., Baranowski, J., and Pernet, A. G. Mechanism of inhibition of DNA gyrase of quinolone antibacterials: Specificity and cooperativity of drug binding to DNA. Biochemistry. **28:** 3879–85, 1989.

31. Shen, L. L., Mitscher, L. A., Sharma, P. N., O'Donnell, T. J., Chu, D. W. T., Cooper, C. S., Rosen, T., and Pernet, A. G. Mechanism of inhibition of DNA gyrase by quinolone antibacterials: A cooperative drug-DNA binding model. Biochemistry. **28:** 3886–94, 1989.

32. Shen, L. L. and Pernet, A. G. Mechanism of inhibition of DNA gyrase by analogues of naldixic acid: The target of the drugs is

DNA. Proc. Natl. Acad. Sci. USA. **82:** 307–11, 1985.

33. Muller, M. T., Spitzner, J. R., DiDonato, J. A., Mehta, V. B., Tsutsui, K., and Tsutsui, K. Single-strand DNA cleavages by eukaryotic topoisomerase II. Biochemistry **27:** 8369–79, 1988.

34. Riou, J-F., Multon, E., Vilaren, M-J., Larsen, C-J., and Riou, Guy. *In vivo* stimulation by antitumor drugs of the topoisomerase II induced cleavage sites in c-myc protooncogene. Biochem. Biophys. Res. Commun. **137:** 157–60, 1986.

35. Sander, M. and Hsieh, T-S. *Drosophilia* topoisomerase II double-strand DNA cleavage: Analysis of DNA sequence homology at the cleavage site. Nucleic Acids Res. **13:** 1057–72, 1985.

Chapter 17

The Mechanism of Antitumor Drug Action in a Simple Bacteriophage Model System

ANNE C. HUFF

AND KENNETH N. KREUZER

DNA CLEAVAGE BY THE TYPE II TOPOISOMERASES

The type II topoisomerase reaction mechanism involves the passage of one duplex segment of DNA through a transient double-strand break in another segment (for reviews, see 3–6). A presumptive reaction intermediate consists of a topoisomerase–DNA complex with the enzyme covalently attached to each of the $5'$ phosphate groups at the double-strand DNA cleavage site (7–9). The covalent protein–DNA complex is detectable after the addition of protein denaturant (e.g., sodium dodecyl sulfate—SDS), which is thought to disrupt noncovalent interactions between enzyme subunits. Prior to SDS addition, topoisomerase apparently forms a bridge that conceals the DNA break. The enzyme–DNA complex that accumulates prior to SDS addition has been termed the "cleavable complex" (10,11).

The cleavable complex has been observed in two situations. First, a very low level of covalent enzyme–DNA complexes can be detected when uninhibited topoisomerase reactions are terminated by the addition of SDS (12–14). These complexes are thought to represent the fraction of enzyme molecules that are transiently in the intermediate state described above. Second, treatment with certain topoisomerase inhibitors (e.g., $4'$-(9-acridinylamino) methanesulfon-m-anisidide—m-AMSA) results in the efficient production of cleavable complexes (11,15). The simplest explanation for cleavable complex production is that the inhibitors block the DNA resealing step in the topoisomerase reaction cycle, thereby stabilizing the covalent enzyme–DNA reaction intermediate. Specific models for the molecular mechanism of action of the topoisomerase inhibitors will be considered in the Discussion.

The DNA sites cleaved by topoisomerases in either the presence or absence of inhibitors are quite specific; however, the rules governing site selection are not known (6,15). Addition of a topoisomerase inhibitor such as m-AMSA can influence the DNA cleavage pattern generated by the topoisomerase (1,16), suggesting that DNA site recognition by both the enzyme and the inhibitor might be important.

The production of cleavable complexes *in vivo* appears to be critical in the physiological response to a variety of topoisomerase inhibitors (11,15). Several models that relate drug-dependent cytotoxicity to the production of cleavable complexes are described in detail elsewhere (for reviews, see 11,17,18).

THE BACTERIOPHAGE T4 MODEL SYSTEM

Bacteriophage T4 has numerous features that make it amenable to both genetic and biochemical analyses. This simple bacteriophage is relatively independent of host functions and is one of the best-characterized organisms with respect to classical genetics. A precise genetic map of the T4 genome has been constructed (19) and a wide variety of phage mutants are available. Novel phage mutants, such as the *m*-AMSA[R] (*m*-AMSA resistant) phage described below, can be easily and rapidly isolated. Complementing these genetic approaches, biochemical studies are facilitated by the fact that most viral proteins are produced in large amounts during phage infection (20). Consequently, it has been possible to analyze the viral topoisomerase and many other phage proteins involved in nucleic acid metabolism (20).

The T4–encoded type II DNA topoisomerase is strikingly similar to the corresponding eukaryotic enzyme. Several *in vitro* properties of the phage enzyme are nearly identical to those of the eukaryotic/mammalian topoisomerase, but quite distinct from those of the related bacterial enzyme, DNA gyrase (6,21). Both the T4 and eukaryotic enzymes catalyze ATP-dependent DNA relaxation, while only DNA gyrase is able to introduce negative superhelical turns into closed circular DNA. Single-strand DNA inhibits the phage and eukaryotic topoisomerases, but does not affect DNA gyrase (21–23). Most importantly, the mammalian and T4 enzymes, but not DNA gyrase, are sensitive to the antitumor drug *m*-AMSA. For both sensitive enzymes, *m*-AMSA treatment results in the accumulation of cleavable complexes, suggesting a similar mechanism of inhibition (10,24). Surprisingly, wild-type T4 topoisomerase is sensitive to representatives of at least three other chemical classes of antitumor agents known to inhibit the mammalian type II DNA topoisomerase (24a).

Several other aspects of nucleic acid metabolism in T4–infected bacterial cells also resemble those in eukaryotic cells. The T4 DNA polymerase shares greater homology with the mammalian DNA polymerase α than with *Escherichia coli* DNA polymerases (25,26). As in eukaryotic cells, introns processed at the level of mRNA are contained in several T4 genes (27–29). Further, the yeast *RAD52* gene product has been reported to substitute for the phage gene 46/47 proteins in T4 DNA metabolism (30). Given the numerous technical advantages and the similarities to mammalian systems, bacteriophage T4 is an inexpensive, convenient, and valuable model system for the analysis of antitumor drug action.

TOPOISOMERASE-MEDIATED FRAMESHIFT MUTAGENESIS

Antitumor agents that inhibit the mammalian type II topoisomerase are strongly mutagenic (31–34), and this property may prove to be important in the design and clinical use of these compounds. An investigation of *m*-AMSA–induced mutagenesis in the phage T4 model system has suggested a general class of models for mutagenesis by topoisomerase inhibitors (2).

The possible involvement of the T4 topoisomerase in the generation of frameshift mutations was first suggested by the unusual nature of a drug-induced frameshift mutation hotspot in the *r*IIB gene of T4. Both proflavin and *m*-AMSA induced a variety of small deletions and duplications that were tightly clustered and, in general, were not predicted by classical models for frameshift mutagenesis (2,35). Interestingly, each of the recurring mutations at this hotspot had an endpoint at one of two phosphodiester bonds that were spaced 4 basepairs apart on opposite strands of the DNA helix. The spacing of 4 basepairs suggested that the topoisomerase cleavable complex might be involved in mutagenesis *in vivo;* a similar 4-basepair spacing is detected after topoisomerase-mediated DNA cleavage *in vitro*.

If the cleavable complex is involved in mutagenesis, then the frameshift mutation hotspot should also be a T4 topoisomerase cleavage site. In fact, the DNA sequence location of the mutation hotspot coincides with the strongest site of topoisomerase-mediated cleavage in the relevant segment of the *r*II genes (2). Furthermore, a phage mutant deficient in topoisomerase activity is also deficient in acridine-promoted frameshift mutagenesis (2). Finally, a DNA sequence change in the region of the hotspot abolishes both frameshift mutagenesis and topoisomerase-mediated DNA cleavage (L. Ripley and K.N.K., unpublished data). These results strongly implicate the T4 topoisomerase in the generation of both proflavin- and *m*-AMSA–induced frameshift mutations. Since these two drugs result in the accumulation of the cleavable complex *in vitro*, intracellular processing of the trapped reaction intermediate is presumably responsible for the production of frameshift mutations. The possible involvement of nuclease and DNA polymerase activities in the processing of the cleavable complex are discussed elsewhere (2).

BACTERIOPHAGE T4 MUTANTS RESISTANT TO *m*-AMSA

Antitumor agent *m*-AMSA inhibits the T4 topoisomerase *in vitro* and also blocks phage growth. The involvement of topoisomerase in the generation of frameshift mutations implies that the enzyme is at least one of the intracellular targets of *m*-AMSA, but does not establish topoisomerase as the sole, or even the most important, intracellular target. We therefore began to explore the drug sensitivity of phage growth by isolating T4 mutants that are resistant to *m*-AMSA. The *m*-AMSA^R mutant phage were selected simply by plating hydroxylamine-mutagenized T4 on lawns of *E. coli* in the presence of *m*-AMSA (1). The drug-resistant mutant phage create easily visible plaques overnight,

$-m$-AMSA $+m$-AMSA

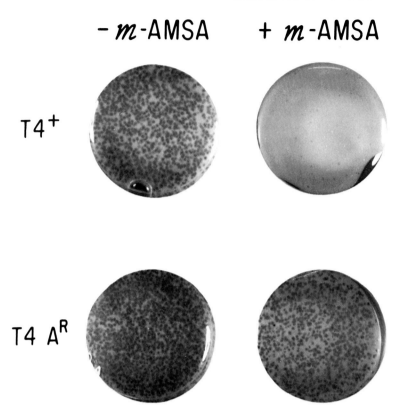

Figure 17.1. m-AMSA–resistant mutant of bacteriophage T4. Lawns of the *E. coli* host were prepared in the absence ($-$) or presence ($+$) of m-AMSA (100 µg/ml), with approximately 1000 plaque-forming units of either wild-type (T4$^+$) or m-AMSA^R (T4 A^R) phage. The few small plaques formed by T4$^+$ phage in the presence of m-AMSA presumably result from m-AMSA–induced drug-resistance mutations; m-AMSA is a potent frameshift mutagen in the T4 system (2).

whereas the drug-sensitive parental T4 phage form essentially no plaques (Fig. 17.1). The success of this approach was dependent on the fact that the bacterial host is refractory to m-AMSA; normal bacterial lawns were observed in the presence of drug (see Fig. 17.1).

Two strongly m-AMSA^R mutant phage were characterized by standard genetic analyses (1,35a). For each mutant, drug resistance was found to be due to a single point mutation (or very closely linked multiple mutations). Because we suspected that T4 topoisomerase is the target of m-AMSA, we also tested for linkage of each m-AMSA^R mutation to known amber mutations in the topoisomerase structural genes. T4 topoisomerase consists of three different subunits encoded by genes *39, 52,* and *60.* Interestingly, these two mutations are widely separated in the T4 genome; mapping experiments revealed that one drug-resistance mutation lies in or very near topoisomerase gene *39* (or the neighboring gene *60*), while the second is in or near gene *52* (1,35a). Together with the results described below, these genetic analyses demonstrate that high level *m*-AMSA resistance can be conferred by mutational alteration of either the topoisomerase gene *39* or gene *52* subunit. For convenience, we shall refer to the two *m*-AMSA^R mutations as 39-A^R and 52-A^R, respectively.

M-AMSA^R TOPOISOMERASE ACTIVITY

To determine if either *m*-AMSA^R mutant phage directs the production of a drug-insensitive enzyme, we purified T4 topoisomerase from *E. coli* infected with T4 39-A^R or with T4 52-A^R. Wild-type T4 topoisomerase was purified in parallel to provide a drug-sensitive control enzyme. All three enzyme preparations were essentially homogeneous, as judged by SDS polyacrylamide gel electrophoresis (1,35a).

As expected from previous studies (24), the DNA relaxation activity of the wild-type enzyme was completely blocked by even a low concentration (5 μg/ml) of *m*-AMSA. However, topoisomerase encoded by either the 39-A^R or the 52-A^R mutant phage exhibited substantial drug-resistant DNA relaxation activity, even with a relatively high concentration (20 μg/ml) of *m*-AMSA (1,35a). The results of DNA cleavage assays corroborated the conclusion that both *m*-AMSA^R mutant phage encode drug-resistant topoisomerases (Fig. 17.2). DNA cleavage by the wild-type enzyme increased at least 50-fold in the presence of *m*-AMSA, whereas DNA cleavage by either mutant enzyme showed little or no increase upon drug addition (1,35a). We therefore conclude that each *m*-AMSA^R mutation confers *m*-AMSA–resistant phage growth and *m*-AMSA–insensitive topoisomerase activity. Because a single mutation can render both the topoisomerase and the phage infection drug-resistant, the T4 topoisomerase must be the only significant intracellular target of *m*-AMSA in T4–infected *E. coli*.

In the absence of *m*-AMSA, DNA cleavage by the two drug-resistant mutant enzymes was quantitatively and qualitatively distinct from cleavage by the control wild-type enzyme (Fig. 17.2). Quantitatively, both mutant enzymes mediated approximately fivefold more drug-independent DNA cleavage than did the wild-type enzyme. Qualitatively, the DNA cleavage pattern generated by each mutant enzyme was different from that generated by the wild-type enzyme; the specificities of the two mutant enzymes were also distinct from each other. It seems quite likely that these surprising alterations in DNA cleavage properties are intimately related to the mechanism of drug resistance conferred by the *m*-AMSA^R mutations (see Discussion).

We also analyzed the drug-resistant mutant enzymes to determine if either *m*-AMSA^R mutation resulted in an amino acid substitution that led to a net charge alteration. Using nonequilibrium pH-gradient gel electrophoresis, the gene *39* subunit of the 39-A^R mutant enzyme was shown to be more positively charged than the wild-type gene *39* subunit (1). This result, together with the genetic analyses described above, clearly indicates that the 39-A^R mutation involves an alteration in the amino acid sequence of the gene *39* subunit. In contrast to these results with the 39-A^R mutant enzyme, the pH-gradient gel migration pattern of the 52-A^R mutant topoisomerase matched that of the wild-

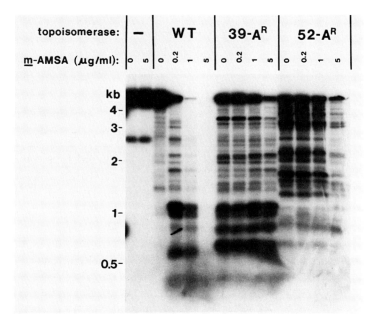

Figure 17.2. DNA cleavage activities of the 39-A^R and 52-A^R mutant topoisomerases are insensitive to *m*-AMSA. Uniquely end-labeled, linear pBR322 DNA was incubated with 1 μg of wild-type, 39-A^R, or 52-A^R topoisomerase in the presence of increasing concentrations of *m*-AMSA. Cleavage products were resolved by agarose gel electrophoresis, and an autoradiogram of the gel is shown. A molecular mass scale (kb, kilobase), generated from the migration of pBR322 DNA restriction fragments, is given in the lefthand margin. The approximately 2700-basepair fragment visible in the untreated substrate control (lefthand lane; also present in some other lanes) is a byproduct of the pBR322 DNA linearization reaction. The exposed areas at the left edge of the untreated substrate control lane (lefthand lane) are from an adjacent lane (not shown) containing labeled sizing markers.

type enzyme (35a). Therefore, the amino acid substitution in the 52-A^R mutant enzyme did not detectably change the overall charge of the gene *52* subunit. Determination of the exact amino acid substitutions that provide drug resistance awaits DNA sequencing analyses of the mutant genes.

WILD-TYPE T4 TOPOISOMERASE IS SENSITIVE TO ADDITIONAL ANTITUMOR AGENTS

Numerous structurally distinct antitumor agents inhibit the mammalian type II DNA topoisomerase, resulting in the accumulation of cleavable complexes (11,15). In addition, the quinolone antibacterials (e.g., nalidixic and oxolinic acids) trap bacterial DNA gyrase in a cleavable complex (3–6). Because such a wide variety of agents results in similar cleavable complexes involving type II topoisomerases, it seems likely that these agents share a common mecha-

Table 17.1. Comparison of Effective Inhibitor Concentrations

Inhibitor	Approximate Concentration (μM) for 90% DNA Cleavage[a]	Concentration Difference[b]
Mitoxantrone	0.2	—
m-AMSA	3	15X
Ellipticine	8	40X
VP-16	40	200X
Oxolinic acid	2000	10,000X

[a]Effective concentrations were derived from experiments similar to that shown in Figure 17.2.
[b]Difference values were calculated relative to mitoxantrone.

nism of action. To begin to investigate this mechanism using the bacteriophage model system, we tested the sensitivity of the T4 topoisomerase to several inhibitors of mammalian or bacterial type II topoisomerases.

The antitumor agents doxorubicin, ellipticine, mitoxantrone, and epipodophyllotoxins VM-26 and VP-16, as well as the antibacterial oxolinic acid, were each tested for the induction of DNA cleavage mediated by the wild-type T4 topoisomerase. To our surprise, ellipticine, mitoxantrone, and VP-16 each induced a high level of topoisomerase-mediated DNA cleavage (24a). As expected from previous studies (24,36), oxolinic acid at very high concentrations also induced DNA cleavage by the T4 topoisomerase. In comparison, very little DNA cleavage was detected in response to doxorubicin or VM-26 addition.

The drug concentrations required to induce cleavage of approximately 90% of the DNA substrate varied greatly (Table 17.1). Generally, the mammalian and bacteriophage enzymes do not show the same relative sensitivities to topoisomerase inhibitors. For example, the mammalian enzyme is more sensitive to VM-26 than VP-16 (37), while the T4 topoisomerase is substantially more sensitive to the latter drug.

The multidrug sensitivity of the T4 topoisomerase is provocative. Initial results indicating that both the mammalian and bacteriophage enzymes are sensitive to m-AMSA could have been considered fortuitous. However, the fact that at least four structurally distinct agents attack both enzymes cannot be as easily discounted. It is most interesting that the amino acid sequence of the T4 enzyme shares only limited homology with the corresponding mammalian topoisomerase (38–40; Nolan et al., this volume). Therefore, several structurally dissimilar drugs are able to inhibit two structurally distinct enzymes, in all cases resulting in the production of cleavable complexes. These results argue strongly that the drug binding site and the precise mechanism of inhibition have been highly conserved in the evolution of type II topoisomerases.

CROSS-RESISTANCE OF MUTANT TOPOISOMERASES

We next analyzed the sensitivity of the m-AMSA^R mutant topoisomerases to those drugs that inhibited the wild-type T4 enzyme. The 39-A^R and 52-A^R mutant topoisomerases were tested for the induction of DNA cleavage in the pres-

Table 17.2. Inhibitor Sensitivities of Mutant T4 DNA Topoisomerases[a]

| Inhibitor | Mutant Topoisomerases | |
	39-A^R	52-A^R
Mitoxantrone	R	r
m-AMSA	R	R
Ellipticine	=	R
VP-16	US	=
Oxolinic acid	US	r

[a]All sensitivities are relative to wild-type T4 topoisomerase.
R, Strongly resistant; r, resistant; =, similar to wild-type topoisomerase; US, ultrasensitive.

ence of varying concentrations of m-AMSA, mitoxantrone, ellipticine, VP-16, and oxolinic acid. As shown in Table 17.2, the 52-A^R mutant enzyme displayed at least partial cross-resistance to every drug except VP-16, while the 39-A^R mutant enzyme demonstrated cross-resistance to mitoxantrone. Surprisingly, the 39-A^R mutant enzyme proved to be ultrasensitive to VP-16 and oxolinic acid (relative to the wild-type enzyme). Therefore, for each of the drugs tested, one or both m-AMSA^R mutant topoisomerases exhibited a significant alteration in drug sensitivity.

There are several interesting implications of these results. First, a simple mutational alteration of the topoisomerase can simultaneously alter the sensitivity of the enzyme to several structurally distinct inhibitors. These results support the proposal that all of the tested inhibitors act by a common mechanism. Second, the ultrasensitivity of the 39-A^R mutant enzyme to oxolinic acid provides a link between the mechanism of action of the antibacterial quinolones and that of the various antitumor agents under consideration. One way to consider this result is to suppose that the wild-type T4 enzyme has a cryptic sensitivity to quinolones and the 39-A^R mutation has exposed that sensitivity, perhaps by a subtle modification of the drug binding site (also see Discussion). Third, very small changes (presumably single amino acid) in the sequence of the topoisomerase can drastically alter the spectrum of drug sensitivities. This observation suggests that the natural interspecies variation in type II topoisomerase sequences may lead to a variety of sensitivity profiles. Therefore, topoisomerase inhibitors may have currently unrecognized clinical utility. For example, topoisomerase inhibitors may be discovered that exert specific antifungal or antiviral activity (41).

The DNA cleavage patterns observed in these experiments are also worthy of note. Treatment of the wild-type enzyme with topoisomerase inhibitors generally altered the DNA cleavage pattern, and different inhibitors produced distinct patterns. In addition, treatment of either m-AMSA^R mutant enzyme with a drug to which that enzyme was sensitive also introduced variation in the associated DNA cleavage patterns. Recall that each of the m-AMSA^R mutations themselves also altered the DNA cleavage site specificity of the T4 topoisomerase (see m-AMSA^R Topoisomerase Activity). Therefore, DNA site recognition can apparently be altered by either topoisomerase inhibitors or mutations that render the enzyme insensitive to these inhibitors. It is apparent, therefore, that DNA sequence (or sequence-dependent structure) plays some important role in the mechanism of both drug sensitivity and resistance. Various possible DNA–topoisomerase–drug interaction schemes are considered in the Discussion.

DISCUSSION

We are using the simple T4 bacteriophage as a model system to investigate the mechanism of action of m-AMSA and other antitumor agents. Genetic analyses of two m-AMSA^R mutant phage indicated that drug resistance can be conferred by single point mutations in the topoisomerase structural genes. Topoisomerase encoded by drug-resistant mutant phage exhibited m-AMSA–resistant DNA relaxation and m-AMSA–insensitive DNA cleavage activities. Because a single mutation results in both drug-resistant phage growth and a drug-insensitive viral topoisomerase, we conclude that the T4 type II DNA topoisomerase is the physiological target of m-AMSA in phage-infected $E.$ $coli$.

Numerous antibacterial and antitumor agents apparently exert their action through a topoisomerase. Bacterial DNA gyrase, a type II topoisomerase, is the intracellular target of the quinolone class of antibacterials (23,42). Recent studies using a yeast model system demonstrated that eukaryotic type I topoisomerase is the target of the plant alkaloid camptothecin (43). Finally, the mammalian type II topoisomerase is inhibited by members of many important classes of antitumor agents, including aminoacridines, anthracyclines, ellipticines, and epipodophyllotoxins (11,15). There is currently no conclusive evidence that the mammalian type II enzyme is the sole intracellular target for any of these antitumor agents. However, analogy with the T4 system described here strengthens the argument that mammalian topoisomerase is the only significant physiological target of antitumor drug action.

All of the topoisomerase inhibitors mentioned above result in the formation of a cleavable complex between the relevant topoisomerase and DNA. Consistent with their reaction mechanisms, cleavable complexes involving the type I topoisomerase contain single-strand DNA interruptions, and those involving type II enzymes contain double-strand interruptions. The induction of similar cleavable complexes involving these different topoisomerases and a wide variety of inhibitors suggests a unified mechanism of inhibition. This suggestion is supported by the oxolinic acid sensitivity of the 39-A^R T4 topoisomerase. The unexpected sensitivity to a gyrase inhibitor provides a direct link between the mechanism of action of quinolones and that of antitumor agents that inhibit type II topoisomerases.

The Inhibitor Binding Site

Before we discuss possible models for inhibition, the nature of the inhibitor binding site will be considered. What have we learned about this site from our studies with phage T4? The fact that m-AMSA^R mutations concurrently alter sensitivity to m-AMSA, ellipticine, mitoxantrone, VP-16, and oxolinic acid argues that all of these compounds bind to overlapping or identical site(s). The inference of a common binding site for at least five structurally distinct compounds is quite remarkable. The enzyme and/or associated DNA apparently contains a site able to bind these various inhibitors and yet able to exclude the countless compounds that do not affect topoisomerase. It was also surprising to find that the wild-type phage T4 and mammalian enzymes are commonly sensitive to m-AMSA, ellipticine, mitoxantrone, and VP-16. As already noted, the T4 and mammalian enzymes exhibit little direct amino acid homology (38–40; Nolan et al., this volume), and yet these (and conceivably other) drug sensitivities are conserved. The oxolinic acid sensitivity of the 39-A^R mutant topoisomerase also implies some similarity in the inhibitor binding sites of bacterial DNA gyrase and T4 topoisomerase, two enzymes that are functionally dissimilar.

These results with the phage T4 system therefore imply that the fundamental nature of the inhibitor binding site is highly conserved within diverse type II topoisomerases. This conservation might be compatible with binding of the inhibitor to some functionally critical location on the enzyme, such as a site normally occupied by DNA or by a cofactor. However, there is no evidence favoring this proposal. Alternatively, an inhibitor binding site on the DNA molecule might explain the conservation, since all type II topoisomerases must react similarly with DNA (see below).

Three Models for Inhibition

The inhibitors under discussion each result in the accumulation of a cleavable complex involving DNA, topoisomerase, and presumably the inhibitor itself. It seems likely that the interactions between these components occur in an obligatory sequence, so that one specific binary complex is formed prior to the final ternary complex. If so, there are three possible interaction sequences that may be formulated as general models of inhibition. These three models will be referred to on the basis of their initial binary complex: (1) enzyme–inhibitor; (2) DNA–inhibitor; (3) enzyme–DNA.

The first model proposes that inhibitors are able to bind free enzyme, resulting in a binary enzyme–inhibitor complex competent for binding DNA to create the cleavable complex. According to this model, a well-defined inhibitor binding site exists within free topoisomerase. However, the conserved nature of the inhibitor binding site argues against this possibility (see above). A second drawback of this model is that it fails to explain how various inhibitors alter the DNA cleavage patterns of the type II topoisomerases in different ways (1,16,24a). It is possible to argue that inhibitor binding results in a conformational change within topoisomerase that leads, in turn, to a change in cleavage site selection. However, the fact that each class of inhibitors results in a distinctly different cleavage pattern would necessitate a variety of conformational changes. A final argument against this model is that it does not acknowledge the fact that many or all topoisomerase inhibitors bind DNA (44–46).

The second general model involves an initial inhibitor–DNA complex that is subsequently bound by topoisomerase to form the cleavable complex. This model has several attractive features. Many or all of the type II topoisomerase inhibitors under consideration are DNA-binding agents (44–46), consistent with an inhibitor–DNA binary complex. In addition, each of the inhibitors may have somewhat different binding site preferences along the DNA molecule (see 47–49), possibly relating to the drug-dependent alterations in cleavage site specificity noted above. This model is conceptually pleasing, because the binding of inhibitor to DNA may alter the local DNA conformation so that it is more readily assimilated by topoisomerase into a cleavable complex (Macdonald et al., this volume). Furthermore, if topoisomerase does bind DNA at sites already containing inhibitor, the inhibitor would thereby be placed near the enzyme active site where it could exert its inhibitory effect. In spite of these appealing features, this model suffers an important disadvantage. The various topoisomerase inhibitors do not share a common primary mode of binding to free DNA. Anthracyclines, ellipticines, and acridine derivatives intercalate into duplex DNA, while the quinolones and epipodophyllotoxins apparently prefer binding to single-stranded DNA (44–46).

In the third proposed interaction sequence, a topoisomerase–DNA complex is formed prior to inhibitor binding. Assuming that the cleavable complex is a short-lived reaction intermediate with enzyme covalently attached to cleaved DNA, the inhibitor may bind to this intermediate and simply block the resealing reaction. One version of this model is that, upon formation of the cleavable complex, the enzyme creates the inhibitor binding site on the DNA molecule. By proposing that this inhibitor binding site is created by the action of the enzyme, the unique characteristics of this site can be explained. For example, because each enzyme forms a cleavable complex with DNA as a reaction intermediate, the inhibitor binding sites of all type II topoisomerases would display conservation. The binding of structurally dissimilar compounds to this site might depend on some unique aspect of the DNA structure formed at the active site, because the DNA must be cleaved and transiently denaturated during the strand passage reaction. Even though a conserved inhibitor binding site apparently exists, simple mutational alterations in the topoisomerase can markedly alter drug sensitivities. Therefore, the amino acids near the active site may affect the access of inhibitors to the conserved binding site, or may even form part of the binding site by interacting with functional groups on the inhibitor. Indeed, the alterations in DNA cleavage specificity due to the m-AMSA^R mutations argue that these mutations affect regions of the protein that normally contact DNA. An interesting precedent for this third model is that the binding of resolvase to its specific DNA recognition site creates a novel binding site for the intercalator methidium (50).

As does model two, model three can readily explain the unique alterations in cleavage site specificity caused by various type II topoisomerase inhibitors. As noted earlier, each class of inhibitor may have preferences for particular locations on DNA (47–49). Therefore, each class could stabilize cleavable complexes only at certain topoisomerase recognition sites; topoisomerase bound to other sites would continue to actively cleave and reseal DNA.

It is not yet possible to choose among these three models for the inhibition of type II topoisomerases. Our studies with the phage T4 topoisomerase indi-

cate that the inhibitor binding site is shared by dissimilar drugs and is conserved between diverse topoisomerases. We believe that these findings argue
strongly against model one and are most consistent with model three. However,
more definitive tests are required to distinguish between these general models
and to provide a detailed mechanism of inhibition.

Mechanism of Drug Resistance

Resistance to *m*-AMSA was found to arise from mutation of either T4 gene *39*
or *52*, two of the three topoisomerase structural genes. This result is somewhat
surprising given the apparent functions of the topoisomerase subunits. Gene *52*
product becomes covalently attached to DNA in the presence of *m*-AMSA,
indicating that this subunit catalyzes DNA cleavage and resealing (24; also see
38). The isolated gene *39* product is reported to catalyze ATP hydrolysis, and
the predicted amino acid sequence of this subunit has similarity with the
ATPase subunit of DNA gyrase (39). Therefore, mutational alteration of either
the cleavage–resealing or ATPase subunit of the T4 topoisomerase can alter
drug sensitivity. In the case of bacterial DNA gyrase, high level resistance to
nalidixic acid involves alteration of the cleavage–resealing subunit. However,
as with the T4 enzyme, both gyrase subunits apparently control drug sensitivity: quinolone-resistance mutations in the ATPase subunit have also been reported (51).

 Although the mutational alterations conferring *m*-AMSA resistance are located in distinct subunits of the T4 topoisomerase, the two mutant enzymes
share several important characteristics. First, each mutant enzyme exhibits an
altered pattern of drug-independent DNA cleavage relative to the wild-type
topoisomerase. Second, both mutant enzymes appear to mediate higher levels
of drug-independent DNA cleavage than does the wild-type enzyme. This apparent increase in DNA cleavage activity need not be due to an actual increase
in the rate of DNA cleavage, but could instead be explained by a decreased
rate of DNA resealing. In the latter case, the reaction intermediate consisting
of the cleavable complex has a longer lifetime for the mutant than for the wild-
type enzyme. A similar increase in stability of a cleavable complex has been
reported for a mutant camptothecin-resistant type I topoisomerase (52). Third,
each mutational alteration confers resistance to some, but not all, topoisomerase inhibitors. These similarities between the two *m*-AMSA^R mutant enzymes suggest that the enzymes share a similar mode of drug resistance.

 The mechanism of drug resistance seems to involve some alteration at or
very near the inhibitor binding site. The 39-A^R mutant topoisomerase is resistant to *m*-AMSA and mitoxantrone, but ultrasensitive to oxolinic acid and VP-
16. One simple explanation for this finding is that the drug-resistance mutation
alters the drug binding site to facilitate the binding of some inhibitors but to
reduce the binding of others. Clearly, the inhibitor binding site is not simply
destroyed by the mutational alterations because each mutant enzyme retains
sensitivity to some inhibitors. In the third inhibition model discussed earlier,
most or all of the inhibitor binding site is composed of DNA at the active site
of the enzyme. To comply with this model, the drug-resistance mutations would

alter the enzyme structure near the active site to differentially affect inhibitor binding. Perhaps such alterations near the active site are also responsible for the dramatic changes in DNA cleavage site specificity of the mutant enzymes.

SUMMARY

We have demonstrated that the T4–encoded type II topoisomerase is the physiological target of *m*-AMSA in T4–infected *E. coli*. Powerful genetic and biochemical approaches available in the T4 system have facilitated investigations of the mechanism of action of topoisomerase inhibitors and the mechanism of mutationally induced drug resistance.

Acknowledgments

The work in this laboratory was supported by grants from the Elsa U. Pardee Foundation and the Bristol-Myers Company. A.C.H. was supported by the National Research Service Award 5T32 CA09111-13 from the U.S. Department of Health and Human Services. This work was done during the tenure of an Established Investigatorship from the American Heart Association to K.N.K.

REFERENCES

1. Huff, A. C., Leatherwood, J. K., and Kreuzer, K. N. Bacteriophage T4 DNA topoisomerase is the target of antitumor agent 4′-(9-acridinylamino) methanesulfon-*m*-anisidide (*m*-AMSA) in T4-infected *Escherichia coli*. Proc. Natl. Acad. Sci. USA. **86:** 1307, 1989.

2. Ripley, L. S., Dubins, J. S., deBoer, J. G., DeMarini, D. M., Bogerd, A. M., and Kreuzer, K. N. Hotspot sites for acridine-induced frameshift mutations in bacteriophage T4 correspond to sites of action of the T4 type II topoisomerase. J. Mol. Biol. **200:** 665, 1988.

3. Cozzarelli, N. R. DNA gyrase and the supercoiling of DNA. Science. **207:** 953, 1980.

4. Gellert, M. DNA topoisomerases. Annu. Rev. Biochem. **50:** 879, 1981.

5. Liu, L. F. DNA topoisomerases: Enzymes that catalyze the breaking and rejoining of DNA. CRC Crit. Rev. Biochem. **15:** 1, 1983.

6. Wang, J. C. DNA topoisomerases. Annu. Rev. Biochem. **54:** 665, 1985.

7. Morrison, A. and Cozzarelli, N. R. Site-specific cleavage of DNA by *E. coli* DNA gyrase. Cell. **17:** 175, 1979.

8. Tse, Y-C., Kirkegaard, K., and Wang, J. C. Covalent bonds between protein and DNA. Formation of phosphotyrosine linkage between certain DNA topoisomerases and DNA. J. Biol. Chem. **255:** 5560, 1980.

9. Gellert, M., Fisher, L. M., Ohmori, H., O'Dea, M. H., and Mizuuchi, K. DNA gyrase: Site-specific interactions and transient double-strand breakage of DNA. Cold Spring Harbor Symp. Quant. Biol. **45:** 391, 1981.

10. Nelson, E. M., Tewey, K. M., and Liu, L. F. Mechanism of antitumor drug action: Poisoning of mammalian DNA topoisomerase II on DNA by 4′-(9-acridinylamino)-methanesulfon-*m*-anisidide. Proc. Natl. Acad. Sci. USA. **81:** 1361, 1984.

11. Glisson, B. S. and Ross, W. E. DNA topoisomerase II: A primer on the enzyme and its unique role as a multidrug target in cancer chemotherapy. Pharmacol. Ther. **32:** 89, 1987.

12. Brown, P. O., Peebles, C. L., and Cozzarelli, N. R. A topoisomerase from *Escherichia coli* related to DNA gyrase. Proc. Natl. Acad. Sci. USA. **76:** 6110, 1979.

13. Kirkegaard, K. and Wang, J. C. Mapping the topography of DNA wrapped around gyrase by nucleolytic and chemical prob-

ing of complexes of unique DNA sequences. Cell. **23:** 721, 1981.

14. Fisher, L. M., Barot, H. A., and Cullen, M. E. DNA gyrase complex with DNA: Determinants for site-specific DNA breakage. EMBO J. **5:** 1411, 1986.

15. Drlica, K. and Franco, R. J. Inhibitors of DNA topoisomerases. Biochemistry. **27:** 2253, 1988.

16. Tewey, K. M., Rowe, T. C., Yang, L., Halligan, B. D., and Liu, L. F. Adriamycin-induced DNA damage mediated by mammalian DNA topoisomerase II. Science. **226:** 466, 1984.

17. Drlica, K. Biology of bacterial deoxyribonucleic acid topoisomerases. Microbiol. Rev. **48:** 273, 1984.

18. Ross, W. E. DNA topoisomerases as targets for cancer therapy. Biochem. Pharmacol. **34:** 4191, 1985.

19. Kutter, E. and Ruger, W. Map of the T4 genome and its transcription control sites. In C. K. Mathews, E. M. Kutter, G. Mosig, and P. B. Berget, eds. *Bacteriophage T4*. Washington, D.C.: American Society for Microbiology, 1983, p. 277.

20. Mathews, C. K., Kutter, E. M., Mosig, G., and Berget, P. B. *Bacteriophage T4*. Washington, D.C.: American Society for Microbiology, 1983.

21. Kreuzer, K. N. and Jongeneel, C. V. *Escherichia coli* phage T4 topoisomerase. Methods Enzymol. **100:** 144, 1983.

22. Osheroff, N., Shelton, E. R., and Brutlag, D. L. DNA topoisomerase II from *Drosophila melanogaster*. J. Biol. Chem. **258:** 9536, 1983.

23. Sugino, A., Peebles, C. L., Kreuzer, K. N., and Cozzarelli, N. R. Mechanism of action of nalidixic acid: Purification of *Escherichia coli nalA* gene product and its relationship to DNA gyrase and a novel nicking-closing enzyme. Proc. Natl. Acad. Sci. USA. **85:** 7501, 1977.

24. Rowe, T. C., Tewey, K. M., and Liu, L. F. Identification of the breakage-reunion subunit of T4 DNA topoisomerase. J. Biol. Chem. **259:** 9177, 1984.

24a. Huff, A. C. and Kreuzer, K. N. Evidence for a common mechanism of action for antitumor and antibacterial agents that inhibit type II DNA topoisomerases. J. Biol. Chem., in press.

25. Wong, S. W., Wahl, A. F., Yuan, P-M., Arai, N., Pearson, B. E., Arai, K.-I., Korn, D., Hunkapiller, M. W., and Wang, T.S.-F. Human DNA polymerase α gene expression is cell proliferation dependent and its primary structure is similar to both prokaryotic and eukaryotic replicative DNA polymerases. EMBO J. **7:** 37, 1988.

26. Spicer, E. K., Rush, J., Fung, C., Rhea-Krantz, L. J., Karam, J. D., and Konigsberg, W. H. Primary structure of T4 DNA polymerase. J. Biol. Chem. **263:** 7478, 1988.

27. Schmidt, F. J. RNA splicing in prokaryotes: Bacteriophage T4 leads the way. Cell. **41:** 339, 1985.

28. Belfort, M., Pederson-Lane, J., West, D., Ehrenman, K., Maley, G., Chu, F., and Maley, F. Processing of the intron-containing thymidylate synthase *(td)* gene of phage T4 is at the RNA level. Cell. **41:** 375, 1985.

29. Gott, J. M., Shub, D. A., and Belfort, M. Multiple self-splicing introns in bacteriophage T4: Evidence from autocatalytic GTP labeling of RNA in vitro. Cell. **47:** 81, 1986.

30. Chen, D. S. and Bernstein, H. Yeast gene RAD52 can substitute for phage T4 gene 46 or 47 in carrying out recombination and DNA repair. Proc. Natl. Acad. Sci. USA. **85:** 6821, 1988.

31. DeMarini, D. M., Doerr, C. L., Meyer, M. K., Brock, K. H., Hozier, J., and Moore, M. M. Mutagenicity of *m*-AMSA and *o*-AMSA in mammalian cells due to clastogenic mechanism: Possible role of topoisomerase. Mutagenesis. **2:** 349, 1987.

32. DeMarini, D. M., Brock, K. H., Doerr, C. L., and Moore, M. M. Mutagenicity and clastogenicity of teniposide (VM-26) in L5178Y/TK$^{+/-}$-3.7.2C mouse lymphoma cells. Mutat. Res. **187:** 141, 1987.

33. Moore, M. M., Brock, K. H., Doerr, C. L., and Demarini, D. M. Mutagenesis of L5178Y/TK$^{+/-}$-3.7.2C mouse lymphoma cells by the clastogen ellipticine. Environ. Mutagen. **9:** 161, 1987.

34. Gupta, R. S., Bromke, A., Bryant, D. W., Gupta, R., Singh, B., and McCalla, D. R. Etoposide (VP16) and teniposide (VM26): Novel anticancer drugs, strongly mutagenic in mammalian but not prokaryotic test systems. *Mutagenesis*. **2:** 179, 1987.

35. Ripley, L. S. and Clark, A. Frameshift mutations produced by proflavin in bacteriophage T4: Specificity within a hotspot. Proc. Natl. Acad. Sci. USA. **83:** 6954, 1986.

35a. Huff, A. C., Ward IV, R. E., and Kreuzer, K. N. Mutational alteration of the breakage/resealing subunit of bacteriophage T4 DNA topoisomerase confers resistance to antitumor agent *m*-AMSA. Mol. Gen. Genet. **221:** 27, 1990.

36. Kreuzer, K. N. and Alberts, B. M. Site-specific recognition of bacteriophage T4 DNA by T4 type II DNA topoisomerase and *Escherichia coli* DNA gyrase. J. Biol. Chem. **259:** 5339, 1984.
37. Chen, G. L., Yang, L., Rowe, T. C., Halligan, B. D., Tewey, K. M., and Liu, L. F. Nonintercalative antitumor drugs interfere with the breakage-reunion reaction of mammalian DNA topoisomerase II. J. Biol. Chem. **259:** 13560, 1984.
38. Huang, W. M. The 52-protein subunit of T4 DNA topoisomerase is homologous to the gyrA-protein of gyrase. Nucleic Acids Res. **14:** 7379, 1986.
39. Huang, W. M. Nucleotide sequence of a type II DNA topoisomerase gene. Bacteriophage T4 gene 39. Nucleic Acids Res. **14:** 7751, 1986.
40. Tsai-Pflugfelder, M., Liu, L. F., Liu, A. A., Tewey, K. M., Whang-Peng, J., Knutsen, T., Huebner, K., Croce, C. M., and Wang, J. C. Cloning and sequencing of cDNA encoding human DNA topoisomerase II and localization of the gene to chromosome region 17q21-22. Proc. Natl. Acad. Sci. USA. **85:** 7177, 1988.
41. Kreuzer, K. N. DNA topoisomerases as potential targets of antiviral action. Pharmacol. Ther. **43:** 377, 1989.
42. Gellert, M., Mizuuchi, K., O'Dea, M. H., Itoh, T., and Tomizawa, J.-I. Nalidixic acid resistance: A second genetic character involved in DNA gyrase activity. Proc. Natl. Acad. Sci. USA. **74:** 4772, 1977.
43. Nitiss, J. and Wang, J. C. DNA topoisomerase-targeting antitumor drugs can be studied in yeast. Proc. Natl. Acad. Sci. USA. **85:** 7501, 1988.
44. Waring, M. J. DNA modification and cancer. Annu. Rev. Biochem. **50:** 159, 1981.
45. Shen, L. L. and Pernet, A. G. Mechanism of inhibition of DNA gyrase by analogues of nalidixic acid: The target of the drugs is DNA. Proc. Natl. Acad. Sci. USA. **82:** 307, 1985.
46. Chow, K-C., MacDonald, T. L., and Ross, W. E. DNA binding by epipodophyllotoxins and *N*-acyl anthracyclines: Implications for mechanism of topoisomerase II inhibition. Mol. Pharmacol. **34:** 467, 1988.
47. Dabrowiak, J. C. Sequence specificity of drug-DNA interactions. Life Sci. **32:** 2915, 1983.
48. Robbie, M. and Wilkins, R. J. Identification of the specific sites of interaction between intercalating drugs and DNA. Chem.-Biol. Interact. **49:** 189, 1984.
49. Fox, K. R., Waring, M. J., Brown, J. R., and Neidle, S. DNA sequence preferences for the anti-cancer drug mitoxantrone and related anthraquinones revealed by DNase I footprinting. FEBS Lett. **202:** 289, 1986.
50. Hatfull, G. F., Noble, S. M., and Grindley, N.D.F. The γδ resolvase induces an unusual DNA structure at the recombinational crossover point. Cell. **49:** 103, 1987.
51. Yamagishi, J.-i., Yoshida, H., Yamayoshi, M., and Nakamura, S. Nalidixic acid-resistant mutations of the *gyrB* gene of *Escherichia coli*. Mol. Gen. Genet. **204:** 367, 1986.
52. Kjeldsen, E., Bonven, B. J., Andoh, T., Ishii, K., Okada, K., Bolund, L., and Westergaard, O. Characterization of a camptothecin-resistant human DNA topoisomerase I. J. Biol. Chem. **263:** 3912, 1988.

Chapter 18
Mechanism of the Topoisomerase II–Mediated DNA Cleavage–Religation Reaction: Inhibition of DNA Religation by Antineoplastic Drugs

NEIL OSHEROFF, MEGAN J. ROBINSON,
AND E. LYNN ZECHIEDRICH

DNA topoisomerase II is an essential enzyme (1–4) that is involved in many fundamental cellular processes, including DNA replication, transcription (5–7), chromosome segregation (1,3,4,8,9), and chromosome structure (10–13). Central to the physiological functions of the enzyme is its ability to introduce and reseal site-specific double-stranded DNA breaks in the genome (5–7).

The importance of the topoisomerase II–mediated DNA cleavage–religation cycle has led to the development of an assay that allows this process to be monitored *in vitro* (14,15). In this assay, topoisomerase II and DNA are mixed and allowed to establish a cleavage–religation equilibrium. Enzyme-mediated DNA cleavage products are isolated by the rapid addition of a denaturing detergent, such as sodium dodecyl sulfate (SDS), to the reaction mixture. It has not yet been resolved whether SDS acts by inducing DNA cleavage to take place within an existing precleavage (i.e., "cleavable") topoisomerase II–DNA complex or whether the detergent rapidly denatures (and thereby traps) an existing complex in which the nucleic acid has already been cleaved by the enzyme. However, on the basis of mechanistic comparisons with type I topoisomerases (16–18), the latter would appear to be true. Irrespective of mechanism, the *in vitro* assay is believed to reflect the physiological reaction of the enzyme (19–21). To this point, substrates that contain sites of DNA cleavage defined by the above system display enhanced kinetic and binding affinities for topoisomerase II (22).

Using the *in vitro* assay, several features of the double-stranded DNA cleavage–religation reaction have been characterized. First, the product is a covalent topoisomerase II–DNA complex (14,15) in which the enzyme is attached to the 4 base protruding 5' termini of the cleaved nucleic acid (14,15) *via* an O^4-phosphotyrosyl bond (23). Second, DNA cleavage and religation are in equilibrium with one another. If the equilibrium is shifted toward religation by the addition of salt, the DNA substrate is regenerated in its original topological form (15,24). Third, cleavage is not dependent on the presence of ATP (14), the cofactor required for the enzyme's DNA strand passage reaction (5–7). Finally, the reaction is absolutely dependent on the presence of a divalent cation (14,25). While the physiological cation appears to be magnesium, high levels of enzyme-mediated DNA cleavage can also be promoted by calcium (24). With respect to covalent enzyme–DNA linkage, salt reversibility, and nucleotide specificity of cleavage, products of calcium-promoted reactions are identical to those produced in the presence of magnesium (24).

Beyond its normal cellular activities, topoisomerase II appears to be the primary cellular target for a number of clinically relevant antineoplastic drugs (26–28). The chemotherapeutic activities of these agents correlate with their abilities to stabilize covalent topoisomerase II–DNA cleavage complexes (26–28). Thus, as monitored *in vitro,* these drugs increase levels of enzyme-mediated double- and single-stranded DNA cleavage (26–28). Unfortunately, despite the important role of topoisomerase II in the treatment of human cancers, virtually nothing is known about the mechanism by which antineoplastic drugs alter enzyme function.

One of the major stumbling blocks that has prevented the detailed mechanism of drug action on topoisomerase II from being delineated has been the inability to uncouple the forward DNA cleavage reaction from the reverse religation event. Therefore, while it is possible to demonstrate that antineoplastic agents stimulate enzyme-mediated DNA breakage by shifting the cleavage–religation equilibrium toward cleavage, it is impossible to state with certainty whether these drugs act by enhancing the forward cleavage reaction or by inhibiting DNA religation.

A novel assay has been developed that uncouples religation from DNA cleavage (24). The assay takes advantage of the finding that DNA cleavage products generated by topoisomerase II in the presence of calcium can be trapped in the complete absence of a protein denaturant (24). This allows the covalent enzyme–DNA cleavage complex to be isolated in a kinetically competent form and provides a system in which religation can be examined in the absence of the forward cleavage reaction.

This assay has been employed to examine the kinetic pathway of the topoisomerase II–mediated DNA cleavage–religation reaction as well as the mechanism of antineoplastic drug action. The enzyme appears to produce double-stranded breaks in DNA by making two sequential single-stranded breaks in the nucleic acid backbone. Moreover, both intercalative (4'-(9-acridinylamino)methanesulfon-*m*-anisidide; *m*-AMSA) and nonintercalative (4'-demethylepipodophyllotoxin thenylidene-B-D-glucoside; etoposide) antineoplastic agents stabilize enzyme–DNA cleavage complexes (at least in part) by inhibiting the religation of cleaved DNA.

KINETIC PATHWAY OF THE TOPOISOMERASE II–MEDIATED
DOUBLE-STRANDED DNA CLEAVAGE–RELIGATION REACTION

Invariably, topoisomerase II–mediated DNA cleavage produces not only double-stranded breaks in the nucleic acid backbone but single-stranded breaks (i.e., nicks) as well (15,24,29–31). The substitution of calcium for magnesium ions in reaction mixtures exacerbates this DNA nicking (24). Moreover, the presence of many antineoplastic agents increases both double-stranded and single-stranded DNA cleavage (20,29–32). While the physiological implications of enzyme-mediated DNA nicking are not known, it has been suggested that single-stranded breaks are intermediates in the double-stranded DNA cleavage–religation reaction of topoisomerase II (24).

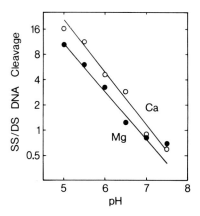

Figure 18.1. pH titration of the DNA cleavage–religation reaction of *Drosophila melanogaster* topoisomerase II. The data are plotted as the ratio of single-stranded (SS) to double-stranded (DS) DNA cleavage. A semilogarithmic plot is shown. The enzyme was isolated from the nuclei of *Drosophila* Kc tissue culture cells by the procedure of Shelton et al. (33). DNA cleavage assays contained 5 nM negatively supercoiled pBR322 plasmid DNA and 100 nM topoisomerase II and were carried out in a total of 20 µl of cleavage buffer (10 mM imidazole, pH 5.0 to 7.5, 50 mM NaCl, 50 mM KCl, 0.1 mM EDTA, and either 2.5% glycerol or 15 µg/ml bovine serum albumin) which contained 5 mM divalent cations. The pH of completed reaction mixtures was confirmed using a Lazar Research Laboratories micro pH electrode (model PHR-146). Samples were incubated at 30°C for 6 min. DNA cleavage products were trapped by the addition of 2 µl of 10% SDS. One microliter of 250 mM EDTA and 2 µl of 0.8 mg/ml proteinase K were added and mixtures were incubated at 45°C for 30 min to digest the topoisomerase II. Products were mixed with 3 µl of loading buffer (60% sucrose, 0.05% bromophenol blue, 0.05% xylene cyanole FF, and 10 mM Tris-HCl, pH 7.9), heated at 75°C for 2 min, and subjected to electrophoresis in 1% agarose (MCB) gels in 40 mM Tris-acetate, pH 8.3, and 2 mM EDTA at 5 V/cm. Following electrophoresis, gels were stained in an aqueous solution of ethidium bromide (1 µg/ml). DNA bands were visualized by transillumination with ultraviolet light (300 nm) and photographed through Kodak Nos. 24A and 12 filters using Polaroid type 665 positive/negative film. The amount of DNA was quantitated by scanning negatives with a Biomed Instruments Model SL-504-XL scanning densitometer. Reactions were carried out in the presence of either 5 mM $MgCl_2$ (filled circle) or 5 mM $CaCl_2$ (open circle).

This suggestion is supported by the results of a pH titration of the DNA cleavage–religation reaction (Fig. 18.1). At neutral to slightly alkaline pH, *Drosophila* topoisomerase II generated predominately double-stranded breaks in negatively supercoiled pBR322 plasmid DNA. This was evidenced by a single-stranded:double-stranded DNA cleavage ratio of less than 1. However, as the pH of the reaction was lowered, the enzyme produced DNA nicks at the near exclusion of double-stranded breaks (single-stranded:double-stranded cleavage ratio ≈ 10 to 20:1 at pH 5). The predominance of DNA nicking was not due to a loss in enzyme activity, as the total amount of topoisomerase II–mediated cleavage (i.e., single-stranded plus double-stranded) remained relatively constant over the pH range tested (not shown).

The finding that topoisomerase II can mediate high levels of DNA nicking provides a strong argument against a reaction mechanism in which the enzyme makes only concerted double-stranded breaks in the nucleic acid backbone. To explore more fully the possibility that nicks represent an intermediate in the double-stranded DNA cleavage–religation reaction, the kinetic pathway of the enzyme-mediated religation reaction was characterized (34). To this end, the DNA religation assay of Osheroff and Zechiedrich (24) was employed. The assay takes advantage of the fact that a kinetically competent covalent topoisomerase II–DNA cleavage complex can be trapped by chelating the divalent

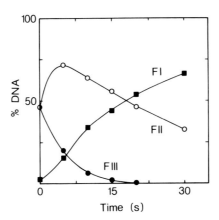

Figure 18.2. Time course of enzyme-mediated religation of cleaved DNA. Assays were carried out as described by Osheroff and Zechiedrich (24). Topoisomerase II (75 nM) and 5 nM negatively supercoiled pBR322 DNA were incubated for 6 min at 30°C in 20 μl of cleavage buffer that contained 5 mM $CaCl_2$ and 10 mM Tris-HCl, pH 7.9, in place of imidazole. Kinetically competent covalent topoisomerase II–DNA cleavage complexes were trapped by the addition of 10 mM EDTA (final concentration). NaCl (200 mM final concentration) was added to prevent recleavage of the DNA during the religation reaction (15,24). Samples were placed on ice to slow reaction rates, and religation was initiated by the addition of cold $MgCl_2$ (7.5 mM final concentration). SDS (2 μl of a 10% solution) was added to terminate religation at various time points up to 30 sec. Samples were digested with proteinase K and were analyzed by electrophoresis as described in the legend on Figure 18.1. Linear form III DNA (FIII, filled circle), nicked form II DNA (FII, open circle), and negatively supercoiled form I DNA (FI, filled box) are plotted as the percentage of the total DNA present in the reaction mixture.

cation from calcium-promoted DNA cleavage–religation reactions (24). By increasing the ionic strength of assay mixtures prior to the back addition of magnesium ions, DNA religation within the covalent enzyme–DNA complex can be monitored in the absence of the forward cleavage reaction.

A time course for topoisomerase II–mediated DNA religation is depicted graphically in Figure 18.2. During the course of the reaction, levels of linear DNA (FIII) dropped rapidly. The drop in linear DNA was accompanied by a transient rise in nicked circular molecules (FII). Following an initial lag, the rate of regeneration of supercoiled plasmids (FI) was proportional to the rate of disappearance of nicked DNA. This reaction profile is diagnostic of a two-step sequential mechanism (35,36) in which nicked circular DNA is an obligatory kinetic intermediate in the topoisomerase II–mediated religation of double-stranded DNA breaks (i.e., FIII→FII→FI).

EFFECTS OF ANTINEOPLASTIC AGENTS ON THE TOPOISOMERASE II–MEDIATED DNA RELIGATION REACTION

Topoisomerase II appears to be the primary cellular target for a number of antineoplastic agents (26–28). These agents can be grouped broadly into two classes: those drugs that are intercalative with respect to DNA (of which the acridine *m*-AMSA is a representative example) and those that are nonintercalative (of which the epipodophyllotoxin etoposide is a representative example). The chemotherapeutic properties of the above drugs correlate with their abilities to stabilize (i.e., increase levels of) covalent topoisomerase II–DNA cleavage complexes (26–28). Although it is widely assumed that these agents act by inhibiting the enzyme's ability to religate cleaved DNA, no direct evidence supporting such a mechanism has been reported. Therefore, the assay system discussed earlier was employed to determine the effects of antineoplastic agents on the religation reaction of *Drosophila* topoisomerase II.

As previously shown for mammalian type II topoisomerases (26–32,37), both *m*-AMSA and etoposide stimulated the formation of DNA cleavage products by the *Drosophila* enzyme (Fig. 18.3). The presence of 60 μM *m*-AMSA increased levels of enzyme-mediated double-stranded and single-stranded DNA cleavage approximately fivefold and twofold, respectively, while 100 μM etoposide increased these values approximately sixfold and fourfold, respectively.

The effects of *m*-AMSA and etoposide on the DNA religation reaction of topoisomerase II are shown in Figure 18.4. The data are presented as a semilogarithmic plot of percent linear DNA versus time. Although Figure 18.4 shows only the effects of antineoplastic agents on the religation of the first strand of DNA (i.e., the FIII→FII reaction), similar results were obtained for the FII→FI event (not shown). As expected for the first order religation reaction, straight lines were obtained. When 60 μm *m*-AMSA was included in assays at the time of cleavage, the rate of enzyme-mediated DNA religation was decreased by 3.5-fold (*left panel*). Similarly, inclusion of 100 μM etoposide decreased the rate of religation by threefold (*right panel*). These results dem-

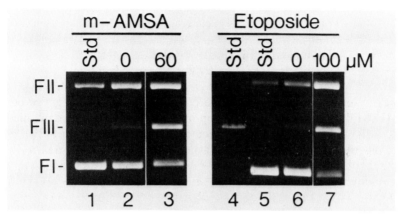

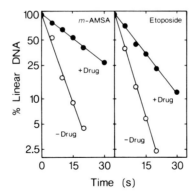

Figure 18.3. Effect of antineoplastic agents on the DNA cleavage–religation reaction of *Drosophila* topoisomerase II. Assays were carried out in cleavage buffer that contained 10 mM Tris-HCl, pH 7.9, in place of imidazole and 5 mM $MgCl_2$ as described in the legend in Figure 18.1. *m*-AMSA (NSC 249992) was the generous gift of Dr. Yves Pommier, Laboratory of Molecular Pharmacology, NCI. The drug was stored at $-20°C$ as a 10 mM solution in 100% dimethylsulfoxide (DMSO). Etoposide (VePesid, VP-16-213) was obtained from Bristol Laboratories. The drug was supplied as a sterile 20 mg/ml solution and was stored at room temperature as per the manufacturer's instructions. Both drugs were diluted to appropriate concentrations with deionized water prior to use. The relative positions of negatively supercoiled (FI), nicked (FII), and linear (FIII) DNA are indicated. Lanes 1, 4, and 5, DNA standards; lanes 2 and 6, control reactions that contained appropriate dilutions of either DMSO or etoposide buffer, respectively, but did not contain drugs; lane 3, reaction contained 60 μM *m*-AMSA; lane 7, reaction contained 100 μM etoposide.

Figure 18.4. Effect of antineoplastic drugs on the rate of topoisomerase II–mediated DNA religation. A semilogarithmic plot of percent linear DNA versus time is shown. Assays were carried out as described in the legend of Figure 18.2. Initial values of linear DNA were normalized to 100%. **Left panel.** Reactions were carried out in the absence (open circle) or presence (solid circle) of 60 μM *m*-AMSA. **Right panel.** Reactions were carried out in the absence (open circle) or presence (solid circle) of 100 μM etoposide. Reactions carried out in the absence of drug contained appropriate dilutions of either DMSO or etoposide buffer.

onstrate for the first time that both intercalative and nonintercalative antineoplastic agents stabilize covalent topoisomerase II–DNA cleavage complexes by inhibiting (at least in part) the enzyme's ability to religate its cleaved nucleic acid intermediate.

DISCUSSION

On the basis of the results presented here, two conclusions can be drawn. First, the enzyme mediates its action on double-stranded DNA by making two coordinated and sequential single-stranded breaks rather than one concerted double-stranded break in the nucleic acid backbone. Second, two potent and clinically relevant antineoplastic agents, m-AMSA and etoposide, stabilize covalent topoisomerase II–DNA cleavage complexes by inhibiting the enzyme-mediated DNA religation reaction.

Drosophila melanogaster topoisomerase II was used for the present study. Of the eukaryotic topoisomerases, the *Drosophila* type II enzyme is by far the most well characterized. In all instances where comparable studies have been carried out, results found for *Drosophila* topoisomerase II were always similar to those determined for other eukaryotic enzymes (including those from mammalian sources) (5–7). Comparisons extend to primary and quaternary structure, enzymological characteristics, nucleotide specificity, cellular regulation, and intracellular location. Thus, it seems likely that the results of the present study will be generally applicable to other eukaryotic type II topoisomerases.

Understanding the molecular mechanism by which a drug mediates its action is critical to rational drug design. Although no supporting evidence has been reported, it has long been assumed that antineoplastic agents stabilize covalent topoisomerase II–DNA cleavage complexes by inhibiting the religation reaction of the enzyme (26–28). The data presented validate this assumption. However, it must be noted that the inhibition of religation observed in the presence of m-AMSA or etoposide (3-fold to 3.5-fold) is somewhat less than the drug-induced stimulation of double-stranded cleavage (fivefold to sixfold). Moreover, since the experimental conditions (i.e., temperature, ionic strength, and divalent cation concentration) employed for the religation assay differ from those utilized in cleavage assays, it is impossible to directly compare results generated by the two systems. Therefore, while it is clear that these drugs inhibit enzyme-mediated DNA religation, it is not yet definitive that this represents their sole mode of action. Indeed, it is quite possible that antineoplastic drugs increase levels of enzyme–DNA cleavage intermediates not only by inhibiting the rate of their disappearance but by stimulating the rate of their formation as well.

Finally, m-AMSA, which is highly intercalative with respect to DNA, and etoposide, which is nonintercalative, represent two very different classes of drugs (26–28). The finding that (relative to their enhancement of DNA cleavage) both inhibit DNA religation to a similar extent argues for a common mechanism of action on topoisomerase II. Future studies will be able to more fully address this important concept.

SUMMARY

The ability to create and religate double-stranded breaks in DNA is central to the physiological functions of topoisomerase II. In addition, this activity serves as the primary target reaction for a number of antineoplastic agents whose chemotherapeutic activities correlate with their abilities to stabilize covalent enzyme–DNA cleavage complexes. Despite the importance of the topoisomerase II–mediated DNA cleavage–religation cycle to the survival of the eukaryotic cell and to the treatment of human cancers, little is known concerning its detailed mechanism. Employing a novel DNA religation assay, both the kinetic pathway of the reaction and the mechanism by which two potent antineoplastic drugs (*m*-AMSA and etoposide) affect the DNA cleavage–religation equilibrium have been characterized. Results indicate that the enzyme mediates DNA cleavage–religation by making two sequential single-stranded breaks rather than one concerted double-stranded break in the nucleic acid backbone. Moreover, antineoplastic agents stabilize the covalent topoisomerase II–DNA cleavage complex (at least in part) by inhibiting the rate of religation of both the first and second strands of cleaved DNA.

NOTE ADDED

This chapter was last revised in October 1989. A recent study on the DNA cleavage–religation reaction of topoisomerase II (38) demonstrated that SDS acts by trapping the enzyme's active DNA cleavage complex.

Acknowledgments

This work was supported by grant GM-33944 from the National Institutes of Health, training grant T32-CA09582 from the National Cancer Institute of the National Institutes of Health, and Faculty Research Award FRA-370 from the American Cancer Society.

The authors wish to thank Susan Heaver and David Sullins for their conscientious preparation of this manuscript, Elizabeth Smith for her assistance in preparing the topoisomerase II employed in this study, and Caroline R. Heise and Katherine F. Prillaman for carrying out preliminary enzymological experiments with *m*-AMSA.

REFERENCES

1. Uemura, T. and Yanagida, M. Isolation of type I and II DNA topoisomerase mutants from fission yeast: Single and double mutants show different phenotypes in cell growth and chromatin organization. EMBO J. **3:** 1737, 1984.
2. Goto, T. and Wang, J. C. Yeast DNA topoisomerase II is encoded by a single-copy, essential gene. Cell. **36:** 1073, 1984.
3. DiNardo, S., Voelkel, K., and Sternglanz, R. DNA topoisomerase II mutant of *Saccharomyces cerevisiae:* Topoisomerase II is required for segregation of daughter molecules at the termination of DNA rep-

lication. Proc. Natl. Acad. Sci. USA. **81:** 2616, 1984.

4. Holm, C., Goto, T., Wang, J. C., and Botstein, D. DNA topoisomerase II is required at the time of mitosis in yeast. Cell. **41:** 553, 1985.

5. Wang, J. C. DNA topoisomerases. Annu. Rev. Biochem. **54:** 665, 1985.

6. Vosberg, H.-P. DNA topoisomerases: Enzymes that control DNA conformation. Curr. Top. Microbiol. Immunol. **114:** 19, 1985.

7. Osheroff, N. Biochemical basis for the interactions of type I and type II topoisomerases with DNA. Pharmacol. Ther. **41:** 223, 1989.

8. Uemura, T., and Yanagida, M. Mitotic spindle pulls but fails to separate chromosomes in type II DNA topoisomerase mutants: Uncoordinated mitosis. EMBO J. **5:** 1003, 1986.

9. Uemura, T., Ohkura, H., Adachi, Y., Morino, K., Shiozaki, K., and Yanagida, M. DNA topoisomerase II is required for condensation and separation of mitotic chromosomes in *S. pombe*. Cell. **50:** 917, 1987.

10. Earnshaw, W. C., Halligan, B., Cooke, C. A., Heck, M. M. S., and Liu, L. F. Topoisomerase II is a structural component of mitotic chromosome scaffolds. J. Cell. Biol. **100:** 1706, 1985.

11. Earnshaw, W. C., and Heck, M. M. S. Localization of topoisomerase II in mitotic chromosomes. J. Cell. Biol. **100:** 1716, 1985.

12. Gasser, S. M., Laroche, T., Falquet, J., Boy de la Tour, E., and Laemmli, U. K. Metaphase chromosome structure: Involvement of topoisomerase II. J. Mol. Biol. **188:** 613, 1986.

13. Berrios, M., Osheroff, N., and Fisher, P. A. *In situ* localization of DNA topoisomerase II, a major polypeptide component of the *Drosophila* nuclear matrix fraction. Proc. Natl. Acad. Sci. USA. **82:** 4142, 1985.

14. Sander, M. and Hsieh, T.-S. Double-stranded DNA cleavage by type II DNA topoisomerase from *Drosophila melanogaster*. J. Biol. Chem. **258:** 8421, 1983.

15. Liu, L. F., Rowe, T. C., Yang, L., Tewey, K. M., and Chen, G. L. Cleavage of DNA by mammalian DNA topoisomerase II. J. Biol. Chem. **258:** 15365, 1983.

16. Been, M. D. and Champoux, J. J. DNA breakage and closure by rat liver type I topoisomerase: Separation of the half-reactions by using a single-stranded DNA substrate. Proc. Natl. Acad. Sci. USA. **78:** 2883, 1982.

17. Halligan, B. D., Davis, J. L., Edwards,

K. A., and Liu, L. F. Intra- and intermolecular strand transfer by HeLa DNA topoisomerase I. J. Biol. Chem. **257:** 3995, 1982.

18. Tse-Dinh, Y.-C. Uncoupling of the DNA breaking and rejoining steps of *Escherichia coli* type I DNA topoisomerase. J. Biol. Chem. **261:** 10931, 1986.

19. Udvardy, A., Schedl, P., Sander, M., and Hsieh, T.-S. Novel partitioning of DNA cleavage sites for *Drosophila* topoisomerase II. Cell. **40:** 933, 1985.

20. Yang, L., Rowe, T. C., Nelson, E. M., and Liu, L. F. *In vivo* mapping of DNA topoisomerase II-specific cleavage sites on SV40 chromatin. Cell. **41:** 127, 1985.

21. Rowe, T. C., Wang, J. C., and Liu, L. F. *In vivo* localization of DNA topoisomerase II cleavage sites on *Drosophila* heat shock chromatin. Mol. Cell. Biol. **6:** 985, 1986.

22. Sander, M., Hsieh, T.-S., Udvardy, A., and Schedl, P. Sequence dependence of *Drosophila* topoisomerase II in plasmid relaxation and DNA binding. J. Mol. Biol. **194:** 219, 1987.

23. Rowe, T. C., Chen, G. L., Hsiang, Y.-H., and Liu, L. F. DNA damage by antitumor acridines mediated by mammalian DNA topoisomerase II. Cancer Res. **46:** 2021, 1986.

24. Osheroff, N. and Zechiedrich, E. L. Calcium-promoted DNA cleavage by eukaryotic topoisomerase II: Trapping the covalent enzyme-DNA complex in an active form. Biochemistry. **26:** 4303, 1987.

25. Osheroff, N. Role of the divalent cation in topoisomerase II mediated reactions. Biochemistry. **26:** 6402, 1987.

26. Glisson, B. S. and Ross, W. E. DNA topoisomerase II: A primer on the enzyme and its unique role as a multidrug target in cancer chemotherapy. Pharmacol. Ther. **32:** 89, 1987.

27. Lock, R. B. and Ross, W. E. DNA topoisomerases in cancer therapy. Anti-Cancer Drug Design. **2:** 151, 1987.

28. Rose, K. M. DNA topoisomerases as targets for chemotherapy. FASEB J. **2:** 2474, 1988.

29. Nelson, E. M., Tewey, K. M., and Liu, L. F. Mechanism of antitumor drug action: Poisoning of mammalian DNA topoisomerase II on DNA by 4'-(9-acridinylamino)methanesulfon-*m*-anisidide. Proc. Natl. Acad. Sci. USA. **81:** 1361, 1984.

30. Tewey, K. M., Chen, G. L., Nelson, E. M., and Liu, L. F. Intercalative antitumor drugs interfere with the breakage-reunion reaction of mammalian DNA topoisomerase II. J. Biol. Chem. **259:** 9182, 1984.

31. Pommier, Y., Schwartz, R. E., Zwelling,

L. A., and Kohn, K. W. Effects of DNA intercalating agents on topoisomerase II induced DNA strand cleavage in isolated mammalian cell nuclei. Biochemistry. **24:** 6406, 1985.

32. Pommier, Y., Schwartz, R. E., Kohn, K. W., and Zwelling, L. A. Formation and rejoining of deoxyribonucleic acid double-strand breaks induced in isolated cell nuclei by antineoplastic intercalating agents. Biochemistry. **23:** 3194, 1984.

33. Shelton, E. R., Osheroff, N., and Brutlag, D. L. DNA topoisomerase II from *Drosophila melanogaster:* Purification and physical characterization. J. Biol. Chem. **258:** 9530, 1983.

34. Zechiedrich, E. L., Christiansen, K., Andersen, A. H., Westergaard, O., and Osheroff, N. Double-stranded DNA cleavage/religation reaction of eukaryotic topo-isomerase II: Evidence for a nicked DNA intermediate. Biochemistry. **28:** 6229, 1989.

35. Segel, I. H. *Enzyme Kinetics.* New York: John Wiley and Sons, 1975.

36. Fersht, A. *Enzyme Structure and Mechanism,* 2nd ed. New York: W.H. Freeman, 1985.

37. Chen, G. L., Yang, L., Rowe, T. C., Halligan, B. D., Tewey, K. M., and Liu, L. F. Nonintercalative antitumor drugs interfere with the breakage-reunion reaction of mammalian DNA topoisomerase II. J. Biol. Chem. **259:** 13560, 1984.

38. Gale, K. C., and Osheroff, N. Uncoupling the DNA cleavage and religation activities of topoisomerase II with a single-stranded nucleic acid substrate: Evidence for an active enzyme-cleaved DNA intermediate. Biochemistry. **29:** 9538, 1990.

Chapter 19
DNA Recombination in Mammalian Cells: Potential Role of Topoisomerases

PIERRE CHARTRAND

Numerous assays have been devised to look at recombination in mammalian cells (see References in 5). So far (excluding site-specific recombination), three distinct recombination mechanisms have been observed: homologous conservative, homologous nonconservative, and nonhomologous (Fig. 19.1). The products of conservative homologous recombination are of two types. In one case there is the formation of two reciprocal homologous junctions that are flanked on one side by sequences originating from one parental molecule and on the other side by sequences originating from the other parental molecule. This process is usually referred to as crossing-over. In the other case there is no crossing-over, but homologous sequences from one parental molecule are nonreciprocally transferred to the other. This process is usually referred to as gene conversion. It is important to note that in both cases there is no net loss of DNA sequences even though certain sequences can be "converted." Nonconservative homologous recombination involves a crossing-over but with the formation of only one homologous junction and is accompanied by the loss of sequences. Finally, nonhomologous recombination involves the formation of nonhomologous junctions.

RELATIVE FREQUENCIES OF THE THREE TYPES OF RECOMBINATION

What is the relative preponderance of these three mechanisms in mammalian cells? To answer this question we devised an intermolecular recombination assay that permitted the simultaneous and quantitative recovery of products from the three types of mechanisms (5). The parental molecules are, on one hand, a eukaryotic vector consisting of an entire polyoma viral genome with a 2 Kbp insert of mouse cellular DNA, and, on the other hand, a prokaryotic vector consisting of a plasmid in which we have cloned the mouse cellular DNA present in the other vector. Thus the two parental molecules share 2 Kbp of homology. They are co-transfected into mouse cells. Recombination between the

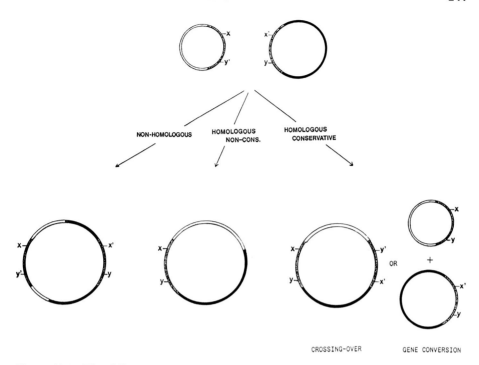

Figure 19.1. The different types of recombination in mammalian cells. X, X' and Y, Y' represent allelic markers. The dotted regions represent homologous sequences, and the open and solid regions represent nonhomologous sequences.

eukaryotic and prokaryotic vectors generates a shuttle vector that can be rescued in an *E. coli* RecA⁻ strain with selection for a marker from the prokaryotic vector. Bacterial colonies containing recombinant molecules are identified by *in situ* hybridization with sequences specific to the eukaryotic vector. Any recombinant that contains the selected prokaryotic vector marker and eukaryotic vector sequences is picked up in this assay.

We have analyzed by restriction mapping hundreds of intermolecular recombinants and found their distribution to be 77% nonhomologous recombinants, 20% homologous nonconservative, and 3% homologous conservative recombinants (5, Desautels et al. (1990) Mol. Cell. Biol., in press). Others have looked at intramolecular recombination and found that homologous and non-homologous recombination occurred at about equal frequencies (7,20,25,26) and that the vast majority of homologous recombinants were nonconservative (1,22). These results are in sharp contrast with bacteria and yeast where by far the predominant mechanism is conservative homologous recombination. It should be noted that our assay did not take into account gene conversion products and thus the total incidence of conservative homologous recombinants is underestimated. Anderson and Eliason (1) have shown, however, that gene conversion in mammalian cells was a rare event in comparison to nonconservative homologous recombination.

CURRENT MODELS OF RECOMBINATION

What are the current models used to explain the formation of the various types of recombinants? The model proposed for homologous conservative recombination in mammalian cells is derived from the one proposed by Szostak et al. (27) for yeast. The main features are the occurrence of a double-strand break in the homologous sequences of one of the parental sequences, followed by exonuclease digestion leading to the formation of a gap. The resulting free ends invade the corresponding homologous sequences of the other parental molecule, which, in turn, are used as template to resynthesize the gap. Depending on how the recombinational intermediate is resolved, this leads to either reciprocal crossing-over or to nonreciprocal gene conversion. There is experimental evidence supporting the implication of a gap repair process in gene conversion in mammalian cells (3). Furthermore, we have recently obtained evidence for a gap repair process in cases of reciprocal crossing-over (Desautels and Chartrand, manuscript in preparation).

A model for nonconservative homologous recombination has been proposed by Lin et al. (17,18). The key steps are double-strand breaks in both parental molecules occurring in or near the homologous sequences such as to create ends sharing an overlap of homologous sequences. This is followed by either single-strand exonuclease digestion (17) or unwinding of the DNA helix (29) to create single-strand complementary ends that can pair together to form a homologous junction. One prediction of this model is that in an intermolecular recombination event, the second junction will be nonhomologous and will have lost the homologous sequences present in the overlap. We found this to be the case for all the homologous nonconservative recombinants we obtained (5).

In the case of nonhomologous recombination, the initial step is thought to be a double-strand break such as to create free ends. These can then be ligated efficiently to other free ends (11,28).

TOPOISOMERASES AND RECOMBINATION

In all three types of recombination mechanisms it is thought that an initial step is a double-strand break in one or both target sequences. Indeed it has been shown repeatedly, with various recombination assays, that double-strand breaks significantly increase the frequency of all three recombination mechanisms (3,7,10,16,17,21,29), suggesting that generation of a double-strand break is an integral step of the recombination process.

One obvious candidate for such an enzymatic activity is topoisomerase II. Ikeda et al. (13) have shown that prokaryotic topoisomerase II could catalyze *in vitro* the formation of nonhomologous recombinants, and they found the recombination sites to be associated with topoisomerase II cleavage sites (8). These authors have proposed that nonhomologous junctions were the result of topoisomerase II–mediated double-strand breaks followed by an exchange of topoisomerase II subunits between free ends. They have recently obtained similar results with mammalian topoisomerase II (2). Sperry et al. (24) have ob-

Table 19.1. Effect of Addition of Exogenous Topoisomerase II on the Recombination Frequency in Mammalian Cells

Exogenous[b] Topo II Added	Frequency of Recombinants[a]		
	Expt 1	Expt 2	Expt 3
Dose 0	0.64	0.10	0.20
Dose 1x	1.24	0.16	0.28
Dose 10x	7.1	0.45	0.71
Dose 100x	1.7	0.57	0.6

[a]Percentage of recombinants per rescued plasmid.
[b]The amount of topoisomerase II representing dose 1 was arbitrarily chosen.

served chromosomal loop deletions in mammalian cells that involved matrix association regions (MAR). These regions contain multiple topoisomerase II cleavage sites. The authors hypothesize that a dysfunction of MARs could lead to nonhomologous recombination mediated by topoisomerase II.

To probe further the involvement of topoisomerase II in DNA recombination in mammalian cells, we modified our recombination assay (5) so as to introduce exogenous topoisomerase II enzymes into the cells along with the parental molecules (L. Desautels, et al., manuscript in preparation). This was done by forming complexes between the DNA and topoisomerase II purified from mammalian cells (12) and then using these complexes in our assay. The results indicate that this can significantly increase the recombination frequency (Table 19.1). The amount of topoisomerase II added in the assay was arbitrarily chosen. We can see in three separate experiments an increase in the frequency of recombination that varies between threefold to tenfold. Thus, the capacity of topoisomerase II to stimulate recombination *in vitro* and *in vivo* suggests that topoisomerase II is directly involved in recombination in mammalian cells.

Topoisomerase I is also most probably involved in recombination in mammalian cells, at least in the case of nonhomologous recombination. Bullock et al. (6) had first noticed the high occurrence of topoisomerase I–trinucleotide recognition sequences at or near the crossing-over sites of nonhomologous recombinants. In a study of 496 previously published nonhomologous junctions, Konopka (14) also found such sites near 92% of the junctions. Furthermore, Shuman (23) has observed that topoisomerase I coded for by the mammalian virus vaccinia, when expressed in *E. coli,* promotes nonhomologous recombination. Thus, the involvement of topoisomerase I (at least in nonhomologous recombination) appears very likely. However, it is not immediately clear how this fits into the current models of recombination.

Recent studies in yeast have shown that topoisomerases (both I and II) could also suppress recombination. Nitiss and Wang (19) have observed that antitumor drugs that presumably interfere with DNA topoisomerases I and II activities induce high levels of homologous recombination. It has also been found that low cellular levels of topoisomerases I and II resulted in highly increased frequencies of rDNA mitotic recombination (9). Interestingly, however, this effect was specific to rDNA. Furthermore, Kim and Wang (15) have demonstrated that low levels of topoisomerases I and II resulted in excision of rDNA, but that when levels were returned to normal, reintegration of rDNA was promoted. Thus the effect appears to be more a modulation of recombination directionality rather than a simple suppression.

CONCLUSION

Current data strongly suggest that topoisomerases are involved in recombination in mammalian cells. Their specific role is unclear but appears to be more complex than the simple generation of free ends. Furthermore, recombination in mammalian cells might yet involve additional topoisomerases, as was shown to be the case in yeast (30).

REFERENCES

1. Anderson, R. A. and Eliason, S. L. Recombination of homologous DNA fragments transfected into mammalian cells occurs predominantly by terminal pairing. Mol. Cell. Biol. **6:** 3246, 1986.
2. Bae, Y. S., Kawasaki, I., Ikeda, H., and Liu, L. F. Illegitimate recombination mediated by calf thymus DNA topoisomerase II in vitro. Proc. Natl. Acad. Sci. USA. **85:** 2076, 1988.
3. Brenner, D. A., Smigocki, A. C., Camerini-Otero, R. D. Effect of insertions, deletions and double-strand breaks on homologous recombination in mouse L cells. Mol. Cell. Biol. **5:** 684, 1985.
4. Brenner, D. A., Smigocki, A. C., and Camerini-Otero, R. D. Double-strand gap repair results in homologous recombination in mouse L cells. Proc. Natl. Acad. Sci. USA. **83:** 1762, 1986.
5. Brouillette, S. and Chartrand, P. Intermolecular recombination assay for mammalian cells that produces recombinants carrying both homologous and nonhomologous junctions. Mol. Cell. Biol. **7:** 2248, 1987.
6. Bullock, P., Champoux, J. J., and Botchan, M. Association of crossover points with topoisomerase I cleavage sites: A model for nonhomologous recombination. Science. **230:** 954, 1985.
7. Chakrabarti, S., Joffe, S., and Seidman, M. M. Recombination and deletion of sequences in shuttle vector plasmids in mammalian cells. Mol. Cell. Biol. **5:** 2265, 1985.
8. Chiba, M., Shimizu, H., Fujomoto, R., Nashimoto, H., and Ikeda, H. Common sites for recombination and cleavage mediated by bacteriophage T4 DNA topoisomerase in vitro. J. Biol. Chem. **264:** 12785, 1989.
9. Christman, M. F., Dietrich, F. S., and Fink, G. R. Mitotic recombination in the rDNA of S. cerevisiae is suppressed by the combined action of DNA topoisomerase I and II. Cell. **55:** 413, 1988.
10. Folger, K. R., Thomas, K., and Capecchi, M. R. Nonreciprocal exchanges of information between DNA duplexes coinjected into mammalian cell nuclei. Mol. Cell. Biol. **5:** 59, 1985.
11. Wong, E. A., Wahl, G., and Capecchi, M. R. Patterns of integration of DNA microinjected into cultured mammalian cells: Evidence for homologous recombination between injected plasmid DNA molecules. Mol. Cell. Biol. **2:** 1372, 1982.
12. Glisson, B. S., Smallwood, S. E., and Ross, W. E. Characterization of VP-16-induced DNA damage in isolated nuclei from L1210 cells. Biochim. Biophys. Acta. **783:** 74, 1984.
13. Ikeda, H., Aoki, K., and Naito, A. Illegitimate recombination mediated in vitro by DNA gyrase of Escherichia coli. Structure of recombinant DNA molecules. Proc. Natl. Acad. Sci. USA. **79:** 3724, 1982.
14. Kanopka, A. K. Compilation of DNA strand exchange sites for non-homologous recombination in somatic cells. Nucleic Acids Res. **16:** 1739, 1988.
15. Kim, R. A. and Wang, J. C. A subthreshold level of DNA topoisomerases leads to the excision of yeast rDNA as extrachromosomal rings. Cell. **57:** 975, 1989.
16. Kucherlapati, R. S., Eves, E. M., Song, K. Y., Morse, B. S., and Smithies, O. Homologous recombination between plasmids in mammalian cells can be enhanced by treatment of input DNA. Proc. Natl. Acad. Sci. USA. **81:** 3153, 1984.
17. Lin, F. L., Sperle, K., and Sternberg, N.

Model for homologous recombination during transfer of DNA into mouse L cells: Role for DNA ends in the recombination process. Mol. Cell. Biol. **4:** 1020, 1984.

18. Lin, F. L., Sperle, K., and Sternberg, N. Extrachromosomal recombination in mammalian cells as studied with single- and double-stranded DNA substrates. Mol. Cell. Biol. **7:** 129, 1987.

19. Nitiss, J. and Wang, J. C. DNA topoisomerase targeting antitumor drugs can be studied in yeast. Proc. Natl. Acad. Sci. USA. **85:** 7501, 1988.

20. Roth, D. B. and Wilson, J. H. Relative rates of homologous and nonhomologous recombination in transfected DNA. Proc. Natl. Acad. Sci. USA. **82:** 3355, 1985.

21. Rubnitz, J. and Subramani, S. Rapid assay for extrachromosomal homologous recombination in monkey cells. Mol. Cell. Biol. **5:** 529, 1985.

22. Seidman, M. M. Intermolecular homologous recombination between transfected sequences in mammalian cells is primarily nonconservative. Mol. Cell. Biol. **7:** 3561, 1987.

23. Shuman, S. Vaccinia DNA topoisomerase I promotes illegitimate recombination in Escherichia coli. Proc. Natl. Acad. Sci. USA. **86:** 3489, 1989.

24. Sperry, A. O., Blasquez, V. C., and Gar-rard, W. T. Dysfunction of chromosomal loop attachment sites: Illegitimate recombination linked to matrix association regions and topoisomerame II. Proc. Natl. Acad. Sci. USA. **86:** 5497, 1989.

25. Stringer, J. R. Recombination between poly [d(GT).d(CA)] sequences in simian virus 40-infected cultured cells. Mol. Cell. Biol. **5:** 1247, 1985.

26. Subramani, S. and Berg, P. Homologous and nonhomologous recombination in monkey cells. Mol. Cell. Biol. **3:** 1040, 1983.

27. Szostak, J. W., Orr-Weaver, T. L., Rothstein, R. J., and Stahl, F. W. The double-strand break repair model for recombination. Cell. **33:** 25, 1983.

28. Wake, C. T., Gudewicz, T., Porter, T., White, A., and Wilson, J. H. How damaged is the biologically active subpopulation of transfected DNA? Mol. Cell. Biol. **4:** 387, 1984.

29. Wake, C. T., Vernaleone, F., and Wilson, J. H. Topological requirements for homologous recombination among DNA molecules transfected into mammalian cells. Mol. Cell. Biol. **5:** 2080, 1985.

30. Wallis, J. W., Chrebet, G., Brodsky, G., Rolfe, M., and Rothstein, R. A hyper-recombination mutation in S. cerevisiae identifies a novel eukaryotic topoisomerase. Cell. **58:** 409, 1989.

PART IV

DRUG RESISTANCE AND TOPOISOMERASES

Chapter 20
Camptothecin-Resistant DNA Topoisomerase I

TOSHIWO ANDOH, EIGIL KJELDSEN,
BJARNE JUUL BONVEN, OLE WESTERGAARD,
KAZUYUKI ISHII, AND KOSUKE OKADA

DNA topoisomerases participate in various aspects of genetic processes by concerted breakage and rejoining of the DNA backbone (1,2). Genetic analysis has been successfully applied to elucidate the biological role of these enzymes in prokaryotes (2) and in lower eukaryotes (3). In higher eukaryotes, however, a similar genetic approach has been hampered owing to the lack of specific screening systems. Since the discovery that topoisomerases are the targets of a number of different anticancer drugs (4–8) a genetic approach to this problem in higher eukaryotes has become feasible by isolating and analyzing mutants resistant to these drugs as candidates of topoisomerase mutants. A cytotoxic plant alkaloid, camptothecin, which is active against a number of experimental tumors (9–14), was shown to be a potent inhibitor of mammalian DNA topoisomerase I (8,15). The inhibitory effect of camptothecin on topoisomerase catalysis was demonstrated to be related to a drug-mediated stabilization of the "cleavable complex," an intermediate covalent enzyme–DNA complex. We have shown previously that a mutant of a human leukemic cell line selected for resistance to high level of camptothecin possessed a biochemically altered drug-resistant form of DNA topoisomerase I (16). The specific alteration of the enzyme in this mutant provides strong evidence that this enzyme is the main cellular target of camptothecin, and that the severe physiological effects of the drug, including cytotoxicity, genome fragmentation, and inhibition of nucleic acid synthesis (9,17–20), are mediated solely by topoisomerase I. In an effort to further characterize enzymatic properties of the mutant enzyme, we have compared the cleavage properties of the camptothecin-resistant topoisomerase I and the corresponding wild-type enzyme. The use of a highly specific topoisomerase I recognition sequence, originally discovered in the rDNA spacers of Tetrahymena (21,22) and recently shown to be a preferred substrate for topoisomerase I cleavage (23,24) and relaxation (25), enabled us to perform quantitative analysis of topoisomerase I–mediated cleavage at a specific site (26).

ISOLATION AND SOME PROPERTIES OF CAMPTOTHECIN-
RESISTANT MUTANT OF HUMAN LEUKEMIC CELLS RPMI 8402

To obtain camptothecin-resistant cells we made use of a hydrophilic derivative of camptothecin, 7-ethyl-10[4-(1-piperidyl)-1-piperidyl]carbonyloxy-campto-thecin, camptothecin-11 (13). Unmutagenized human acute lymphoblastic leukemia cells, RPMI 8402, were exposed to gradually increasing concentrations of camptothecin-11 beginning with 0.1 μg/ml over a period of 10 months. The cells finally obtained were resistant to the drug at 50 μg/ml, and were then cloned. CPT-K5 is one of the clonal isolates and was analyzed. CPT-K5 cells grow slower than the parent cells, with a doubling time of 35 h compared with that of 22 h. Growth of the wild-type cells was inhibited completely with camptothecin at 0.05 μM, whereas the resistant cells were inhibited only slightly even at 20 μM, the resistance index being more than 400. In wild-type cells camptothecin severely inhibited RNA and DNA synthesis, and had no effect on protein synthesis, as reported previously (18,20). In the mutant cells, however, camptothecin had only minimal effects on macromolecular synthesis. The resistance of CPT-K5 cells to camptothecin could in part be due to reduced uptake of the drug. For the study of uptake and efflux kinetics the cells were incubated with [7-ethyl-^{14}C]camptothecin-11 at 10 μM. The uptake and efflux were not appreciably modified in the mutant cells. Therefore we may presume that some changes in the intracellular function seem to have occurred in the generation of CPT-K5 cells from the parental cells.

TOTAL ACTIVITY AND TOTAL AMOUNT OF TOPOISOMERASE I
AND II IN CRUDE EXTRACT

Total cellular activity of topoisomerase I and II in wild-type and CPT-K5 cells was measured in whole cell extracts made with 1M NaCl-containing buffer (Table 20.1). About one-third of the wild-type activity of topoisomerase I was recovered from the mutant cells, whereas the level of topoisomerase II activity as assayed by ATP-dependent catenation of plasmid DNA, and confirmed later by decatenation of kinetoplast DNA and unknotting of knotted DNA of phage P4, was not appreciably changed. We further measured total amount of the enzymes by immunoblotting of the 1M NaCl extract using antisera raised against mouse topoisomerase I and human topoisomerase II (kindly donated by Dr. L. F. Liu), respectively. The content of topoisomerase I in the mutant

Table 20.1. Total Activities of Topoisomerase I and II

	Topoisomerase I (Units/10⁷ Cells)[a]	Topoisomerase II (Units/10⁷ Cells)[b]
RPMI 8402	1.0×10^4	3×10^2
CPT-K5	3.8×10^3	3×10^2

[a]Assayed by relaxation of plasmid DNA.
[b]Assayed by ATP-dependent catenation of plasmid DNA.

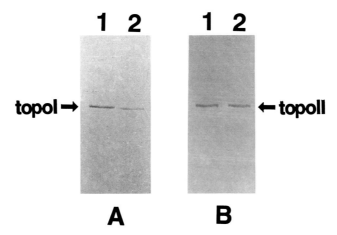

Figure 20.1. Immunoblotting of DNA topoisomerase I and II in extracts from wild-type and CPT-K5 cells. Equivalent amounts of whole cell extract from both cell lines were electrophoresed on SDS-polyacrylamide gels, and the proteins were transferred to nitrocellulose membranes and processed for immunostaining by the peroxidase-coupled biotin–avidin system using antibodies against mouse DNA topoisomerase I (**A**) and human DNA topoisomerase II (**B**). Immunoblots of extracts from wild-type (lane 1) and CPT-K5 cells (lane 2).

cells seems to be reduced to less than half that of the wild-type (Fig. 20.1A), suggesting that the observed reduction in the enzymatic activity was not due to modification of the enzyme changing the activity such as poly(ADP ribosylation), but rather to reduction in the amount of the enzyme. Topoisomerase II, on the other hand, appeared to be unchanged (Fig. 20.1B).

CAMPTOTHECIN SENSITIVITY OF DNA TOPOISOMERASE I PURIFIED FROM WILD-TYPE AND CPT-K5 CELLS

Topoisomerase I was purified from wild-type (topo I–wt) and CPT-K5 (topo I–K5) cells as described previously (27). Both enzymes purified to near homogeneity had an apparent Mr of about 96,000 in SDS-polyacrylamide gel electrophoresis (Fig. 20.2). The differential effect of camptothecin on the wild-type and camptothecin-resistant topoisomerase I is illustrated in Figure 20.3. In this experiment, the influence of enzyme concentration on the rate of DNA relaxation was measured as a function of camptothecin concentration. Figure 20.3A displays an electrophoretic analysis of the reaction products obtained by relaxation of fixed amounts of supercoiled substrate DNA with increasing amounts of topo I–wt. Approximately 2 units of enzyme was required to give complete relaxation within the given reaction period. When a similar enzyme titration experiment was performed in the presence of 5 μM camptothecin, about eightfold more enzyme was needed to achieve complete relaxation (Fig. 20.3B), demonstrating that the wild-type topoisomerase I was sensitive to camptothecin. The inhibitory effect could be overcome by addition of excess amounts of

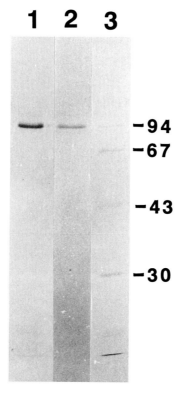

Figure 20.2. SDS-polyacrylamide gel electrophoresis of purified DNA topoisomerase I from wild-type (lane 1) and from CPT-K5 cells (lane 2); lane 3 for marker proteins indicated as Mr $\times$ 10^{-3}: phosphorylase b, 94; bovine serum albumin, 67; ovalbumin, 43; carbonic anhydrase, 30.

enzyme. The enzyme titration profiles recorded with topo I–K5 in the absence (Fig. 20.3C) or presence (Fig. 20.3D) of camptothecin were similar, showing the insensitivity of this enzyme. The observation that the camptothecin inhibition was counterbalanced at high concentrations of topo I–wt raised the question whether the extra amount of enzyme required to neutralize the inhibition was proportional to the concentration of the inhibitor. This problem was addressed by reiteration of the enzyme titration experiments at various concentrations of camptothecin. From these results, the quantity ΔE was calculated for each concentration of camptothecin. (ΔE = the amount of enzyme required to give complete relaxation at a certain inhibitor concentration subtracted by the amount of enzyme giving the same degree of relaxation in the absence of inhibitor.) A plot of ΔE versus the camptothecin concentration is shown in Figure 20.3E. For topo I–wt, ΔE is proportional to the concentration of camptothecin, consistent with the view that this inhibitor interacts with the enzyme or the enzyme–substrate complex rather than the DNA substrate (15). The enzyme titration profiles recorded with the mutant enzyme in the absence or in the presence of camptothecin, however, were similar, emphasizing the insensitivity of this enzyme to the drug.

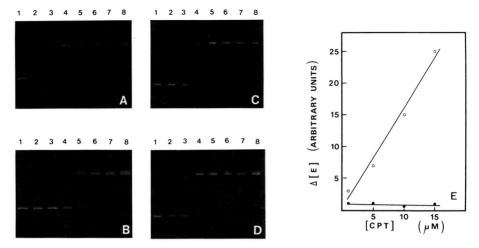

Figure 20.3. The effect of camptothecin on topoisomerase I–mediated DNA relaxation. Aliquots of a dilution series of topoisomerase I were incubated for 15 min at 30°C with 0.5 μg supercoiled plasmid DNA. The reaction products were analyzed on 1% agarose gels and visualized by ethidium bromide staining and UV transillumination. Lower and upper bands represent fully supercoiled and fully relaxed DNA, respectively. The amounts of enzyme added were 0.25, 0.5, 1, 2, 4, 8, 16, 32 units, respectively, for ech of the lanes 1 through 8. **A,** topo I–wt, no camptothecin; **B,** topo I–wt, 5 μM camptothecin present; **C,** topo I–K5, no camptothecin; **D,** topo, I–K5, 5 μM camptothecin present. **E,** the experiments in A through D were repeated at various camptothecin concentrations. The excess of enzyme needed to overcome a certain inhibitor concentration, ΔE (defined in the text), was plotted against the concentration of camptothecin. Open symbols, topo I–wt; closed symbols, topo I–K5; CPT, camptothecin.

CLEAVABLE COMPLEX FORMATION BY TOPOISOMERASE I FROM WILD-TYPE AND CPT-K5 CELLS AT A SPECIFIC RECOGNITION SEQUENCE

Camptothecin was shown to inhibit the activity of topoisomerase I by stabilizing the covalent enzyme–DNA complex (15). To characterize the mutant enzyme further the influence of camptothecin on the cleavage properties of topo I–wt and topo I–K5 was assessed (Fig. 20.4). Cleavage was monitored on a *Hin*dIII-*Pvu*II restriction fragment of the plasmid pNC1 (23). The fragment contains a strong hexadecameric topoisomerase I recognition sequence (21):

-AGACTTAGAAAAATTT-
-TCTGAATCTTTTTAAA-

Incubation of the fragment with topo I–wt in the absence of camptothecin cleavage was confined to the hexadecameric recognition sequence (lane 1). In the presence of camptothecin (1 μM) several additional cleavages were observed on the fragment (lane 2). No further changes in the cleavage pattern

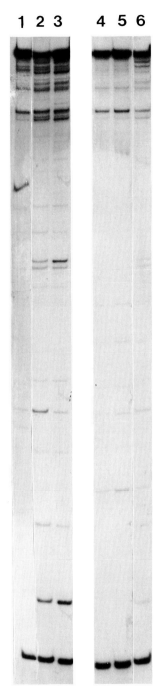

Figure 20.4. Cleavage specificity of topoisomerase I from wild-type and CPT-K5 cells in the presence and absence of camptothecin. Three fmol of end-labeled *Hin*dIII-*Pvu*II fragment of pNC1 containing a strong topoisomerase I recognition sequence was incubated with 75 units of topo I–wt (lanes 1–3) and topo I–K5 (lanes 4–6) in the absence (lanes 1 and 4) or presence of camptothecin at 1 μM (lanes 2 and 5) and 125 μM (lanes 3 and 6). The reaction was terminated with SDS and the samples processed for polyacrylamide gel electrophoresis.

resulted from increasing the concentration of camptothecin to 125 μM (lane 3). Cleavage by topo I–K5 was confined to the recognition sequence irrespective of the presence of camptothecin (Fig. 20.4, lanes 4–6), demonstrating that the mutant enzyme escaped the general alteration of the cleavage pattern elicited by camptothecin. Thus the recognition and cleavage specificity of the mutant enzyme appears to be unaffected by the mutation. Cleavage by the wild-type enzyme was observed only in the presence of Ca^{2+} (23,26), while a considerable amount of cleavage by the mutant enzyme was seen in the absence of the divalent cation. Incubation with Ca^{2+}, however, enhanced cleavage at this site approximately threefold. These findings demonstrate that the change in CPT-K5 topoisomerase I has abolished the absolute requirement for divalent cations in the cleavage exhibited by the wild-type enzyme.

To obtain a quantitative measure of cleavage at the recognition sequence, the end-labeled HindIII-PvuII fragment of pNCl was titrated with both wild-type and mutant topoisomerase I. The amount of cleavage as determined by densitometric scanning of autoradiogram was expressed as percentage of cleavage as a function of the amount of enzyme added. The result shows that 20–25 units of the mutant enzyme and 30–35 units of the wild-type enzyme were required to achieve half-maximal cleavage, demonstrating that both enzymes seem to bind to the recognition sequence with similar affinities with the equilibrium dissociation constant of the range of 10^{-10} M. However, the two enzymes differed with respect to the maximally attainable levels of cleavage. Close to 60% of the substrate was cleaved with saturating amounts of the mutant enzyme as compared to approximately 30% with wild-type enzyme (26). Thus, the cleavable complexes formed by the mutant enzyme appeared to be more stable than that of the wild-type. The relative stabilities of the cleavable complexes formed by the two enzymes were further examined by characterizing the effect of increased ionic strength on the cleavage (24). As the concentration of sodium chloride was increased, residual cleavable complex decreased. The mutant cleavable complex disappeared with slower kinetics, and the equilibrium level of the residual complex was higher (26), again indicating the increased stability of the cleavable complex formed by the mutant enzyme with the recognition sequence.

DISCUSSION

The finding that camptothecin inhibits a mammalian DNA topoisomerase I *in vitro* (15) enabled us to isolate for the first time a topoisomerase I mutant of mammalian cells. The mutant cells, selected for the resistance to camptothecin, grow more slowly and are 400-fold more resistant to the drug, compared to the parent cells. Biochemical analyses of topoisomerase I from wild-type cells and the mutant cells revealed the following important differences. (1) Western blot analysis of topoisomerase I and II in crude extracts demonstrated that the level of topoisomerase I from the mutant cells was reduced to one-half to one-third that of the wild-type enzyme, in parallel with its activity, while the amount of topoisomerase II was the same in both cell types. The reduction in the level of topoisomerase I may be ascribed to an increased instability of the mutant enzyme, since Northern blot analysis of polyA RNA from both cell lines with topoisomerase I cDNA as a probe gave the same signal intensity (unpublished result). (2) The catalytic activity of topoisomerase I purified from the mutant cells was more than 125-fold more resistant to camptothecin compared with the wild-type enzyme, reflecting the cellular resistance to the drug. (3) Specificity of the enzyme in recognition and cleavage of a previously identified recognition sequence (21) was not altered by the mutation. However, while the cleavage pattern of the mutant enzyme was little affected by camptothecin, that of the wild-type enzyme was changed and thus a unique set of novel cleavages were induced in the presence of the inhibitor (24). (4) The K5 mutation conferred a higher intrinsic kinetic stability to the cleavable complex formed by the topo I–K5, which was reflected in altered ionic requirements. The enzyme site(s) or domain(s) affected by camptothecin and the mutation conferring resistance to the drug are determinants of the kinetic stability of the cleavable complex. Conceivably, these site(s) are involved in the second half-reaction of the nicking-closing cycle. The relationship of this site(s) to the active site of the enzyme is currently under investigation. Based on these observations and our present knowledge of the enzymatic mechanism for topoisomerase I, a working model for the drug action on the wild-type and the mutant enzyme is shown schematically in Figure 20.5. We assume as proposed by Hsiang et al. (15) that there are at least two stages of intermediate enzyme–DNA complex, binding (stage

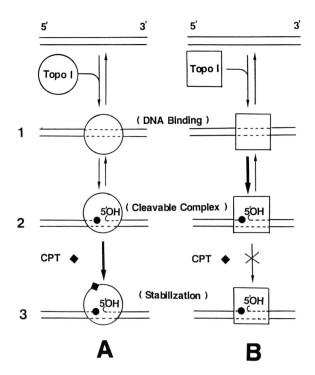

Figure 20.5. A model of catalysis by DNA topoisomerase I from wild-type (**A**) and CPT-K5 (**B**) cells and the action of camptothecin.

1) and cleavable complex formation (stage 2). Exposure of the cleavable complex to SDS results in single-strand breaks of DNA and covalent linkage of the enzyme to phosphoryl end of the breaks of DNA. Camptothecin acting on either stage 1 or 2 stabilizes the cleavable complex (stage 3). In contrast to this mechanism of action of the wild-type enzyme, little binding and stabilization by camptothecin of the mutant enzyme–DNA comlex occur. Furthermore, the cleavable complex formed with the mutant enzyme seems to be more stable than that of the wild-type complex, as illustrated by a thick arrow.

The findings suggest that topoisomerase I is the main cellular target of camptothecin and thus the mutation to acquired resistance to the drug has rescued the cells from the severe physiological effects of the drug, e.g., inhibition of nucleic acid synthesis and genome fragmentation (17–20).

Gupta et al. (28) reported a camptothecin-resistant CHO cell line possessing a drug-resistant topoisomerase I. It is of obvious importance to note that the manifestation of camptothecin resistance was due to the appearance of a qualitatively different topoisomerase I in the two unrelated cell lines. These findings appear to support the notion that topoisomerase I is the sole cellular target of the drug.

SUMMARY

DNA topoisomerase I was purified from a clonal line, CPT-K5, of human lymphoblastic leukemia cells, RPMI 8402, that is resistant to camptothecin and was compared to that of the parent wild-type cells. As assayed by relaxation of supercoiled plasmid DNA, the mutant enzyme was shown to be 125-fold less sensitive to the inhibitory effect of camptothecin than the topo I–wt, reflected as a cellular resistance index of about 400. Thus, the cellular resistance appears to be due to the resistance of the enzyme. The amount of the immunoreactive enzyme protein in whole cell extract appeared to be reduced to less than one-half that of the wild-type enzyme. Camptothecin altered the cleavage pattern of the wild-type but not the mutant enzyme. The cleavable complex formed by the mutant enzyme was stabilized relative to that of the wild-type by several criteria, i.e., efficiency of cleavage and salt sensitivity of the cleavable complex. The mutant enzyme formed the cleavable complex in the absence of divalent cations, which were required for the complex formation by the wild-type enzyme. These results establish that DNA topoisomerase I is the cellular target of camptothecin.

Acknowledgments

This study was supported by the Grant-in-Aid for Cancer Research from the Ministry of Education, Science and Culture of Japan (grant 63010071), the Commission of the European Communities (contract B-6-0170-DK), the Danish Medical Research Council (grant 5.1017.06), the Danish Cancer Society (grant 86-178, 87-025, and 87-088), the National Agency of Technology (contract 1985-133/001-85.521), the Danish Programme of Biotechnology, and the Michaelsen Foundation.

REFERENCES

1. Wang, J. C. DNA topoisomerases. Annu. Rev. Biochem. **54:** 665, 1985.

2. Wang, J. C. Recent studies of DNA topoisomerases. Biochem. Biophys. Acta. **909:** 1, 1987.

3. Yanagida, M. and Wang, J. C. Yeast DNA topoisomerases and their structural genes. *Nucleic Acids and Molecular Biology.* Berlin: Springer-Verlag, 1987, **1:** 196.

4. Chen, G. L. and Liu, L. F. DNA topoisomerases as therapeutic targets in cancer chemotherapy. *Annual Reports in Medicinal Chemistry.* New York: Academic Press, 1986, **21:** 257.

5. Ross, W. E., Sullivan, D. M., and Chow, K. C. Altered function of DNA topoisomerases as a basis for antineoplastic drug action. *Important Advances in Oncology.* Philadelphia: J. B. Lippincott, 1988, p. 65.

6. Drlica, K. and Franco, R. L. Inhibitors of DNA topoisomerases. Biochemistry. **27:** 2253, 1988.

7. Liu, L. F. DNA topoisomerase poisons as antitumor drugs. Annu. Rev. Biochem. **58:** 351, 1989.

8. Zhang, H., D'Arpa, P., and Liu, L. F. A model for tumor cell killing by topoisomerase poisons. Cancer Cells. **2:** 23, 1990.

9. Wall, M. E., Wani, M. C., Cook, C. E., Palmer, K. H., Mcphail, A. T., and Sim, G. A. Plant antitumor agents. I. The isolation and structure of camptothecin, a novel alkaloid leukemia and tumor inhibitor from *Camptotheca acuminata.* J. Am. Chem. Soc. **88:** 3888, 1966.

10. Wall, M. E. and Wani, M. C. Camptothecin. *Anticancer Agents Based on Natural Product Models.* New York: Academic Press, 1980, p. 417.

11. Hutchinson, C. R. Camptothecin: Chemistry, biogenesis and medicinal chemistry. Tetrahedron Report Number **105:** 1047, Pergamon Press, 1981.

12. Gallo, R. C., Whang-Peng, J., and Adamson, R. H. Studies on the antitumor activity, mechanism of action, and cell cycle effects of camptothecin. J. Natl. Cancer Inst. **46:** 789, 1971.

13. Nitta, K., Yokokura, T., Sawada, S., Takeuchi, M., Tanaka, T., Uehara, N., Baba, H., Kunimoto, T., Miyasaka, T., and Mutai, M. Antitumor activity of a new derivative of camptothecin. *Recent Advances in Chemotherapy.* Tokyo: University of Tokyo Press, 1985, p. 28.

14. Tsuruo, T., Matsuzaki, T., Matsushita, M., Saito, H., and Yokokura, T. Antitumor effect of CPT-11, a new derivative of camptothecin, against pleiotropic drug-resistant tumors *in vitro* and *in vivo.* Cancer Chemother. Pharmacol. **21:** 71, 1988.

15. Hsiang, Y.-H., Hertzberg, R., Hecht, S., and Liu, L. F. Camptothecin induces protein-linked DNA breaks via mammalian DNA topoisomerase I. J. Biol. Chem. **260:** 14873, 1985.

16. Andoh, T., Ishii, K., Suzuki, Y., Ikegami, Y., Kusunoki, Y., Takemoto, Y., and Okada, K. Characterization of a mammalian mutant with a camptothecin-resistant DNA topoisomerase I. Proc. Natl. Acad. Sci. USA. **84:** 5565, 1987.

17. Bosmann, H. B. Camptothecin inhibits macromolecular synthesis in mammalian cells but not in isolated mitochondria of *E. coli.* Biochem. Biophys. Res. Commun. **41:** 1412, 1970.

18. Horwitz, M. S. and Horwitz, S. B. Intracellular degradation of HeLa and adenovirus type 2 DNA induced by camptothecin. Biochem. Biophys. Res. Commun. **45:** 723, 1971.

19. Kessel, D. Some determinants of camptothecin responsiveness in leukemia L1210 cells. Cancer Res. **31:** 1883, 1971.

20. Spataro, A. and Kessel, D. Studies on camptothecin-induced degradation and apparent reaggregation of DNA from L1210 cells. Biochem. Biophys. Res. Commun. **48:** 648, 1972.

21. Bonven, B. J., Gocke, E., and Westergaard, O. A high affinity topoisomerase I binding sequence is clustered at DNase I hypersensitive sites in *Tetrahymena* R-chromatin. *Cell.* **41:** 541, 1985.

22. Christiansen, K., Bonven, B. J., and Westergaard, O. Mapping of sequence-specific chromatin proteins by a novel method: Topoisomerase I on *Tetrahymena* ribosomal chromatin. J. Mol. Biol. **193:** 517, 1987.

23. Thomsen, B., Mollerup, S., Bonven, B. J., Frank, R., Bloecker, H., Nielsen, O. F., and Westergaard, O. Sequence specificity of DNA topoisomerase I in the presence and absence of camptothecin. EMBO J. **6:** 1817, 1987.

24. Kjeldsen, E., Mollerup, S., Thomsen, B., Bonven, B. J., Bolund, L., and Westergaard, O. Sequence-dependent effect of camptothecin on human topoisomerase I DNA cleavage. J. Mol. Biol. **202:** 333, 1988.

25. Busk, H., Thomsen, B., Bonven, B. J., Kjeldsen, E., Nielsen, O. F., and Westergaard, O. Preferential relaxation cf super-

coiled DNA containing a hexadecameric recognition sequence for topoisomerase I. Nature. **327:** 638, 1987.

26. Kjeldsen, E., Bonven, B. J., Andoh, T., Ishii, K., Okada, K., Bolund, L., and Westergaard, O. Characterization of a camptothecin-resistant human DNA topoisomerase I. J. Biol. Chem. **263:** 3912, 1988.

27. Ishii, K., Hasegawa, T., Fujisawa, K., and Andoh, T. Rapid purification and characterization of DNA topoisomerase I from cultured mouse mammary carcinoma FM3A cells. J. Biol. Chem. **258:** 12728, 1983.

28. Gupta, R. S., Gupta, R., Eng, E., Lock, R. B., Ross, W. E., Hertzberg, R. P., Caranfa, M. J., and Johnson, R. K. Camptothecin-resistant mutants of Chinese hamster ovary cells containing a resistant form of topoisomerase I. Cancer Res. **48:** 6404, 1988.

Chapter 21
Multidrug Resistance Associated with Alterations in Topoisomerase II

WILLIAM T. BECK

AND MARY K. DANKS

We now have a good understanding of the essential features of the biochemistry, pharmacology, and molecular biology of multidrug resistance (MDR) associated with P-glycoprotein (Pgp) overexpression, the details of which have been studied over the past decade (1–4). Of considerable interest is the observation that this form of MDR may occur in some clinically resistant tumors (5–7). However, because Pgp overexpression cannot be detected in all or even in the majority of them (5–7), other mechanisms of MDR probably exist. Recent laboratory studies support this hypothesis: [1] MDR cells having an accumulation–retention defect *without* overexpression of the Pgp have been described (8,9); [2] alterations in glutathione metabolism in some cell lines may account for their resistance (10); [3] other cell lines have been described that display neither an accumulation defect nor overexpression of Pgp, but are cross-resistant to many natural product drugs known to interfere with DNA topoisomerase II activity (11,12); and [4] some cell lines have been reported that appear to have more than one of these forms of MDR (13,14).

In our initial descriptions of our VM-26–resistant cell line, CEM/VM-1, we suggested that it displayed an "atypical" form of MDR (at-MDR; 11,12). We did this to distinguish it from the well-characterized MDR cell lines associated with Pgp overexpression (Pgp-MDR). Since the CEM/VM-1 and similar cell lines show a broad cross-resistance to a variety of "natural product" compounds, they are clearly "multidrug resistant," a term that had already been used by Glisson, Ross, and colleagues to describe their etoposide-resistant Chinese hamster cell line (15,16). We now have considerable evidence that our CEM/VM-1 cells and a more resistant subline derived from it are altered in some functions of topoisomerase II (17). We still call this type of resistance "at-MDR," with the term *"at"* now connoting *"altered topoisomerase II"* to distinguish this form of MDR from that associated with Pgp overexpression (Pgp-MDR).

Our goal in this paper is to summarize our knowledge about the biochemistry of at-MDR, determined primarily from studies of our two human leukemic lymphoblastic cell lines selected for increasing resistance to teniposide (VM-26), to compare our cell lines with others that display apparent at-MDR, and to propose several mechanisms based on the actions of topoisomerase II that might result in this phenotype.

MATERIALS AND METHODS

Cells and Culture Conditions

We have selected and grown sublines of CCRF-CEM human leukemic T-lymphoblasts for progressive resistance to VM-26, as detailed elsewhere (11,17). Resistance and cross-resistance data have also been reported (11,17).

Strand-Passing Assays

Unknotting of P4 DNA and catenation of pBR322 DNA were modifications of the methods of Liu et al. (18), as detailed (17).

Stabilization of Enzyme–DNA Complexes ("Cleavable Complex Formation")

Modification of the method of Liu et al. (19) was followed to precipitate [^{32}P]-labeled pBR322 DNA–protein complexes with K-SDS, as detailed elsewhere (17).

Removal of Endogenous ATP from Nuclear Extracts

Endogenous ATP that may have been extracted simultaneously with topoisomerase II from nuclei of CEM, CEM/VM-1, and CEM/VM-1-5 cells was removed by passing the extracts through Sephadex G-50 spin columns, using a modification of the methods of Neal and Florini (20) and Fry et al. (21). The method is detailed elsewhere (21a), but as done in our laboratory, molecules with apparent molecular weights less than ≈15,000 were retained by the columns. By Western blot analysis no topoisomerase II was retained by the columns.

RESULTS AND DISCUSSION

Comparison of Pgp-MDR and at-MDR

It is now well established that at-MDR is a distinct entity from Pgp-MDR (11,12,22). We have shown that two human leukemic cell lines, selected for primary resistance to either vinblastine (VLB; CEM/VLB$_{100}$) or teniposide (VM-26; CEM/VM-1), are about equally resistant and cross-resistant to the epipodophyllotoxins and anthracyclines (11,12). However, the mechanisms of resistance for these two lines are entirely different. Table 21.1 summarizes in

Table 21.1. Properties of Cell Lines with P-Glycoprotein (Pgp)-Associated and Altered Topoisomerase II (at)-Associated Multidrug Resistance Phenotypes[a]

	Change[b]	
	Pgp-MDR	at-MDR
Cytotoxicity of		
Anthracyclines	↓	↓
Epipodophyllotoxins	↓	↓
Aminoacridines	↓	↓
Vinca alkaloids	↓	N.C./↓
Effect of "modulators"	↑	N.C.
(verapamil, chloroquine, etc.)		
Cell pharmacology		
Drug accumulation	↓	N.C.
Drug retention	↓	N.C.
P-glycoprotein gene		
Amplification	N.C./↑	N.C.
Expression	↑	N.C.
Product (P170, Pgp)	↑	N.C.
Topoisomerase II activities	N.C.	↓
Topoisomerase II gene		
Expression	N.C.	↓
Product (topo II)	N.C.	N.C./↓
Phenotype	Dominant or codominant[c]	Recessive

[a]Determined primarily with CEM/VLB$_{100}$ and CEM/VM-1 cells, respectively (11,12).
[b]Relative to drug-sensitive parent cell line: ↑, increase; ↓, decrease; N.C., no change.
[c]Shown for other Pgp-MDR cell lines (26,27), and most likely true for CEM/VLB$_{100}$ cells.

general terms features of both types of MDR drawn primarily but not exclusively from our studies. As will be shown later, not all of the characteristics listed in the table are present in all of the at-MDR cell lines. Despite these few inconsistencies (which may be due to assay differences), it is clear that at-MDR cells express a broad cross-resistance to many natural product drugs (see also Table 21.2). An important distinguishing feature, however, is that several of these lines are either not cross-resistant or are minimally cross-resistant to the Vinca alkaloids (11,15,23). Moreover, we showed (12) that modulators of Pgp-MDR, such as verapamil and chloroquine, were unable to enhance the cytotoxicity of anticancer drugs in our CEM/VM-1 cells. "Pure" at-MDR cell lines do not have defects in drug accumulation (11), nor do they overexpress Pgp or its mRNA (12). We have found in our at-MDR cell lines little or no change in amount of salt-extractable nuclear topoisomerase II (17), but preliminary results revealed decreases in topoisomerase II mRNA, compared to either Pgp-MDR cells or drug-sensitive cells (Beck et al., unpublished results). Nuclear extracts from these at-MDR cell lines commonly exhibit a decrease in topoisomerase II–associated activities or functions, and this will be detailed subsequently. Finally, cell fusion studies indicate that the at-MDR phenotype is expressed recessively (16,24,25); in contrast, Pgp-MDR is expressed in a dominant or codominant manner (26,27).

The central message from Table 21.1 is that at-MDR is clearly a distinct entity from Pgp-MDR. A corollary of this finding is that cell lines can be equally resistant to a given natural product drug by two different mechanisms. This observation has consequences for studies of clinical MDR, since [1] commonly used anticancer drugs can clearly select for very different drug-resistant tumor cell populations, and [2] examination of patient tumors for markers of "MDR" will require probes for at-MDR as well as those already in use to detect Pgp-MDR.

Resistance and Cross-Resistance Properties of at-MDR Cell Lines

Compared with Pgp-MDR cell lines (28), there have been few at-MDR cell lines described to date, and they are listed in Table 21.2. Of the nine cell lines, five appear to have no alteration in drug transport or expression of Pgp or its mRNA. For the purposes of the present discussion, we may consider these to be "pure" at-MDR cell lines. The drugs used most frequently to select these lines were the aminoacridine, m-AMSA, and the epipodophyllotoxins, VM-26 and VP-16-213, all three of which are known to interact with topoisomerase II (36,37). It should be noted that an L1210 MDR cell line selected for VM-26 resistance was shown to overexpress Pgp (38), and two Chinese hamster cell lines selected for resistance to VP-16 are thought to express both a topoisomerase II-dependent and -independent mechanism of resistance (38a). Also, cell lines selected for resistance to adriamycin frequently have mixed phenotypes of both at-MDR and Pgp-MDR (13,14). Thus, it is not always possible to predict the type of resistance that will be obtained, and this may reflect the cytotoxic targets of the agent used, the solubility of the drug, and the method by which these cells were selected for resistance.

Effects of Drugs and ATP on Topoisomerase II–Associated Activities in at-MDR Cell Lines

Table 21.3 summarizes the effects of antitopoisomerase II drugs on both strand passing and DNA–protein binding as reported in several at-MDR cell lines. The DNA–enzyme binding was reported as single-strand breaks, double-strand breaks, or stabilized ("cleavable") DNA–protein complexes. In general, where comparisons can be made, drugs are less effective in increasing DNA–protein binding or stimulating cleavable complex formation in all of the at-MDR cell lines reported. It may be important to the underlying molecular mechanism(s) of at-MDR that this decreased effect of topoisomerase II–active drugs on enzyme–DNA binding and cleavage is the only feature thus far reported that is common to all the at-MDR lines.

These differences in drug effects are also reflected in strand passing reactions (Table 21.3). For example, VM-26 decreases unknotting activity of nuclear extracts from our sensitive cell line at a lower concentration than an equal activity from the resistant cell lines (17). We note that although we saw differences among our cell lines in effect of drug on strand-passing activity, this

Table 21.2. Features of at-MDR Cell Lines

Parent Line	Resistant Line	Selecting Agent (fold-resistance)	Cross-resistance (x-fold)	Accumulation Defect or Pgp Expression	Reference
CHO	Vpm^R-5	VP-16 (20)	m-AMSA (3) mitoxantrone (5) adriamycin (5) vinblastine (1.5)	−	15,29
DC3F	DC3F/9-OHE	9-hydroxy-ellipticine	m-AMSA 2-me-9-OHE VP-16 adriamycin	+	24
Wt20	A20	amsacrine (20)	teniposide (10) bisantrine (200) ellipticine (5) dactinomycin (10) mitomycin C (2.5) vinblastine (10)	+/−	30,31
HL-60	HL-60/AMSA	m-AMSA (70)	VP-16 (11) adriamycin (1.8) vinblastine (1.3)	−	23,32
CEM	CEM/VM-1	VM-26 (50)	VP-16 (40) doxorubicin (15) m-AMSA (20) actinomycin D (3) vinblastine (1.4) vincristine (1.5)	−	11,12

CEM	CEM-VM-1-5	VM-26 (140)	VP-16 (130) doxorubicin (115) m-AMSA (85) actinomycin D (10) vinblastine (1) vincristine (7)	–	17, and unpublished observation
K562	K/VP.5	VP-16 (11)	VM-26 (11) m-AMSA (13) doxorubicin (5) mitoxantrone (5) vinblastine (1) vincristine (1)	–	33
GLC$_4$	GLC$_4$/ADR	adriamycin (45)	vincristine (5) vindesine (30) VP-16 (38) actinomycin D (0.9)	+	34
MCF-7	ADR^R	adriamycin (125–300)	VP-16 (100) VCR (>250) VLB (375) actD (175)	+	35

Table 21.3. Effects of Antitopoisomerase II Drugs on Topoisomerase II Activity (Strand Passing and DNA–Protein Binding) in at-MDR Cell Lines

at-MDR Cell Line	Strand Passing		DNA–Protein Binding[a] (+ Drug)	Reference
	− Drug	+ Drug		
CEM/VM-1	↓ (P4)[b]	↓ (P4; pBR)	↓	17
CEM/VM-1-5	↓ (P4)	↓ (P4; pBR)	↓	17
Vpm^R-5	N.C. (kDNA)	N.C. (kDNA)	↓	16
DC3F/9-OHE	N.C. (kDNA)	—	↓	39
A20	↓ (P4)	—	↓	31
HL-60/ AMSA	N.C. (kDNA)	—	↓	40
K/VP.5	↓ (P4)	—	↓	41
GLC₄/ADR	—	—	↓	34
ADR^R	—	—	↓	14

[a]Measured as protein-associated single-strand breaks, double-strand breaks, or stabilized ("cleavable") DNA–protein complexes; N.C., no change; ↓, decreased compared with drug-sensitive controls.
[b]Terms in parentheses represent assays used: P4, P4 DNA unknotting; kDNA, kinetoplast DNA decatenation; pBR, pBR322 DNA catenation.

phenomenon has not been a consistent finding among all the lines reported (Table 21.3). This may be due to differences in assays (e.g., decatenation of kDNA versus unknotting of P4 DNA), assay conditions, or source of enzyme used in measuring topoisomerase activity. These diminished drug effects on topoisomerase-II activity from at-MDR cells permit the suggestion that the resistance-associated lesion(s) may be in a drug-binding site on the enzyme, and not in some essential DNA recognition site, since the cells appear to function relatively normally in the absence of drug.

To expand on these general findings, we examined the effects of drugs on several topoisomerase II–associated functions or activities in isolated nuclei or nuclear extracts from our cell lines. We found that isolated nuclei of CEM/VM-1 cells were relatively resistant to VM-26–induced strand breaks in an alkaline elution filter assay, compared to nuclei from both the drug-sensitive CEM cells and the Pgp-MDR cell line, CEM/VLB$_{100}$ (42). We also found that both VM-26 (Table 21.4) and m-AMSA (21a) were less able to stabilize DNA–enzyme complexes by nuclear extracts from our two at-MDR cell lines compared to the drug-sensitive CEM cells. It is clear that the degree of resistance is inversely related to formation of drug-stabilized complexes, and this has not been shown before in at-MDR cell lines of progressively increasing resistance. Other recent results support these findings: the effect of these drugs on isolated nuclear matrix was decreased in the resistant cells in comparison with their effect on that of the CEM parent line (42a). This decreased drug effect is associated with a selective decrease in amount of immunoreactive topoisomerase II in the nuclear matrix of the drug-resistant versus drug-sensitive cells (42a).

It is also worth noting that ATP influences cleavage of DNA, cleavage being measured indirectly by assays that quantitate formation of covalent protein–DNA complexes in response to drugs that affect topoisomerase II. While formation of these drug-stabilized enzyme–DNA complexes occurs in the ab-

Table 21.4. Effects of VM-26 on Stabilization of Enzyme–DNA Complexes[a]

| | [32P] Counts Precipitated[b] | | | |
| | No Drug | | + 100 μM VM-26 | |
Nuclear Extract From	− ATP	+ ATP	− ATP	+ ATP
CEM	558	649	2,505	13,940
C/VM-1	565	560	1,010	7,159
C/VM-1-5	489	440	614	2,114

[a]"Cleavable complex formation."
[b]Precipitation of single-stranded protein-associated [32P]3′ end-labeled pBR322 DNA was done according to the method of Liu et al. (19), as detailed elsewhere (17). Because the specific activity of the substrate decreases with time, experiments cannot be averaged and so a representative experiment is shown. The experiment was done at least three times. The numbers shown are the averages of duplicates.

sence of ATP, it is clearly increased by 1 mM ATP. This stimulation is seen with VM-26 (17; Table 21.4) as well as with *m*-AMSA (21a). We speculate that ATP may expose more drug binding sites on topoisomerase II or increase the affinity of the enzyme for DNA. Taken together, these data suggest that there is an essential alteration in the way the topoisomerase II–acting drugs bind to the enzyme or interact with the enzyme–DNA complex in the at-MDR cells.

Alterations in Topoisomerase II–Associated Activities in the Absence of Drugs

We have found differences in strand passing (unknotting) and rates of strand passing (catenation) mediated by nuclear extracts of our VM-26–resistant CEM cell lines even in the absence of drug. For example, we showed in a P4 unknotting assay that strand-passing activity was decreased in nuclear extracts from the drug-resistant cells (17; Table 21.3). Similar results have been observed in VP-16–resistant K562 cells (41; Table 21.3) and in *m*-AMSA–resistant P388 cells (31; Table 21.3). All these studies used a P4 unknotting assay to measure enzyme activity. Three other studies found no difference in topoisomerase II activity in the absence of drug (Table 21.3); these studies measured enzyme activity with a kDNA decatenating assay. Interestingly, while nuclear extracts of the DC3F/9-OHE cell line were unaltered in maximum decatenating activity compared with controls (39), the *rates* of decatenation using this same assay were decreased 3.5-fold (43).

Similarly, we have observed resistance-associated alterations in rates of ATP-dependent catenation of pBR322 DNA with nuclear extracts from our drug-resistant cells (17). For example, Figure 21.1 demonstrates that ATP-dependent catenation of pBR322 DNA by nuclear extracts of CEM cells is essentially completed by 1 min, but it takes about 5 min to complete the reaction with extracts from the CEM/VM-1 nuclei, and 20–30 min to complete the reaction by nuclear extracts from the more resistant CEM/VM-1-5 cells. While other factors may be involved in catenation, these results are comparable with those of Charcosset et al. (43) using the kDNA decatenation assay. The contrasting results in strand-passing assays with the various at-MDR cell lines may

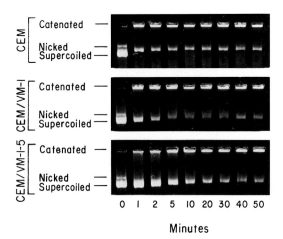

Minutes

Figure 21.1. Time course of catenating activity of nuclear extracts from CEM, CEM/VM-1, and CEM/VM-1-5 cells. pBR322 DNA (0.3 μg) and 1.7 μg of 1.0 M NaCl nuclear extract from each of the cell lines were incubated for the indicated times. The reactions were stopped with SDS and run on a 1% agarose gel. ATP was included in all the reactions. Methods are detailed in Danks et al. (17). The figure is reprinted with permission of the American Chemical Society.

reflect different mechanisms of resistance or simply different assay conditions. It would seem that more than one measure of topoisomerase II activity, probably at more than one time point, would allow us to make more definitive statements when characterizing each enzyme activity.

Effects of ATP on Topoisomerase II Activity

How the differences in topoisomerase II activity relate to the resistance of the cells remains to be determined, but other studies from our laboratory may be informative. We have found that there are differences in requirements for ATP by nuclear extracts of our two at-MDR lines compared with the drug-sensitive parent line. It can be seen in Figure 21.2 that the ATP requirement for P4 unknotting is in the order: CEM/VM-1-5 > CEM/VM-1 > CEM, suggesting that there may be resistance-related differences in ATP utilization or binding by components in the nuclear extracts (possibly topoisomerase II itself) that are required for strand passing. To test this hypothesis, we repeated the experiment in Figure 21.2, but added 200 μM or 400 μM novobiocin, a competitive inhibitor of ATP binding to topoisomerase II (44), to the reaction mixture. As seen in Table 21.5, we found a resistance-related increase in the concentration of ATP required for half-maximal stimulation of unknotting activity of nuclear extracts from CEM, CEM/VM-1, and CEM/VM-1-5 cells. In other results (21a), we noted differences in interaction with AMP-PNP, a nonhydrolyzable analog of ATP, suggesting that ATP binding is impaired in the topoisomerase II of the drug-resistant cells. While these results do not prove that the ATP site of topoisomerase II is altered in the at-MDR cells, they do show that alterations in interaction of ATP with the enzyme or enzyme–DNA complex are coincident with the resistance of these cells to topoisomerase II–acting drugs.

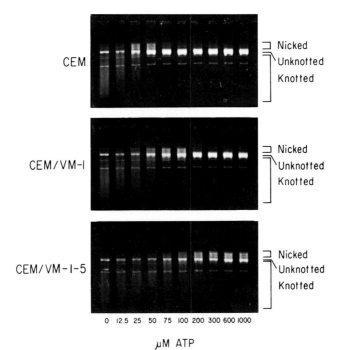

0   12.5 25   50   75 100 200 300 600 1000

μM ATP

Figure 21.2. ATP requirement for unknotting of P4 DNA by nuclear extracts of CEM, CEM/VM-1, and CEM/VM-1-5 cells. Topoisomerase II was extracted from nuclei with 1.0 M NaCl, as described (17). Endogenous ATP was removed by a mini "spincolumn" method, as indicated in Materials and Methods. These extracts (1.0 μg protein) were incubated with ATP at the indicated concentration and 0.75 μg of P4 knotted DNA for 30 min. The samples were treated with SDS-proteinase K and electrophoresed on a 0.7% agarose gel. A representative of seven separate experiments is shown. The figure is reprinted with permission of Pergamon Press.

Possible Mechanisms of at-MDR

Summarized in Table 21.6 are the alterations in topoisomerase II activity that we have found in the CEM/VM-1 and CEM/VM-1-5 cells. Decreases in drug-induced strand-breaks, drug-stabilized enzyme–DNA complex formation, and drug effect on nuclear matrix suggest that there is an essential alteration in the

Table 21.5. Effect of Novobiocin on the ATP Concentration Required for Half-maximal Stimulation of Unknotting of P4 DNA by Nuclear Extracts from CEM, CEM/VM-1, and CEM/VM-1-5 Cells[a]

| | ATP Producing Half-maximal Unknotting (μM) | | |
Novobiocin (μM)	CEM	CEM/VM-1	CEM/VM-1-5
0	38	67	300
200	92	227	942
400	148	869	>1,000

[a]Amounts of unknotted P4 DNA were computed with an image analyzer, and ATP concentrations required for half-maximal stimulation of catalytic activity were calculated by interpolation of the data in Figure 21.2 and from experiments with 200 μM and 400 μM novobiocin (not shown). Reprinted from ref. 21a with permission of Pergamon Press.

Table 21.6. Changes in Topoisomerase II and Topoisomerase II-Associated Activities in CEM/VM-1 and CEM-VM-1-5 Cell Lines

Assay	Effect Compared with Drug-Sensitive Controls[a]	Reference
Drug-induced strand-breaks in whole cells and nuclei	↓	42
Drug-induced stabilization of enzyme–DNA complexes	↓	17
Drug effects on strand passing	↓	17
Immunoreactive topoisomerase II		
Nuclear, salt extractable	N.C.	17, 42a
Nuclear, matrix	↓	42a
Strand passing	↓	17
Rate of catenation	↓	17
ATP requirement	↑	21a
Drug effect on nuclear matrix	↓	42a

[a] ↑, Increased; ↓, decreased; N.C., no change.

way the topoisomerase II–acting drugs bind to the enzyme or enzyme–DNA complex in the at-MDR cells. However, the resistance-associated differences in strand-passing activities, rates of catenation, and ATP requirements seen in the absence of drug suggest that any proposed alterations in drug interaction may in fact be secondary to some more fundamental alteration such as might be seen if, for example, a mutation in the ATP-binding site were involved. In this regard, we note that Liu (45) showed that metabolic inhibitors, which decreased cellular ATP levels, also decreased VP-16 cytotoxicity, essentially producing a metabolically "resistant" cell. It must be remembered that in the absence of drug, the cells behave normally, save for a slight decrease in growth rate. While it is clear that enzyme–DNA complex formation and unknotting of P4 DNA *in vitro* are influenced by ATP (17, 21a), we do not know if the intranuclear ATP concentration limits catalytic activity or enzyme–DNA binding in the at-MDR cells *in vivo*. We do note that *in vitro* (Table 21.5) there is an approximate 2- to 10-fold difference in effective ATP concentration among the three cell lines. It is possible, however, that the increased requirement for ATP, the decreased rates of catenation (also ATP-dependent), and decreased drug effect reflect an alteration in an ATP binding site on topoisomerase II that affects drug binding, ATP hydrolysis, or topoisomerase II phosphorylation. Finally, we (42a) have recently found that decreased drug binding to the nuclear matrix from resistant cells correlates with a selective decrease in the amount of topoisomerase II in the nuclear matrix of CEM/VM-1 versus CEM cells. Since the cytotoxic effect of VM-26 involves its interaction with this form of the enzyme, then a change in the type or amount of topoisomerase II incorporated into the nuclear matrix would change the cytotoxic effect of the drug.

The list of possible mechanisms of resistance in Table 21.7 is an attempt to incorporate all this information, including results with drugs and the data of others. It is not yet clear whether, in the several cell lines that exhibit at-MDR, the underlying mechanism(s) leading to this phenotype is the same. It seems

Table 21.7. at-MDR May Be Due to Alterations in:

Drug binding site(s)
Amount or distribution of topo II (matrix vs. soluble)
ATP utilization (binding or hydrolysis)
Phosphorylation of topo II
Modulator or cofactor interaction
Any of the steps involved in strand passing (46):
  Recognition–binding
  Strand cleavage
    Covalent attachment of enzyme to cleaved 5′ termini
  Passage of second strand
    Dependent on ATP binding but not hydrolysis
  Religation of cleaved DNA
  Enzyme turnover
    Requires ATP hydrolysis

reasonable that any one of the changes listed in Table 21.7 could result in a similar phenotype of at-MDR. As outlined by Osheroff (46), there appear to be five sequential steps in the action of topoisomerase II: [1] binding of topoisomerase II to the double-stranded DNA substrate; [2] double-stranded DNA cleavage, which is accompanied by subsequent covalent attachment of the enzyme to the cleaved 5′ termini; [3] passage of another double-stranded DNA through the break in the nucleic acid backbone, a function that is dependent on ATP binding, but not hydrolysis; [4] religation of the cleaved DNA; and [5] enzyme turnover, i.e., the ability to reinitiate catalysis, which requires hydrolysis of ATP. Alterations in topoisomerase II might affect any one or all of these steps and yield cells with an at-MDR phenotype. Similarly, drugs such as VM-26, VP-16, and m-AMSA might interfere with any of these steps, and alterations in, for example, a drug-binding site could also yield at-MDR cells. Although Osheroff has recently suggested that VP-16 works primarily on the last steps by either inhibiting religation of the DNA strand(s) or blocking enzyme turnover after cleavage (47), the precise mechanism by which these drugs work and by which cells might express at-MDR remains to be determined.

SUMMARY

We have described here features of our VM-26–resistant human leukemic cell lines, suggesting that the basis for their resistance is an alteration in the function of the enzyme topoisomerase II. We have compared our results with those of others and found that while many different types of lesions have been described among the several at-MDR cell lines, the feature common to all of them is a decrease in the ability of drugs to promote strand-breakage.

   We have shown by several assays that resistance-related alterations in topoisomerase II activities can be demonstrated in the absence as well as the presence of drug. Of potential importance are our findings of decreased rates of catenation of pBR322 DNA and increased ATP requirements for unknotting

P4 DNA *in vitro* by nuclear extracts from cells of increasing resistance to VM-26. These results suggest that any putative altered drug-binding site on topoisomerase II or on the topoisomerase II–DNA complex may affect a site that is essential for the proper functioning of the enzyme, possibly either the ATP-site or a site required for interaction of a modulator of the enzyme. We also feel that a significant aspect of our work relates to the fact that we have shown that MDR cell lines, selected for resistance to two different agents, can express the same degree of resistance or cross-resistance to several natural product componds, yet the mechanism of this resistance can be due to two entirely different mechanisms, at-MDR and Pgp-MDR. These findings are important to ongoing clinical studies of MDR markers, since present assays are only screening, at the protein or mRNA level, for Pgp overexpression. That at-MDR cells can express resistance and cross-resistance to many of the same agents as Pgp-MDR cells may afford a partial explanation for some of the negative results in the Pgp assays (6,7) in the face of clear clinical MDR. Knowledge of the biochemical basis of at-MDR will likely produce insights and tools with which to address these problems.

Acknowledgments

This work was supported in part by research grants CA 30103 and CA 40570; CORE grant CA 21765, all from the National Cancer Institute, DHHS, Bethesda, MD; and by American Lebanese Syrian Associated Charities (ALSAC). We are grateful to our colleagues in our laboratory for their tireless and cheerful efforts in helping us understand what at-MDR is all about—Carla Schmidt, Margaret Cirtain, and Judy Wolverton; and we appreciate the helpful comments of our collaborator, Parker Suttle. We are indebted to Warren Ross for his early interest in and preliminary studies of our cell lines. We thank Fabrienne Holloway and Vicki Gray for their excellent secretarial efforts, and salute the Biomedical Communications people—especially Dani Harris, Klo Speilshaus, and John Zacker—for their cheerful accommodation of our many requests for "one last change" in the figures.

REFERENCES

1. Beck, W. T. The cell biology of multiple drug resistance. Biochem. Pharmacol. **36:** 2879–2887, 1987.
2. Pastan, I. and Gottesman, M. Multiple-drug resistance in human cancer. N. Engl. J. Med. **316:** 1388–1397, 1987.
3. Moscow, J. A. and Cowan, K. H. Multidrug resistance. J. Natl. Cancer Inst. **80:** 14–20, 1988.
4. Bradley, G., Juranka, P. F., and Ling, V. Mechanism of multidrug resistance. Biochim. Biophys. Acta. **948:** 87–128, 1988.

5. Bell, D. R., Gerlach, J. H., Kartner, N., Buick, R. N., and Ling, V. Detection of P-glycoprotein in ovarian cancer: A molecular marker associated with multidrug resistance. J. Clin. Oncol. **3:** 311–315, 1985.
6. Gerlach, J. H., Bell, D. R., Karakousis, C., Slocum, H.K., Kartner, N., Rustum, Y. M., Ling, V., and Baker, R. M. P-glycoprotein expression in human sarcoma: Evidence for multidrug resistance. J. Clin. Oncol. **5:** 1452–1460, 1987.
7. Fojo, A. T., Ueda, K., Slamon, D. J.,

Poplack, D. G., Gottesman, M. M., and Pastan, I. Expression of a multidrug-resistance gene in human tumors and tissues. Proc. Natl. Acad. Sci. USA. **84:** 265–269, 1987.

8. Marsh, W. and Center, M. S. Adriamycin resistance in HL60 cells and accompanying modification of a surface membrane protein contained in drug-sensitive cells. Cancer Res. **47:** 5080–5086, 1987.

9. Bhalla, K., Hindenburg, A., Taub, R. N., and Grant, S. Isolation and characterization of an anthracycline-resistant human leukemic cell line. Cancer Res. **45:** 3657–3662, 1985.

10. Kramer, R. A., Zakher, J., and Kim, G. Role of the glutathione redox cycle in acquired and de novo multidrug resistance. Science. **241:** 694–697, 1988.

11. Danks, M. K., Yalowich, J. C., and Beck, W. T. Atypical multiple drug resistance in a human leukemic cell line selected for resistance to teniposide (VM-26). Cancer Res. **47:** 1297–1301, 1987.

12. Beck, W. T., Cirtain, M. C., Danks, M. K., Felsted, R. L., Safa, A. R., Wolverton, J. S., Suttle, D. P., and Trent, J. M. Pharmacological, molecular, and cytogenetic analysis of "atypical" multidrug-resistant human leukemic cells. Cancer Res. **47:** 5455–5460, 1987.

13. Fairchild, C. R., Ivy, S. P., Dao-Shan, C.-S., Whang-Peng, J., Rosen, N., Israel, M., Melera, P. W., Cowan, K., and Goldsmith, M. E. Isolation of amplified and overexpressed DNA sequences from adriamycin-resistant human breast cancer cells. Cancer Res. **47:** 5141–5148, 1987.

14. Sinha, B. K., Haim, N., Dusre, L., Kerrigan, D., and Pommier, Y. DNA strand breaks produced by etoposide (VP-16,213) in sensitive and resistant human breast tumor cells: Implications for the mechanism of action. Cancer Res. **48:** 5096–5100, 1988.

15. Glisson, B., Gupta, R., Smallwood-Kentro, S., and Ross, W. Characterization of acquired epipodophyllotoxin resistance in a Chinese hamster ovary cell line: Loss of drug-stimulated DNA cleavage activity. Cancer Res. **46:** 1934–1938, 1986.

16. Glisson, B., Gupta, R., Hodges, P., and Ross, W. Cross-resistance to intercalating agents in an epipodophyllotoxin-resistant Chinese hamster ovary cell line: Evidence for a common intracellular target. Cancer Res. **46:** 1939–1942, 1986.

17. Danks, M. K., Schmidt, C. A., Cirtain, M. C., Suttle, D. P., and Beck, W. T. Altered catalytic activity of and DNA cleavage by DNA topoisomerase II from human leukemic cells selected for resistance to VM-26. Biochemistry. **27:** 8861–8869, 1988.

18. Liu, L. F., Davis, J. L. and Calendar, R. Novel topologically knotted DNA from bacteriophage P4 capsids: Studies with DNA topoisomerases. Nucleic Acids Res. **9:** 3979–3989, 1981.

19. Liu, L. F., Rowe, T. C., Yang, L., Tewey, K. M., and Chen, G. L. Cleavage of DNA by mammalian DNA topoisomerase II. J. Biol. Chem. **258:** 15365–15370, 1983.

20. Neal, M. W. and Florini, J. R. A rapid method for desalting small volumes of solution. Anal. Biochem. **55:** 328–330, 1973.

21. Fry, D. W., White, J. C., and Goldman, I. D. Rapid separation of low molecular weight solutes from liposomes without dilution. Anal. Biochem. **90:** 809–815, 1978.

21a. Danks, M. K., Schmidt, C. A., Deneka, D. A., and Beck, W. T. Increased ATP requirement for activity of and complex formation by DNA topoisomerase II from human leukemic CCRF-CEM cells selected for resistance to teniposide. Cancer Commun. **1:** 101–109, 1989.

22. Beck, W. T., Danks, M. K., Yalowich, J. C., Zamora, J. M., and Cirtain, M. C. Different mechanisms of multiple drug resistance in two human leukemic cell lines. In P. Wolley and K. Tew, eds. *Mechanisms of Drug Resistance in Neoplastic Cells.* New York: Academic Press, 1988, pp. 211–222.

23. Beran, M. and Anderson, B. S. Development and characterization of a human myelogenous leukemia cell line resistant to 4'-(9-acridinylamino)-3-methane-sulfon-m-anisidide. Cancer Res. **47:** 1897–1904, 1987.

24. Remy, J.-J., Belehradek, J., and Jacquemin-Sablon, A. Expression of drug sensitivity between 9-hydroxyellipticine-sensitive and -resistant cells. Cancer Res. **44:** 4587–4593, 1984.

25. Wolverton, J. S., Danks, M. K., Schmidt, C. A., and Beck, W. T. Genetic characterization of the multidrug-resistant phenotype of VM-26-resistant human leukemic cells. Cancer Res. **49:** 2422–2426, 1989.

26. Ling, V. and Baker, R. M. Dominance of colchicine resistance in hybrid CHO cells. Somatic Cell Genet. **4:** 193–200, 1978.

27. Akiyama, S-I., Fojo, A., Hanover, J. A.,

Pastan, I., and Gottesman, M. M. Isolation and genetic characterization of human KB cell lines resistant to multiple drugs. Somatic Cell Genet. **11**: 117–126, 1985.

28. Beck, W. T. and Danks, M.K. Characteristics of multidrug resistance in human tumor cells. In I. B. Roninson, ed. *Molecular and Cellular Biology of Multidrug Resistance in Tumor Cells.* New York: Plenum Press (in press, 1989).

29. Gupta, R. S. Genetic, biochemical, and cross-resistance studies with mutants of Chinese hamster ovary cells resistant to the anticancer drugs, VM-26 and VP-16-213. Cancer Res. **43**: 1568–1574, 1983.

30. Johnson, R. K. and Howard, R. S. Development and cross-resistance characteristics of a subline of P388 leukemia resistant to 4′-(9-acridinylamino)-methanesulfon-*m*-anisidide. Eur. J. Clin. Oncol. **18**: 479–487, 1982.

31. Per, S. R., Mattern, M. R., Mirabelli, C. K., Drake, F. H., Johnson, R. K., and Crooke, S. T. Characterization of a subline of P388 leukemia resistant to amsacrine: Evidence of altered topoisomerase II function. Mol. Pharmacol. **32**: 17–25, 1987.

32. Odaimi, M., Andersson, B. S., McCredie, K. B., and Beran, M. Drug sensitivity and cross-resistance of the 4′-(9-acridinylamino)methanesulfon-*m* - anisidide-resistant subline of HL-60 human leukemia. Cancer Res. **46**: 3330–3333, 1986.

33. Yalowich, J. C., Roberts, D., Benton, S., Parganas, E. Resistance to etoposide (VP-16) in human leukemia K562 cells is associated with altered DNA topoisomerase II (TOPO II) activity and rapid reversal of drug-induced DNA damage. Proc. Am. Assoc. Cancer Res. **28**: 277, 1987.

34. Zjilstra, J. G., de Vries, E. G. E., and Mulder, N. H. Multifactorial drug resistance in an adriamycin-resistant human small cell lung carcinoma cell line. Cancer Res. **47**: 1780–1784, 1987.

35. Batist, G., Tulpule, A., Sinha, B. K., Katki, A. G., Myers, C. E., and Cowan, K. H. Overexpression of a novel anionic glutathione transferase in multidrug-resistant human breast cancer cells. J. Biol. Chem. **261**: 15544–15549, 1986.

36. Tewey, K. M., Chen, G. L., Nelson, E. M., and Liu, L. F. Intercalative antitumor drugs interfere with the breakage-reunion reaction of mammalian DNA topoisomerase II. J. Biol. Chem. **259**: 9182–9187, 1984.

37. Chen, G. L., Yang, L., Rowe, T. C., Halligan, B. D., Tewey, K. M., and Liu, L. F. Nonintercalative antitumor drugs interfere with the breakage-reunion reaction of mammalian DNA topoisomerase II. J. Biol. Chem. **259**: 13560–13566, 1984.

38. Vasanthakumar, G., and Roberts, D. Isolation of an amplified DNA sequence in multidrug-resistant L1210 mouse leukemia cells. Proc. Am. Assoc. Cancer Res. **28**: 289, 1987.

38a. Spiridonidis, C. A., Chatterjee, S., Petzold, S. J., and Berger, N. A. Topoisomerase II-dependent and -independent mechanisms of etoposide resistance in Chinese hamster cell lines. Cancer Res. **49**: 644–650, 1989.

39. Pommier, Y., Kerrigan, D., Schwartz, R. E., Swack, J. A., and McCurdy, A. Altered DNA topoisomerase II activity in Chinese hamster cells resistant to topoisomerase II inhibitors. Cancer Res. **46**: 3075–3081, 1986.

40. Estey, E. H., Silberman, L., Beran, M., Andersson, B. S., and Zwelling, L. A. The interaction between nuclear topoisomerase II activity from human leukemia cells, exogenous DNA, and 4′ - (9-acridinylamino)methanesulfon-*m*-anisidide (*m*-AMSA) or 4-(4,6-*O*-ethylidene-β-D-glucopyranoside) (VP-16) indicates the sensitivity of the cells to the drugs. Biochem. Biophys. Res. Commun. **144**: 787–793, 1987.

41. Yalowich, J. C. and Benton, S. Effects of nucleotides on VP-16-induced DNA damage in nuclei from human leukemia K562 cells sensitive and resistant to VP-16. Proc. Am. Assoc. Cancer Res. **29**: 317, 1988.

42. Yalowich, J. C., Danks, M. K., Cirtain, M. C., Benton, S., Zamora, J. M., and Beck, W. T. Cellular pharmacology of "atypical" multiple drug resistance (at-MDR) in human leukemic cells selected for resistance to teniposide (VM-26). Proc. Am. Assoc. Cancer Res. **28**: 289, 1987.

42a. Fernandes, D. J., Danks, M. K., and Beck, W. T. Decreased nuclear matrix topoisomerase II in human leukemia cells resistant to VM-26 and *m*-AMSA. Biochemistry. **29**: 4235–4241, 1990.

43. Charcosset, J.-Y., Saucier, J.-M., and Jacquemin-Sablon, A. Reduced DNA topoisomerase II cleavage activity and drug-stimulated DNA cleavage in 9-hydroxyellipticine resistant cells. Biochem. Pharmacol. **37**: 2145–2149, 1988.

44. Sugino, A., Higgins, N. P., Brown, P.

O., Peebles, C. A., and Cozzarelli, N. R. Energy coupling in DNA gyrase and mechanism of action of novobiocin. Proc. Natl. Acad. Sci. USA. **75**: 4838–4842, 1978.

45. Kupfer, G., Bodley, A. L., and Liu, L. F. Involvement of intracellular ATP on cytotoxicity of topoisomerase II-targeting antitumor drugs. NCI Monogr. **4**: 37–40, 1987.

46. Osheroff, N. Eukaryotic topoisomerase II. Characterization of enzyme turnover. J. Biol. Chem. **261**: 9944–9950, 1986.

47. Osheroff, N. and Gale, K. C. Effect of etoposide on the DNA cleavage/religation reaction of topoisomerase II: Analysis of drug action. FASEB J. **2**: A1761, 1988.

Chapter 22

Reconstitution of Drug Sensitivity in Vpm^R-5 Somatic Cell Hybrids

BONNIE S. GLISSON, WARREN E. ROSS, AND

MICHAEL J. SICILIANO

The Vpm^R-5 cell line was established by mutagenizing wild-type (WT) Chinese hamster ovary (CHO) cells with ethylmethane sulfonate and selecting for resistance to teniposide in a single step (1). This cell line has now been analyzed in detail (2) and the data indicate that multidrug resistance of the Vpm^R-5 line may be mediated through a qualitative alteration in topoisomerase II that confers resistance to drug-induced DNA cleavage activity. Resistance of Vpm^R-5 cells to etoposide and intercalating agents (m-AMSA, mitoxantrone, and Adriamycin) is well correlated with loss of drug-induced DNA strand-breaking activity that is not associated with altered drug accumulation. Neither are there quantitative differences in topoisomerase II content in Vpm^R-5 cells compared with WT in immunoblots. Purified enzyme from Vpm^R-5 cells has normal decatenating activity that is equally sensitive to inhibition by etoposide relative to WT enzyme. Strikingly, however, topoisomerase II from Vpm^R-5 cells is quite resistant to etoposide- and m-AMSA–induced DNA cleavage activity. Based on studies with a somatic cell hybrid line, the product of fusion of Vpm^R-5 cells with drug-sensitive CHO line, EOT-3, drug sensitivity is a dominant trait. M$_1$J$_2$7 cells retain only a twofold level of resistance to the cytotoxic effects of etoposide (1) and exhibit a parallel diminution in resistance to etoposide-mediated strand-breaking activity (3). Assuming expression of both the Vpm^R-5 and the EOT-3 topoisomerase II genes in the hybrid cells, these data suggest that conversion to a drug-sensitive phenotype occurs when a normal enzyme becomes available for recruitment by drug to form "cleavable complexes."

The work presented herein represents an effort to define the genetic basis for resistance of the Vpm^R-5 line by studying Vpm^R-5 × human lymphocyte somatic cell hybrids for reconstitution of drug sensitivity and for human chromosomal complement. We hoped to identify a human chromosome whose presence was consistently associated with drug sensitivity and whose absence was associated with stable resistance. If our original hypothesis was correct, this would also map the gene for topoisomerase II.

METHODS

A stable HPRT (hypoxanthine guanine phosphoribosyltransferase)-deficient subline of Vpm^R-5, Vtgm-6, was selected for resistance to 6-thioguanine after mutagenesis with ethylmethane sulfonate. HPRT deficiency was confirmed by HPRT assay (4) as well as low reversion frequency cloning in HAT (hypoxanthine, aminopterin, thymidine)-supplemented medium. Vtgm-6 cells were fused with mitogenized human lymphocytes (5) in the presence of 45% PEG-1000. Hybrid clones selected in HAT-supplemented medium were harvested and expanded into cell lines. Drug-induced DNA single-strand breaks and cytotoxicity were assayed by alkaline elution and clonogenic potential, respectively, as previously described (3). Human chromosomal complement was determined using a combination of isoenzyme and molecular markers (6–7). The c-DNA probe for the human topoisomerase II gene was a generous gift from Dr. Leroy Liu of The Johns Hopkins University, Baltimore, Md. Topoisomerase II content was estimated by immunoprecipitation of whole cell lysates with monoclonal antibody raised to the purified protein from CCRF-CEM cells (8). Steady state concentrations of radiolabeled etoposide and daunomycin were determined as described (3).

RESULTS

Developing a stable 6-thioguanine–resistant HPRT-deficient subline of Vpm^R-5 required mutagenesis with ethylmethane sulfonate. Nine such sublines were developed; the Vtgm-6 subline was chosen for use in the fusion experiments based on its low HAT-reversion frequency and a doubling time equal to that of Vpm^R-5 cells. In direct comparison with Vpm^R-5, Vtgm-6 cells exhibit no significant differences as regards sensitivity to etoposide, m-AMSA, mitoxantrone, or 5-iminodaunorubicin-induced cytotoxic or strand-breaking activities.

Sixteen Vtgm-6 × lymphocyte hybrid lines have been tested and three (HL-8, HL-10, and HL-17) have been chosen for further study based on partial reconstitution of sensitivity to etoposide compared to Vtgm-6 cells. These three lines have also lost resistance to the cytotoxic effects of the anthracyclines, Adriamycin and 5-iminodaunorubicin. HL-8 and HL-10 are also sensitive to mitoxantrone, but all 16 lines have retained full resistance to m-AMSA. Detailed analysis of the HL-8 line indicates that enhanced sensitivity to the cytotoxic effects of etoposide and mitoxantrone is accompanied by a parallel increase in sensitivity to the drugs' strand-breaking activities (Table 22.1). However, cytotoxic effects are dissociated from DNA single-strand breaks when HL-8 cells are studied with regard to the anthracyclines (Table 22.1). Despite an approximate fourfold and twofold reduction in resistance to Adriamycin and 5-iminodaunorubicin, respectively, HL-8 cells exhibit the same DNA single-strand break frequency as Vtgm-6 cells upon exposure to these drugs.

Analysis of human chromosomal complement in all 16 lines failed to identify a chromosome whose presence was consistently associated with drug sen-

Table 22.1. Dose Modification Factors[a]

	Etoposide		Mitoxantrone		Adriamycin		5-ID	
	SSB	D_{50}	SSB	D_{50}	SSB	D_{50}	SSB	D_{50}
Vtgm-6:WT	40	14	22	5.5	14	7.2	2.8	2
HL-8:WT	15	6	14	3.3	13	1.7	2.6	0.85
Vtgm-6:HL-8	2.7	2.3	1.6	1.7	1.1	4.2	1.1	2.3

[a]Factor by which drug dose must be multiplied to achieve equitoxic effect (for DNA strand breaking and cytotoxic activities)

sitivity and whose absence was associated with stable resistance. However, the tendency of human chromosomes to fragment in CHO hybrid cells does not allow complete exclusion of shared and unique chromosomal material in the HL-8, 10, and 17 lines. Computer-assisted concordant segregation analysis of a human lymphocyte-CHO hybrid clone panel indicates that a cDNA probe for the human topoisomerase II gene hybridizes to a sequence on human chromosome 17. In a similar experiment, we identified no hybridizing sequences to the same cDNA probe in any of the 16 Vtgm-6 hybrid lines.

Further, partial loss of drug resistance in the HL lines 8, 10, and 17 is not accompanied by enhanced accumulation of radiolabeled etoposide or daunomycin at steady state as compared to levels in Vtgm-6, Vpm^R-5, and WT.

DISCUSSION

We have identified partial reconstitution of drug sensitivity in 3/16 Vtgm-6 × human lymphocyte hybrid lines. While the precise mechanism for this loss of resistance remains unknown, we have ruled out altered drug accumulation, or presence of the human topoisomerase II gene as contributing to this phenomenon. Increased topoisomerase II content remains a possible explanation for this partial loss of drug resistance; these experiments are in progress. The absence of identifiable common and unique human chromosomal material in the three sensitive hybrid lines suggests that each line may have lost resistance owing to somewhat different factors. In fact, preliminary analysis of data from HL-10 and HL-17 indicates that all three cell lines are somewhat different from each other as regards the degree of altered resistance to each drug and whether this effect is correlated with changes in drug-induced DNA strandbreaks.

The dissociation of anthracycline-induced single-strand breaks from cytotoxic effects in HL-8 cells was unexpected. It should be noted, however, that both adriamycin and 5-iminodaunorubicin produce relatively more doublestrand than single-strand breaks (9) and that double-strand breaks induced by *m*-AMSA and 5-iminodaunorubicin are better correlated with cytotoxic effects (10). Work is in progress to determine Adriamycin and 5-iminodaunorubicin–induced double-strand break frequencies in HL-8, WT, and Vtgm-6 cell lines to resolve this issue. If increased drug-induced double-strand breaks cannot be demonstrated in HL-8 cells relative to Vtgm-6, we are faced with two alternative explanations. Either loss of resistance to these drugs in the HL-8 line is completely independent of topoisomerase II–mediated effects or there is an alteration in cellular responses distal to cleavable complex formation.

The excellent correlation of enhanced cytotoxic and DNA strand-breaking activity of both etoposide and mitoxantrone in the HL-8 line indicates, that at least for these two agents, loss of resistance is related to increased cleavable complex formation. This may be related to an increased quantity of enzyme, or the protein may be modulated by other unknown factors which increase its potential for forming cleavable complexes upon exposure to drug. Alternatively it is conceivable, though we believe unlikely, that chromatin is more accessible to the drugs, the enzyme, or the drug–enzyme complex in HL-8 cells. Answering these questions will obviously require additional biochemical characterization.

The location of the human topoisomerase II gene on chromosome 17 is somewhat unfortunate as CHO $\times$ human hybrids containing this chromosome are only rarely viable. This phenomenon probably explains the complete absence of 17 markers in all 16 Vtgm-6 hybrids that we analyzed. To test more directly the hypothesis that expression of a normal topoisomerase II gene in the milieu of the Vpm^R-5 cell will reconstitute drug sensitivity, we are currently exploring a method that will select for chromosome 17 in Vpm^R-5 hybrid lines. We plan to use microcell-mediated DNA transfer of a mouse cell line carrying human chromosome 17 linked to the dominant selectable marker pSV$_2$ *neo* (11). We will then select Vpm^R-5 hybrids in the antibiotic G418 (geneticin) and again analyze for drug sensitivity and confirm the presence of the 17th chromosome and the human topoisomerase II gene with molecular probes.

Acknowledgments

This work was supported in part by CA-01225 from the National Cancer Institute, National Institutes of Health (B.S.G.). The authors gratefully acknowledge the technical expertise of Janet Woodward, Billie White, Jeanette Siciliano, and Michael Latham.

REFERENCES

1. Gupta, R. S. Genetic, biochemical, and cross-resistance studies with mutants of Chinese hamster ovary cells resistant to the anticancer drugs, VM-26-, and VP-16-213. Cancer Res. **43:** 1568–1574, 1983.
2. Glisson, B. S., Sullivan, D. M., Gupta, R. S., and Ross, W. E. Mediation of multidrug resistance in a Chinese hamster ovary cell line by a mutant type II topoisomerase. NCI Monographs **4:** 89–94, 1987.
3. Glisson, B. S., Gupta, R. S., Smallwood-Kentro, S., and Ross, W. E. Characterization of acquired epipodophyllotoxin resistance in a Chinese hamster ovary cell line: Loss of drug-stimulated DNA cleavage activity. Cancer Res. **46:** 1934–1938, 1986.
4. Gillen, F. D., Roufa, D. J., Beaudet, A. L., and Cashey, C. T. 8-Azaguanine resistance in mammalian cells deficient in hypoxanthine-guanine phosphoribosyltransferase. Genetics. **72:** 239–252, 1972.
5. Edwards, C. M., Glisson, B. S., King, C. K., Kentro-Smallwood, S., and Ross, W. E. Etoposide-induced DNA cleavage in human leukemia cells. Cancer Chemother. Pharmacol. **20:** 162–168, 1987.

6. Siciliano, M. J., Adair, G. M., Atkinson, N. E., and Humphrey, R. M. In M. C. Ratazzi, J. S. Scandaliss, and G. S. Whitt, eds. *Isozymes: Current Topics in Biological and Medical Research.* New York: Alan R. Liss, **10**: 313–321, 1983.

7. Southern, E. M. Detection of specific sequences among DNA fragments separated by gel electrophoresis. J. Mol. Biol. **98**: 503–517, 1985.

8. Springer, T. A. Analysis of proteins. In *Current Protocols in Molecular Biology,* Brooklyn, NY: Greene Publishing Assoc., 1988, pp. 1–10.

9. Pommier, Y., Schwartz, R. E., Kohn, K. W., and Zwelling, L. A. Formation and rejoining of DNA double strand breaks in isolated cell nuclei by antineoplastic intercalating agents. Biochemistry. **23**: 3194–3201, 1984.

10. Pommier, Y., Zwelling, L. A., Chien-Song, K., Whang-Peng, J., and Bradley, M. O. Correlations between intercalator-induced DNA strand breaks and sister chromatid exchanges, mutations, and cytotoxicity in Chinese hamster cells. Cancer Res. **45**: 3143–3149, 1985.

11. McNeill, C. A. and Brown, R. L. Microcell-mediated transfer of normal human chromosomes into recipient mouse cells. Proc. Natl. Acad. Sci. USA. **77**: 5394–5398, 1980.

PART V

DEVELOPMENT AND CLINICAL USE OF TOPOISOMERASE INHIBITORS

Chapter 23
Semisynthetic Congeners of Doxorubicin and Daunorubicin: DNA Topoisomerase II–Mediated Interaction with DNA

ANNETTE BODLEY, LEROY F. LIU, MERVYN ISRAEL,
RAMAKRISHNAN SESHADRI, ROBERT SILBER,
AND MILAN POTMESIL

Mammalian DNA topoisomerase II (topo II), a nuclear enzyme that alters the topological state of DNA and is essential for cell replication and viability (reviewed in 1–3), appears to be the principal target for several groups of anticancer agents (1,4–6). A covalent complex between topo II and DNA is an obligatory intermediate in the catalysis of DNA topoisomerization. Stabilization of this complex by natural products of microbial or plant origin and their analogs presents an initial event that leads to cell death. The stabilization of the complex can interfere with vital functions involving DNA replication and resulting in drug-exerted cytotoxicity (4–6). This interaction plays a substantial role in the cytotoxicity exerted by anthracyclines. The precise nature of the process, however, remains obscure. It has been proposed that the formation of a ternary complex drug–topo II–DNA can be a prerequisite for the stabilization of DNA "cleavable complexes" (7). It remains unclear whether the intercalative mode of drug–DNA binding or just an increased concentration of drug molecules around topo II–DNA adducts is essential for this step. Also, the role of drug metabolism in the process remains to be investigated.

We have studied four groups of analogs of doxorubicin (adriamycin) (DXR) or daunorubicin (daunomycin) (DNR), which differ by the substitution pattern on the chromophore as well as on the sugar moiety (see Fig. 23.1–23.4 for structural formulas). In addition to the clinically important parent drugs DXR and DNR, the test compounds included several potentially useful compounds. Some of the analogs such as 4′epidoxorubicin (epirubicin) (4′epiDXR), 4-demethoxydaunorubicin (4-dmxDNR), or N-trifluoroacetyladriamycin-14-valerate (AD32) have been investigated in clinical trials; others are being screened in initial or advanced preclinical tests (8,9). In this review some of the structural

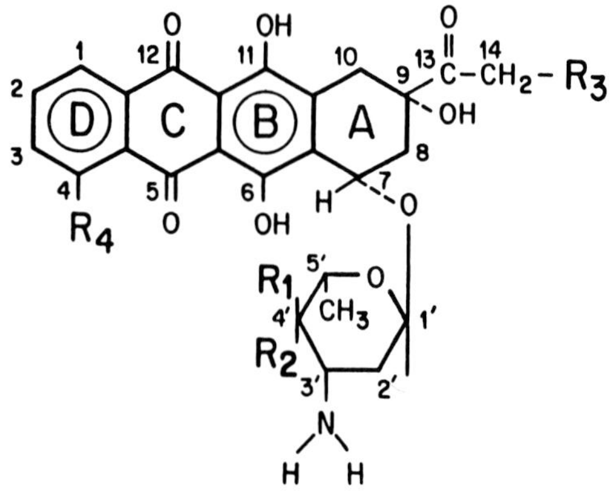

Figure 23.1. 3'-N-Unsubstituted Anthracyclines

Type of Analog/Name Mol. Weight	Abbrev. or Code#	R1	R2	R3	R4
Doxorubicin (Adriamycin) 543.57	DXR	H	OH	OH	OCH$_3$
Daunorubicin (daunomycin) 527.57	DNR	H	OH	H	OCH$_3$
14-Methoxydaunorubicin[a] 557.6	AD121	H	OH	OCH$_3$	OCH$_3$
Adriamycin-14-thio-valerate[a] 680.23	AD268	H	OH	SCO(CH$_2$)$_3$CH$_3$	OCH$_3$
4-Demethoxydaunorubicin 497.54	4-dmxDNR	H	OH	H	H
4'-Epidoxorubicin 543.57	4'epiDXR	OH	H	OH	OCH$_3$
4'Deoxydoxorubicin 527.57	4'deoDXR	H	H	OH	OCH$_3$
4'-Deoxy-4'-iododoxorubicin 653.57	4'd4'IDX	H	I	OH	OCH$_3$

[a]C14 position substituted (R3)

properties connected with DNA intercalation and/or topo II inhibition have been identified. The studies also show that several biologically active intercalating agents apparently do not interact with this enzyme.

BACKGROUND INFORMATION

A series of investigations has identified various anthracyclines, acridine derivatives, and epipodophyllotoxins as topo II–targeted drugs (9–12). The most extensively studied inhibitor of topo II has been DXR (6,8,13), an anthracycline with a broad utility in clinical oncology. An effective therapy of human cancers by topo II–directed drugs, as with most of other cancer therapy, has been derived empirically by trial and error (14). DXR remains the drug of choice in soft tissue sarcomas, and the drug is included in all effective protocols of their combination chemotherapy or multimodal treatment.

DXR is commonly given to patients with acute lymphocytic and nonlym-

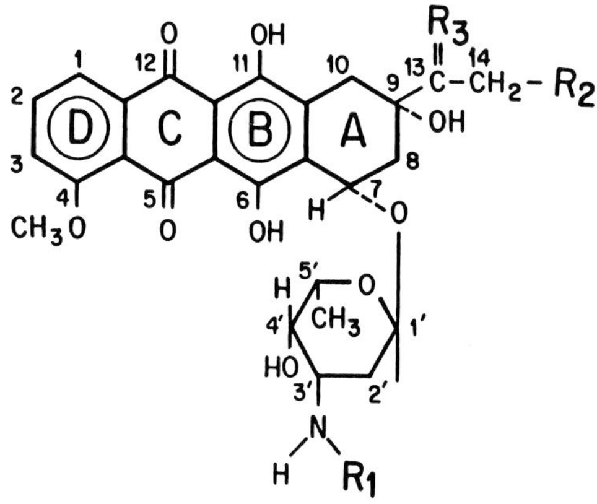

Figure 23.2. 3'-N-Acylanthracyclines

Name Mol. Weight	Abbrev. or Code#	R1	R2	R3
N-trifluoroacetylAdriamycin-14- valerate[a] 723.71	AD32	COCF$_3$	OCO(CH$_2$)$_3$CH$_3$	O
N-trifluoroacetyl-14- methoxydaunorubicin[a] 653.61	AD120	COCF$_3$	OCH$_3$	O
N-acetylAdriamycin-14-valerate[a] 669.74	AD133	COCH$_3$	OCO(CH$_2$)$_3$CH$_3$	O
N-trifluoroacetylAdriamycin-14-O- hemiadipate[a] 767.72	AD143	COCF$_3$	OCO(CH$_2$)$_4$COOH	O
N-acetylAdriamycin 585.61	AD38	COCH$_3$	OH	O
N-trifluoroacetylAdriamycin 639.58	AD41	COCF$_3$	OH	O
N-trifluoroacetylAdriamycinol 641.60	AD92	COCF$_3$	OH	H,OH
N-pentafluoropropionylAdriamycin 689.59	AD115	COCF$_2$CF$_3$	OH	O

[a]C14 position substituted (R3)

phocytic leukemia. Treatment protocols also include an epipodophyllotoxin, VM-26 (teniposide) together with DXR. DXR alone or in a combination with VP-16 (etoposide) is used as part of effective regimens in advanced stages of Hodgkin's disease, as salvage therapy of relapsing patients, and as a first-line treatment in aggressive non-Hodgkin's lymphomas (14). Some of the protocols are highly effective. A combination of DXR and six other drugs induces complete remissions in almost 100% of patients with advanced Hodgkin's disease, and can achieve a disease-free long-term survival in 90% (15).

Combination chemotherapy with DXR regimens continues to be the best primary drug treatment for metastatic breast cancer. There has been interest in intravesical and intraperitoneal application of DXR in patients with urinary bladder or ovarian cancer. DXR has also found use in several protocols for patients with advanced or recurrent epithelial type of ovarian cancer. Combination therapy including DXR, VP-16, and VM-26 is the mainstay in the treatment of small-cell ("oat" cell) lung carcinoma. However, a vast array of cancers remain that are unresponsive to DXR chemotherapy (14). This leaves a

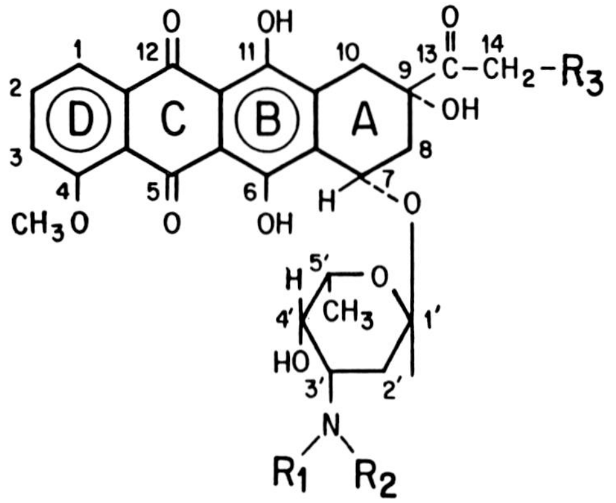

Figure 23.3. 3'-N-Alkylanthracyclines

Name Mol. Weight	Abbrev. or Code#	R1	R2	R3
N-(n-butyl)Adriamycin-14-valerate[a] 683.82	AD194	n–C_4H_9	H	$OCO(CH_2)_3CH_3$
N-benzylAdriamycin-14-valerate[a] 717.83	AD198	$CH_2C_6H_5$	H	$OCO(CH_2)_3CH_3$
N,N-dimethyl Adriamycin-14-valerate[a] 655.77	AD199	CH_3		$OCO(CH_2)_3CH_3$
N,N-di(n-butyl) Adriamycin-14-valerate[a] 739.9	AD202	n–C_4H_9	n–C_4H_9	$OCO(CH_2)_3CH_3$
N,N-dibenzylAdriamycin-14-valerate[a] 807.96	AD206	$CH_2C_6H_5$		$OCO(CH_2)_3CH_3$
N,N-dimethylAdriamycin 571.63	AD280	CH_3		OH
N-(n-butyl)Adriamycin 599.69	AD284	n–C_4H_9	H	OH
N,N-di(n-butyl) Adriamycin) (655.81	AD285	n–C_4H_9	n–C_4H_9	OH
N-benzylAdriamycin 633.69	AD288	$CH_2C_6H_5$	H	OH
N,N-dibenzylAdriamycin 723.82	AD289	$CH_2C_6H_5$		OH

[a]C14 position substituted (R3)

wide latitude for the design and development of new anthracycline agents with improved anticancer efficacy.

3'-N-UNSUBSTITUTED ANTHRACYCLINES

Drug effectiveness of tested compounds in experimental systems is reviewed in Table 23.1, and the structural formulas are shown in Figures 23.1–23.4. The compounds have been divided into four groups according to the substitution pattern at the 3' nitrogen function of the daunosamine moiety. Figure 23.1 re-

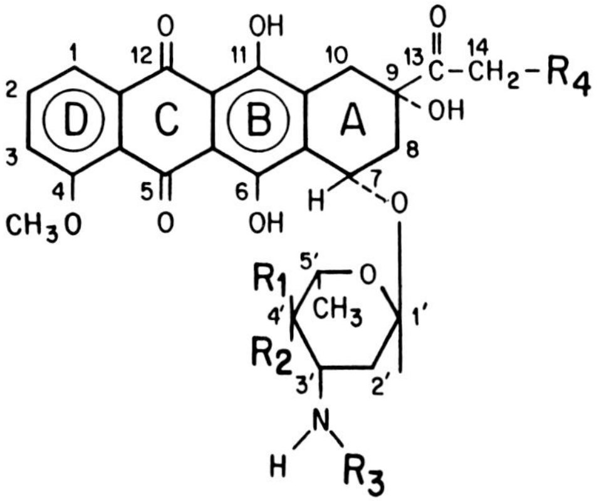

Figure 23.4. Nitrosoureidoanthracyclines

Name Mol. Weight	Abbrev. or Code#	R1	R2	R3	R4
2-Chloroethylureidodaunomycin 633.11	AD307	H	OH	C–NHCH$_2$CH$_2$Cl $\parallel$ O	H
N-nitroso-2-chlorethylureidodaunomycin 662.11	AD312	H	OH	C–NCH$_2$CH$_2$Cl $\parallel$ $\vert$ O NO	H
2-ChloroethylureidoAdriamycin 649.11	AD346	H	OH	C–NHCH$_2$CH$_2$Cl $\parallel$ O	OH
N-nitroso-2-chlorethylureidoAdriamycin 678.11	AD347	H	OH	C–NCH$_2$CH$_2$Cl $\parallel$ $\vert$ O NO	OH
2-Chlorethylureido-4′epidoxorubicin 649.11	AD391	OH	H	C–NHCH$_2$CH$_2$Cl $\parallel$ O	OH
N-nitroso-2-chlorethylureido-4′epidoxorubicin 678.11	AD392	OH	H	C–NCH$_2$CH$_2$Cl $\parallel$ $\vert$ O NO	OH

views the structures of the 3′-N-unsubstituted anthracyclines (group 1) including parent drugs DXR and DNR. Except for 14-methoxydaunorubicin (AD121) and adriamycin-14-thiovalerate (AD268), the anthracycline molecule of other 3′-N-unsubstituted analogs is modified either at the 4′ position of the daunosamine (R1 and R2) or at the C4 position of the chromophore (R4). AD268 is the only analog of this group with a C14-position bulky acyl side chain (R3), whereas AD121 contains a nonhydrolyzable 14-0-methyl ether function. As shown in Figure 23.1, a single dose of 3′-N-unsubstituted analogs on day 1 improved, to a varying degree (81–320% increase in life span relative to untreated controls [ILS]), the survival of mice implanted a day earlier with P388 leukemia. The drugs were also effective against CEM *in vitro*. All compounds of this group are stable in various biological systems, both *in vivo* and *in vitro*, except for AD268, which undergoes esterase-mediated deacylation. The rate of conversion into forms with reduced biological activity such as the C13-

Table 23.1. Doxorubicin and Daunorubicin Analogs: *In Vivo* and *In Vitro* Activity

Drug	P388[a] *In Vivo* (cures or %ILS)[b]	CEM *In Vitro* (ID50 μM)[c]	L1210 *In Vitro* (LD90 μM)[d]
3'-N-unsubstituted anthracyclines			
DXR	320% ILS	0.05	0.31
DNR	100% ILS	0.03	0.9
AD121[e]	81% ILS	0.32	2.0
AD268[e]	130% ILS	0.45	
4-dmxDNR	161% ILS	0.003	0.23
4'epiDXR	270% ILS	0.03	0.42
4'deoDXR	300% ILS	0.03	0.32
4'd4'IDXR	300% ILS	0.009	0.18
3'-N-acylanthracyclines			
AD32[e]	100% cures	0.3	8.3
AD120[e]	63% ILS	3.57	15.2
AD133[e]	81% ILS	2.5	8.8
AD143[e]	100% cures	0.26	7.0
AD38	27% ILS	1.2	12.3
AD41	481% ILS	0.21	7.2
AD92	100% ILS	1.03	10.4
AD115	372% ILS	0.44	4.4
3'-N-alkylanthracyclines			
AD194[e]	>475% ILS	0.11	2.9
AD198[e]	100% cures	0.11	4.6
AD199[e]	72% ILS	0.02	3.3
AD202[e]	>770% ILS	2.1	7.1
AD206[e]	145% ILS	>5.3	>49.5
AD280	164% ILS	0.3	5.1
AD284		0.08	9.8
AD285		0.4	37.0
AD288	85% ILS	0.5	10.2
AD289	75% ILS	>5.0	>55.4
Nitrosoureidoanthracyclines			
AD307	40% ILS	0.43	0.52
AD312	100% cures 100% cures[f]	0.09	0.26
AD346		0.09	1.03
AD347	>500% ILS	0.005	0.58
AD391		0.08	0.9
AD392		0.005	0.53

[a]P388, intraperitoneal mouse leukemia; CEM, tissue-culture line of a human leukemia; P388 and L1210, tissue-culture lines of mouse leukemias.
[b]%ILS, increase in life span, optimal drug doses qd 1 (3'-N-unsubstituted drugs except AD268) or qd 1–4 (the rest of the drugs).
[c]ID50, median inhibition dose, 48-h drug exposure.
[d]LD90, a dose killing 90% of clonogen, 1-h drug exposure.
[e]C14-position substituted analogs.

hydroxy derivatives of 4-dmxDNR, 4'deoxydoxorubicin (4'deoDXR), or 4'deoxy-4-iododoxorubicin (4'd4'IDXR) is small and apparently has no biological significance.

Drug Interaction with DNA

The intercalative drug binding to DNA was measured using an assay in which both supercoiled and relaxed DNA are incubated with the drug in the presence of DNA topo I, and allowed to come to an equilibrium. The inclusion of both topological forms of DNA insures that any inhibitory effect that the drugs may exert on topo I will be detectable and could be compensated for in the assay conditions (16). Figure 23.5 shows some of the gels with assayed drug intercalation. The results were expressed numerically as the relative strength of drug intercalation. The rating ranged, on a relative scale, from 0 (no intercalation) to 9 (strong intercalation). It appears that the 32 anthracyclines tested in these studies could be divided into three categories, strong, weak, and nonintercalating compounds. Of the 3'-N-unsubstituted drugs, both parent drugs, DXR and DNR, as well as all other analogs proved to be strong DNA intercalators.

Topo II–Mediated DNA Cleavage

Drug induction of the topo II–related cleavage of plasmid DNA was tested in cell-free systems (7,17). DXR, DNR, and other C14-unsubstituted analogs inhibit topo II and induce DNA cleavage. The most striking feature of the 10 analogs with three types of C14 substituents was their inability to inhibit topo II. The removal of a thiovalerate, valerate, or 0-hemiadipate changes the 3'-N-unsubstituted anthracyclines (group 1) and 3'-N-acylanthracyclines (group 2) from inactive into active inhibitors of topo II.

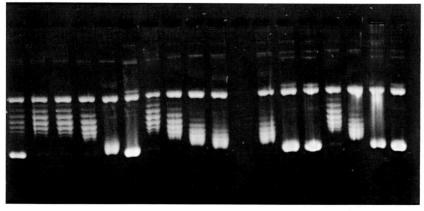

Figure 23.5. DNA unwinding assay. Lane a, PC15 DNA; b, DNA and topoI; c–f, DNA, topo I, and DXR; g–j, DNA, topoI, AD312; k–n, DNA, topoI, AD346; o–r, DNA, topoI, AD347; s–v, DNA, topoI, AD307. Drug concentrations 0.1, 0.5, 2.5, and 12.4 μg/ml.

"Background" DNA Cleavage

Incubation of the 3' end-labeled DNA with purified topo II in the absence of a drug results in slight DNA breakage. This low level of activity has been termed "background" cleavage (18). DXR stimulates topo II–mediated cleavage of plasmid DNA at the concentration range of 0.04–0.92 µM, but at a concentration of 4.6 µM and higher the cleavage reaction including the background cleavage is either diminished or totally abolished (9). The rest of 3'-N-unsubstituted DXR analogs, except AD268, stimulated the cleavage with efficacy comparable to DXR. AD268, a C14-substituted analog, did not mediate topo II–DNA cleavage, yet it effectively abolished the background cleavage reaction (7,17).

3'-N-ACYLANTHRACYCLINES

Group 2, the 3'-N-acyl analogs, is characterized by an acyl function attached to the nitrogen of the daunosamine (Fig. 23.2, **R1**). Four of the analogs included in this group also have C14 position side chain substitution (R2). The *in vivo* treatment of P388 leukemia (Table 23.1) was based on an established optimal treatment schedule (qd 1-4) in terms of cures or ILS. The treatment schedule was consistent with the more extensive metabolism and greater elimination rates of 3'-N-acyl drugs when compared to 3'-N-unsubstituted analogs. Both C14 position substituted and unsubstituted analogs are represented by highly effective [AD32, N-trifluoroacetylAdriamycin-14-O-hemiadipate (AD143), N-trifluoroacetylAdriamycin (AD41) or N-pentafluoropropionyl-Adriamycin (AD115)] or less potent compounds [N-trifluoroacetyl-14-methoxydaunorubicin (AD120), N-acetylAdriamycin-14-valerate (AD133), N-acetylAdriamycin (AD38), and N-trifluoroacetylAdriamycinol (AD92)]. The differential efficacy of the 3'-N-acyl analogs is further confirmed by the results of the *in vitro* CEM and L1210 screens (17). A comparable *in vitro* growth inhibition of CEM cells by the most active 3'-N-acyl analogs requires 3.5-fold (AD41) to 7.3-fold (AD115) higher concentration than that of DXR. In the L1210 system, the difference in cell kill is approximately 13–28-fold. Drug metabolic studies (7,17) have established that the C14 position substituted 3'-N-acyl analogs AD32 and AD143 are largely converted into the C14-unsubstituted congener AD41 and, to a small extent, into AD92. The metbolic conversion of AD133 results in AD38.

Drug Interaction with DNA

Analogs of group 2 are weak DNA intercalators, with the relative strength <5 except for AD32. There was no evidence obtained that indicated this drug's strength of intercalation. Within group 2, there is no apparent correlation between the strength of intercalation and antitumor activity (compare active compounds AD32, AD143, AD41, and AD115 with the less active AD133, AD38, or AD92) (7,17).

Topo II–Mediated DNA Cleavage

There is a straightforward relationship between drug structure and topo II interaction: All C14-substituted analogs, whether biologically active or not, do not inhibit the enzyme. Conversely, C14-unsubstituted drugs mediate topo II–DNA cleavage (17).

"Background" DNA Cleavage

The C14 position unsubstituted analogs of the 3'-N-acyl group did not show the background inhibition. For such effects, substantially higher drug concentrations may be required than those used in the assay (7,9,17).

3'-N-ALKYLANTHRACYCLINES

The analogs of group 3 are modified by mono- or di-alkyl substitution at the sugar nitrogen (Fig. 23.3), **R1**, or **R1** and **R2**). In some of the compounds, there is also a valerate side chain substitution at C14 **(R3).** Analogs of this group include both biologically effective as well as ineffective drugs. Among the C14 position substituted drugs, N-(*m*-butyl)Adriamycin-14-valerate (AD194), N-benzylAdriamycin-14-valerate (AD198), and N,N-di(*n*-butyl)Adriamycin-14-valerate (AD202) are highly effective *in vivo* against P388 leukemia and *in vitro* against CEM and L1210 cell lines (Table 23.1). N,N-dimethylAdriamycin-14-valerate (AD199), despite modest *in vivo* activity, shows marked activity in the *in vitro* assays. In the CEM growth-inhibition assay, AD199 is threefold more active than DXR. N,N-dimethylAdriamycin (AD280) and N-benzyl-Adriamycin (AD288), the respective C14-unsubstituted analogs of AD199 and AD198, are effective *in vitro*. *In vivo*, AD280 shows a modest enhancement in antitumor activity compared to AD199, while AD288 is significantly less effective than AD198. N-(*n*-butyl)Adriamycin (AD284), a C14-unsubstituted analog of AD194, is almost as effective against CEM leukemia as DXR and AD199. N,N-dibenzylAdriamycin (AD289) and its C14-substituted congener N,N-dibenzylAdriamycin-14-valerate (AD206) remain without major effectiveness against tumors *in vivo* as well as *in vitro* (17).

The C14-substituted 3'-N-alkylanthracyclines AD198 and AD199 are partially transformed into the C14-unsubstituted products AD288 or AD280, respectively. AD280 or AD288 appear stable, and no further biotransformation has been detected *in vitro* (17,19). AD206 is metabolically converted into AD289 and AD288 *in vivo*, but not *in vitro*.

Drug Interaction with DNA

With the exception of AD202 and its C14-unsubstituted congener N,N-di(*n*-butyl)Adriamycin (AD285), all biologically active 3'-N-alkylanthracyclines tested are strong intercalators. The two biologically inactive derivatives AD206 and AD289 do not interact with DNA (17,19).

Topo II–Mediated DNA Cleavage

Among the C14-unsubstituted drugs of group 3, neither biologically active AD280 and AD288 nor inactive AD289 have shown any topo II–mediated DNA cleavage. AD285 has marginal biological activity and is the only drug among the 3′-N-alkyl analogs that induces topo II–mediated cleavage. In terms of DNA intercalation and interaction with topo II, AD285 behaves more like an analog of group 2 (17).

"Background" DNA Cleavage

AD198, AD199, AD280, or AD288, biologically active drugs of the third group, effectively abolished the background cleavage reaction in the absence of topo II–mediated DNA cleavage.

NITROSOUREIDOANTHRACYCLINES

Three parental drugs were converted into hybrid nitrosoureidoanthracyclines: DNR, DXR, and 4′epiDXR (Fig. 23.4, **R1, R2,** and **R4**). The N-nitroso-2-chlorethyl compounds AD312, AD347, and AD392 were compared to 2-chlorethylureido analogs that lack the N-nitroso function. AD312, AD347, and AD392 are significantly more effective *in vitro,* on μM basis, against CEM or L1210 leukemia cells than their 2-chlorethylureido congeners. AD312 is more effective than parent compound DNR against P388 leukemia (100% cures) (Table 23.1). This should be compared with 100% ILS for DNR. AD312 is also highly effective against a DXR-resistant subline of P388 (100% cures) (20,21).

Drug Interaction with DNA

A bulky alkylnitrosourea substituent at the 3′-N-position of the daunosamine does not prevent DNA intercalation. It is shown in Figure 23.5 that AD312 and AD347 are strong intercalators, comparable with the effects of DNR and DXR.

Topo II–Mediated DNA Cleavage

All tested N-nitroso-2-chlorethylureidoanthracyclines inhibit, to a various degree, topo II and induce DNA cleavage (Fig. 23.6). There was, however, no detectable induction of DNA cleavage resulting from the exposure of purified topo II to the three 2-chlorethylnitrosoureido analogs (21, 22).

"Background" DNA Cleavage

AD312, AD347, and AD392, the N-nitroso-2-chlorethylureidoanthracyclines, did not show any background inhibition. Similar to N-acylanthracyclines, sub-

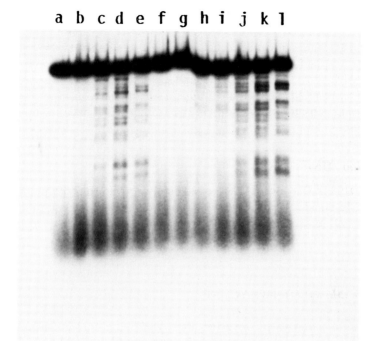

Figure 23.6. Drug-induced topo II–mediated DNA cleavage. Lane a, PMC41 DNA end-labeled with (α-P_{32})dATP; b, DNA and topo II; c–g, DNA, topo II, and DXR; h–l, DNA, topo II, and AD392. Drug concentrations 0.02, 0.1, 0.5, 2.5, and 12.5 μg/ml.

stantially higher drug concentrations may be required than those used in the reported study. The three 2-chlorethylureido analogs did not mediate topo II–DNA cleavage and effectively abolished the background cleavage reaction (21,22).

DNA Alkylation

AD312 and AD307 were studied using an ethidium bromide fluorescence assay of DNA crosslinking (D. B. Yarosh and M. Potmesil, unpublished observations). Unlike AD307, the N-nitroso congener AD312 initiated the production of DNA–DNA interstrand crosslinks, which continued over several hours in a drug-free medium. Such continuing reaction is consistent with the presence of long-lived precursors of the crosslinks, similar to those generated by classical chlorethylnitrosoureas. Purified O^6-alkylguanine DNA transferase blocks crosslink formation by AD312. In another approach, a competition assay measuring the production of DNA adducts was applied (D. B. Yarosh and M. Potmesil, unpublished observations). AD312, and to a lesser extent AD307, produced DNA adducts that serve as a substrate for the action of O^6-alkylguanine DNA transferase.

DRUG EFFECTS ON INTACT CELLS

The experiments in cell-free systems were compared with assays studying drug effects on intact cells. Drugs of group 1 and 2 induced protein-associated DNA breaks (PAB), identical with topo II–DNA cleavable complexes (6). Biologically inactive 3'-N-alkyl-anthracyclines AD206 and AD289 did not induce a significant number of PAB in treated cells (17). The presence of a protein, covalently bound to cleaved DNA in cells treated with active 3'-N-alkyl derivatives, remains unexplained.

Nitrososoureidoanthracyclines AD312 and AD392 (group 4) cause a significant level of PAB in L1210 cells. These lesions may indicate drug-induced inhibition of topo II. Furthermore, DNA–DNA crosslinks, products of alkylation, were detected in cells treated with AD347 and AD392, but not with DXR. Human chronic lymphocytic leukemia cells were shown to have undetectable levels of topo II (24). Accordingly, DXR or AD347 did not induce significant levels of PAB. AD347, however, caused elevated levels of DNA–DNA crosslinks (25).

DISCUSSION

DNA Intercalation of Test Drugs

The extent of DNA intercalation seems to depend on the substitution of the daunosamine nitrogen. The 3'-N-unsubstituted analogs (group 1) are strong intercalators. Analogs bearing one or two N-alkyl substituents such as N-(*n*-butyl), N-benzyl, N,N-dimethyl (group 3) or N-nitroso-2-chlorethylureido and 2-chlorethylureido (group 4) also intercalate strongly. Some of these associations with DNA could be at variance with that of DXR–DNA binding (19). N-dibenzylation, as in AD206 or AD289, and N-dibutylation, as in AD202 or AD285, appear to interfere significantly with or preclude DNA interaction sterically. The 3'-N-acylanthracyclines (group 2) have either N-acetyl, N-trifluoroacetyl, or N-pentafluoropropionyl substitution. All analogs of this group have shown a weak DNA intercalation. The data for AD32 suggest that the bulky C14 substituent may further affect the weakened DNA binding caused by the 3'-N-trifluoroacetyl substitution.

Drug Effects on Topoisomerase II–Mediated DNA Cleavage

It is conclusively documented that the C14 position substitution by a thiovalerate (AD268), valerate (AD32 and AD133), hemiadipate (AD143), or O-methyl ether (AD120 and AD121) prevents the analogs from interacting with topo II. Regardless whether the 3'-nitrogen is substituted or not, the metabolic cleavage of a hydrolyzable C14 position acyl substituent by plasma esterases converts, *in vivo* as well as *in vitro*, AD32 or AD143 into AD41. AD92 can be formed from AD41 by aldo-keto reductase activity. Similarly, AD133 is converted into AD38, while AD268 is deesterified, presumably to 14-thiaDXR and its disulfide. All C14 position unsubstituted 3'-N-acylanthracyclines stimulate the topo II–mediated cleavage. Thus, the study lends support for the conclusion that metabolic activation of 3'-N-acyl C14 substituents *in vivo* or in tissue-culture cells precedes their interaction with topo II. This also becomes applicable to the 3'-N-alkyl compound AD202.

For all active 3'-N-unsubstituted, 3'-N-acyl and N-nitrosoureido anthracyclines (group 1,2, and 4), the strength of topo II–mediated DNA cleavage paralleled the strength of drug intercalation. The three 3'-N-alkyl analogs (group 3), AD280, AD284, and AD288, are C14-unsubstituted DNA intercalators that do not, however, stimulate the topo II–mediated DNA cleavage. Although cytotoxic *in vitro,* they exhibit only moderate *in vivo* antitumor activity.

Inhibition of "Background" DNA Cleavage

Previous study (9) has shown that high concentrations of DXR not only inhibit the drug-induced DNA cleavage but also the background cleavage. It appears that, among 3'-N-unsubstituted and 3'-N-alkyl analogs, the inhibition of the background cleavage is a function of the ability of a drug to intercalate into DNA. This applies to both C14-substituted and unsubstituted analogs. However, AD280, AD284, and AD288, the C14-unsubstituted 3'-N-alkylanthracyclines (group 3), do not cleave DNA in the presence of topo II, yet the drugs are able to inhibit the background cleavage effectively. Similar interaction can be suggested for 2-chlorethylnitrosoureido analogs (group 4), which also failed to interact with purified topo II.

Ethidium bromide, a strong intercalator with minimal cytotoxicity, is known to inhibit background cleavage as well as DNA cleavage induced by other drugs (9). Unlike ethidium bromide, AD280 and AD288, as well as their C14-substituted congeners AD199 and AD198, induce PAB in cells and are cytotoxic *in vitro* or *in vivo.* Taken together, the observations suggest that, following the treatment with 3'-N-alkylanthracyclines, a different mode of drug–topo II–DNA interaction occurs. It is also possible that the analogs kill the cell by other mechanism(s), independent of topo II.

Drug Structure and Cytotoxicity

The side chain C14 substitution in AD32 and AD143 is important for various biological properties, including those connected with intracellular partitioning of the drug (reviewed in 7). The actual effectors of topo II–related cytoxicity are the C14-unsubstituted metabolites of these compounds, mainly AD41. The topo II–mediated DNA cleavage by 3'-N-acylanthracyclines is comparable among the four C14-unsubstituted analogs. However, AD38 and its C14-substituted congener are only marginally active in biological systems. While the 3'-N-acetyl substitution of the two compounds has little effect on the tests conducted in cell-free systems, it may diminish in some way the cell kill efficacy. The 13-OH forms of anthracyclines such as AD92 are generally credited with lower cytotoxicity relative to their parent drugs.

Some of the 3'-N-unsubstituted (DXR, 4-dmxDNR) and the 3'-N-alkyl analogs (for example AD198, AD199, AD280, and AD288) have shown a disparity between their *in vivo* and *in vitro* effectiveness. In either case, other topo II–unrelated mechanism(s) may participate to a various degree *in vivo* and *in vitro* and contribute to the overall cytotoxicity. A unique combination of drug cytotoxicity has been suggested for a nitrosoureidoanthracycline AD312. The drug, a 3'-N-nitroso-2-chlorethylureidodaunorubicin shows not only the interaction with topo II but also DNA alkylation, which leads to the formation of DNA interstrand crosslinks.

The study of anthracycline analogs suggests that there are two domains of the anthracycline molecule that may determine some of the essential biological properties of the congeners. The first is localized at the C14 position of the chromophore ring A. The side chain attached to the chromophore, be it acyl or nonhydrolyzable ether, may prevent the formation of a ternary complex drug–topo II–DNA. Consequently, topo II is not stabilized and the cleavable complex is not formed. The second domain, important for anthracycline intercalation, is localized at the 3'-nitrogen of the daunosamine moiety. The intercalative mode seems to be advantageous for the drug interaction with topo II–DNA complexes. While the daunosamine sugar of the drug molecule is positioned along the minor grove of DNA (26,27), the C14 domain of the chromophore can be presented for further interaction with binding sites of the enzyme molecule. With the increasing number of the intercalated drug molecules, the interaction may reach a saturation level and result in the inhibition of background cleavage. Since the background inhibition is also present in C14-substituted drugs that do not stabilize the cleavable complex, these compounds may exert topo II inhibition, which differs from the trapping of the cleavable complex.

Summary

Four groups of DXR and DNR analogs, differing by their substituents on the chromophore and sugar moieties, were used in the reviewed studies. The 3'-N-unsubstituted (group 1), 3'-N-acyl (group 2), 3'-N-alkyl (group 3), and nitrosoureidoanthracyclines (group 4) were tested for (1) *in vivo* and *in vitro* cytotoxicity, (2) cellular or tissue uptake and metabolic conversion, (3) strength of DNA intercalation, and (4) interaction with topo II. Compounds of *group 1* were cytotoxic, strong intercalators, and, except for those with C14 side chain substitution, induced the formation of topo II–DNA cleavable complexes. The esterolysis of C14-acyl substituents was required to yield a metabolite that can interact with topo II in the purified system. The C14-substituted compounds of *group 2* and their C-14 unsubstituted metabolites were cytotoxic. These drugs were weak intercalators, and the C14-unsubstituted congeners induced cleavable complex formation in the purified system, but with reduced potency relative to DXR. The type of the 3'-N-position substituent determined whether *group 3* analogs were cytotoxic and strong intercalators, cytotoxic and weak intercalators, or inactive and nonintercalating. All of the C14-unsubstituted intercalators of group 3 did not form cleavble complexes in the purified system, but were cytotoxic. Finally, biologically active hybrid nitrosoureidoanthracyclines *(group 4)* were strong DNA intercalators as well as inhibitors of topo II. The drugs have also shown DNA interaction compatible with their alkylating function.

The studies show that DNA intercalation, be it of high or low strength, is required but not sufficient for the activity by topo II–targeted anthracyclines. In addition to the planar chromophore that is involved in intercalation, two other domains of the anthracycline molecule are important for the interaction with topo II: (1) substitution on the C14 position totally inhibits drug activity in the purified system, but enhances cytotoxicity by aiding drug uptake and presumably acting on other cellular targets, (2) substitutions on the 3′-N position of the sugar ring can, depending on the nature of the substituent, inhibit intercalation and/or topo II–targeting activity. These findings may provide guidance for anthracycline taxonomy and for the synthesis and development of new active analogs.

Acknowledgments

This work was supported in part by Public Health Service grants CA-37082, CA-37209, CA-11655, and CA-39662 from the National Cancer Institute, National Institutes of Health, Departments of Health and Human Services, by grant CH-348C from the American Cancer Society, and grants from Farmitalia Carlo Erba and Marcia Slater Society for Research in Leukemia.

REFERENCES

1. Wang, J. C. DNA topoisomerases. Annu. Rev. Biochem. 54: 665, 1985.
2. Vosberg, H. P. DNA topoisomerases: Enzymes that control DNA conformation. Curr. Top. Microbiol. Immun. 114: 19–102, 1985.
3. Potmesil, M. and Ross, W. E. eds. *Proceedings, The First Conference on DNA Topoisomerases in Cancer Chemotherapy.* NCI Monogr. 4, 1987.
4. Liu, L. F. DNA topoisomerase poisons as antitumor drugs. Annu. Rev. Biochem. 58: 351–375, 1989.
5. Chen, G. L. and Liu, L. F. DNA topoisomerases as targets in cancer chemotherapy. In D. M. Bailey, ed. Annu. Rep. Medicin. Chem., Vol. 21. New York: Academic Press, 1986.
6. Potmesil, M. DNA topoisomerase II as an intracellular target in cancer chemotherapy by anthracyclines. In J. W. Lown, ed. *Anthracyclines and Anthracenedione Based Anticancer Agents.* Amsterdam: Elsevier, 1988, pp. 447–474.
7. Silber, R., Liu, L. F., Israel, M., Bodley,

A. L., Hsiang, Y.-H., Kirschenbaum, S., Sweatman, T. W., Seshadri, R., and Potmesil, M. Metabolic activation of N-acyl-anthracyclines precedes their interaction with DNA topoisomerases II. In M. Potmesil and W. E. Ross, eds. *Proceedings, The First Conference on DNA Topoisomerases in Cancer Chemotherapy.* NCI Monogr. 4: 111–115, 1987.
8. Green, M. D., Muggia, F. M., and Blum, R. H. A perspective from recent clinical trials. In J. W. Lown, ed. *Anthracyclines and Anthracenedione Based Anticancer Agents.* Amsterdam: Elsevier, 1988, pp. 667–714.
9. Tewey, K. M., Rowe, T. C., Yang, L., Halligan, B. D., and Liu, L. F. Adriamycin induced DNA damage by mammalian DNA topoisomerase II. Science. 226: 466–468, 1984.
10. Nelson, E. M., Tewey, K. M., and Liu, L. F. Mechanism of antitumor drug action: Poisoning of mammalian DNA topoisomerase II on DNA by 4′-(9-acridinyl-amino)-methanesulfon-m-anisidine. Proc.

Natl. Acad. Sci. USA. **81:** 1361–1365, 1984.

11. Yang, L., Rowe, T. C., Nelson, E. M., and Liu, L. F. In vivo mapping of DNA topoisomerase II-specific cleavage sites on SV40 chromatin. Cell. **41:** 127–132, 1984/1985.

12. Yang, L., Rowe, T. C., and Liu, L. F. Identification of DNA topoisomerase II as an intracellular target of antitumor epipodophyllotoxins in simian virus 40-infected monkey cells. Cancer Res. **45:** 5872–5876, 1985.

13. Crooke, S. T. The anthracyclines. In S. T. Crooke and A. W. Prestayko, eds. *Cancer and Chemotherapy.* Vol. **3.** New York: Academic Press, 1981, pp. 111–132.

14. Pinedo, H. M., Chabner, B. A., and Longo, D. L., eds. *Cancer Chemotherapy and Biol. Response Modif.,* Annual 10. Amsterdam: Elsevier Science Publ., 1988.

15. Klimo, P. and Connors, J. M. An update on the Vancouver experience in the management of advanced Hodgkin's disease treated with the MOPP/ABV hybrid program. Semin. Hematol. 25, Suppl. **2:** 34–40, 1988.

16. Chen, G. L., Yang, L., Rowe, T. C., Halligan, B. D., Tewey, K. M., and Liu, L. F. Nonintercalative antitumor drugs interfere with the breakage reunion reaction of mammalian DNA topoisomerase II. J. Biol. Chem. **259:** 13560–13566, 1984.

17. Bodley, A., Liu, L. F., Israel, M., Seshadri, R., Koseki, Y., Giuliani, F. C., Kirschenbaum, S., Silber, R., and Potmesil, M. DNA topoisomerase II-mediated interaction of doxorubicin and daunorubicin congeners with DNA. Cancer Res. **49:** 5969–5978, 1989.

18. Halligan, B. D., Edwards, K. A., and Liu, L. F. Purification and characterization of type II DNA topoisomerase from bovine calf thymus. J. Biol. Chem. **260:** 2475–2482, 1985.

19. Traganos, F., Israel, M., Seshadri, R., Kirschenbaum, S., and Potmesil, M. Effects of new N-alkyl analogs of adriamycin on *in vitro* survival and cell cycle progression of L1210 cells. Cancer Res. **45:** 6273–6279, 1985.

20. Israel, M., Seshadri, R., Koseki, Y., Kirschenbaum, S., and Potmesil, M. New potent anthracycline nitrosourea derivatives. Proc. Am. Assoc. Cancer Res. **29:** 280, 1988 (Abstract).

21. Israel, M., Seshadri, R., Koseki, Y., Bodley, A., Liu, L. F., Kirschenbaum, S., Silber, R., and Potmesil, M. Novel topoisomerase-II directed nitrosoureidoanthracyclines. *Second Conference on DNA Topoisomerases in Cancer Chemotherapy.* Program and Abstracts, 1988, p. 32 (Extended abstract).

22. Israel, M., Seshadri, R., Koseki, Y., Bodley, A., Liu, L. F., Kirschenbaum, S., Silber, R., and Potmesil, M. Novel topoisomerase II-directed nitrosoureidoanthracyclines. Proc. Am. Assoc. Cancer Res. **30:** 619, 1989.

23. Israel, M., Seshadri, R., Koseki, Y., Potmesil, M., Kirschenbaum, S., Silber, R., Bodley, A., Liu, L. F., and Brent, T. P. New anthracycline analogues directed against DNA topoisomerase II. In H. Tapaiero, J. Robert, and T. J. Lampidis, eds. *Anticancer Drugs.* Colloque INSERM, John Libbey Eurotext Ltd., Montrouge, France. Vol. **191,** 1989, pp. 39–47.

24. Potmesil, M., Hsiang, Y.-H., Liu, L. F., Bank, B., Grossberg, H., Kirschenbaum, S., Penziner, A., Kanganis, D., Knowles, D., Traganos, F., and Silber, R. Resistance of human leukemic and normal lymphocytes to drug-induced DNA cleavage and low levels of DNA topoisomerase II. Cancer Res. **48:** 3537–3543, 1988.

25. Quigley, G. J., Wang, A.H.-J., Ughetto, G., van der Marel, G., van Boom, J. H., and Rich, A. Molecular structure of an anticancer drug-DNA complex: Daunomycin plus d(CpGpTpApCpG). Proc. Natl. Acad. Sci. USA. **77:** 7204–7208, 1980.

26. Patel, D. J., Kozlowski, S. A., and Rice, J. A. Hydrogen bonding, overlap geometry, and sequence specificity in anthracycline antitumor antibiotic-DNA complexes in solution. Proc. Natl. Acad. Sci. USA. **78:** 3333–3337, 1981.

27. Wang, A.H.-J., Ughetto, G., Quigley, G. J., and Rich, A. Interaction between an anthracycline and DNA: Molecular structure of daunomycin complexed to d(CpGpTpApCpG) at 1.2-A resolution. Biochemistry. **26:** 1152–1163, 1987.

Chapter 24
Preclinical Studies of DNA Topoisomerase I–Targeted 9-Amino and 10,11-Methylenedioxy Camptothecins

MILAN POTMESIL, BEPPINO C. GIOVANELLA, LEROY F. LIU,
MONROE E. WALL, ROBERT SILBER, JOHN S. STEHLIN,
YAW-HUEI HSIANG, AND MANSUKH C. WANI

The objective of the studies reviewed is to improve chemotherapy of colon cancer. Carcinoma of the large bowel is one of the most common malignancies among the Western population. Approximately 1 of 25 Americans will develop this disease, and only half will be cured by surgery (1). The most significant progress in the treatment of this cancer has come through improved operative and perioperative care, including the "no-touch" technique, better anesthesia, monitoring, and the use of antibiotics (2). Unfortunately, at the time of diagnosis half of the patients have advanced disease which has poor prognosis.

The most commonly used grading of colon cancer progression is the Astler-Coller modification of the Dukes' staging system (Table 24.1) (3). The staging takes into consideration the degree of cancer growth through the colonic wall, the cancerous involvement of the lymph nodes, and metastatic spread. Management of patients with advanced cancer of the colon (stages C1–C3,D) has been one of the most difficult areas of clinical oncology. Although chemotherapy with 5-fluorouracil (5-FU), or with other fluorinated pyrimidines, remains the standard treatment of advanced disease, the drugs produce objective responses in only 15% of the patients, without any evidence of improved survival (1). Over the past two decades, there were numerous phase II clinical trials that tested the activity of single agents as well as drug combinations. None of the trials showed better results than the treatment with 5-FU alone (1,4). More recently, biochemical modulation of tumor cell metabolism came into focus. Attempts were made to increase the selective cytotoxicity of 5-FU by co-treatment, among others, with bacillus Calmette-Guerin, *C. parvum*, or folinic acid (leucovorin). The latter approach, combined with 5-FU alone (5,6) or with 5-FU plus methotrexate (7), marginally improves patient survival. The best results so far were obtained with levamisole, originally an anthelminthic drug, combined with 5-FU (8). This adjuvant treatment increases

Table 24.1. Modified Dukes' Classification of Colorectal Cancer[a]

Stage	Depth of Invasion of the Colon/Rectum	Lymph Node Involvement
A	Muscularis mucosa	0
B1	To muscularis propria	0
B2	Through muscularis propria or serosa	0
B3	Through muscularis propria or serosa, invasion of contiguous organ	0
C1	To muscularis propria	+
C2	Through muscularis propria or serosa	+
C3	Through muscularis propria or serosa, invasion of contiguous organ	+
D	Distant metastases	

[a]Astler and Coller (3)

the number of patients with completely resected stage C colon cancer who will remain disease-free for 5 years after the surgery by 11%. This small subset of patients has a reduced risk of dying of recurrent colon cancer.

Drugs inhibiting DNA topoisomerase II, doxorubicin (DXR) and actino-mycin C, were tested as single agents or in combination treatments of colon cancer (4,9). None of the protocols matched the meager effectiveness of 5-FU. DXR alone or in combination chemotherapy had a disappointing response rate of less than 20% of short-term remissions. This situation has not been improved by the introduction of new analogs, such as 4'epidoxorubicin (10). In a randomized study, this drug induces short-term remissions in only 3% of treated patients. The multitude of therapeutics tested and the results obtained reflect the need for improvement in the treatment of colon cancer.

In the early 1970s, camptothecin, a plant alkaloid isolated from *Campto-theca acuminata* of the Nyssaceae plant family (11), was briefly introduced into phase I–II clinical trials (12,13). Myelosuppression became the dose-limiting toxicity in cancer patients treated with camptothecin sodium salt, and cystitis the most prominent nonhematopoietic complication. Since the purpose of phase I trials is to establish drug toxicity, therapeutic responses could be eval-uated only in some patients. Responses were recorded among patients with advanced gastrointestinal cancer, refractory to other treatments. Although the median duration of remissions was slightly over 2 months, the performance status was improved in most of the patients treated with a weekly schedule (12,13). No responses, however, were registered among patients with a daily schedule (14). In *in vitro* screens, camptothecin sodium salt is less active than camptothecin lactone or some of the new camptothecin analogs (14,15). Its relatively small activity is apparently due to a pH-dependent cyclization of the sodium salt to the lactone ring.

It was recently found that camptothecin interferes with the DNA break-age–reunion reaction, a biological function exerted by DNA topoisomerase I (topo I), by trapping the enzyme–DNA intermediate termed the "cleavable complex" (16,17). In this complex, topo I is linked to the 3' phosphoryl end of the broken DNA backbone. The event occurs in cell-free systems as well as in mammalian cells. Collision of the cleavable complex with the DNA replicative machinery stops fork elongation. This may represent the first step of a process that irreversibly inhibits DNA synthesis and ultimately leads to cell death (18).

There are several compelling reasons for the development of camptothecin analogs as anticancer agents: [1] new camptothecin compounds with improved effectiveness against experimental leukemia and cancer have been synthesized (19–25); [2] topo I has been identified as a target not only for camptothecin but also for all active analogs tested (14,15); and [3] relatively high levels of the target enzyme, topo I, are present in several types of human cancer and leukemia (26–29).

SCREENING OF CAMPTOTHECIN ANALOGS

New synthetic analogs of camptothecin and their parent compound camptothecin and its sodium salt were screened in cell-free, tissue culture, and *in vivo* systems (14). The screens included the measurements of [1] the cleavage of DNA substrate in the presence of purified topo I; [2] drug-induced trapping of topo I in a covalent complex with DNA, and [3] protein-associated DNA breaks in drug-treated leukemia cells. The results showed that 9-amino-20(RS)-camptothecin, 10,11-methylenedioxy-20(RS)-camptothecin and its sodium salt, drugs effective against murine L1210 leukemia *in vivo*, stabilize topo I–DNA cleavable complexes in a purified system and in leukemic cells. Other analogs, inactive against L1210 leukemia *in vivo*, were totally inactive in topo I–directed screens. The study demonstrated that the analog-induced accumulation of enzyme–DNA cleavable complexes is directly proportional to drug cytotoxicity and antitumor activity.

TOPO I LEVELS IN MALIGNANCIES

Compared to normal tissues, elevated levels of topo I were present in specimens obtained from patients with several types of leukemia and cancer. It was shown (26,27) that, compared to normal lymphocytes, topo I levels are moderately elevated in cells of chronic lymphocytic leukemia as well as in several types of lymphoma. Human colon cancer was selected as a model for solid tumors of epithelial origin. Figure 24.1 presents the results of Western blot analysis in primary colon adenocarcinomas of 38 untreated patients (28,29). The disease was evaluated as [1] an early stage, with tumors confined to the primary site and with various depth of colonic-wall penetration (stages B1–B3, Table 24.1); [2] an advanced stage, with various depth of wall penetration and lymph node involvement (stages C1–C3); and [3] with tumor metastases to distant organs (stages C1–C3,D). On average, topo I levels (normalized DNA content) were 14-fold (patients' stages C1–C3; P <0.01) or 16-fold (stages C1–C3, D; P <0.01; t-test with Bonferroni correction used in both cases) higher in cancerous tissue than in normal colonic mucosa. Our studies revealed that the

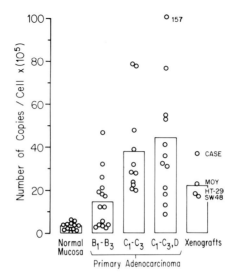

Figure 24.1. DNA topo I levels in surgical specimens of normal human mucosa of the colon, primary adenocarcinoma of the colon, and in human colon cancer xenografts. Under the supervision of a pathologist, tissues of colonic tumors and of normal mucosa were frozen in liquid nitrogen within 1 h after the surgery and stored in multiple aliquots at −80°C for further analysis. Specimens were also obtained from four lines of colon cancer xenografts, growing 10–14 days in NCI-1 immunodeficient mice. The immuno-blot analysis for topo I was performed as described previously (27). DNA content of specimens was used for the normalization of enzyme levels, which were expressed as number of copies per cell with DNA content of a HeLa cell line. Circles show enzyme levels in individual specimens, and the histograms indicate the means of the number of topo I copies/cell. By permission, reprinted from Science (29).

levels of topo I in surgical specimens generally increase with disease progression. The levels significantly surpass the enzyme levels in normal colon mucosa. Topo I was also measured in 10–14-day xenograft implants of human colon cancer into NCI-1 immunodeficient ("nude") mice (Fig. 24.1) (29). The results show that topo I levels in the four xenograft lines examined correspond to enzyme levels in colon cancer of advanced clinical stages.

TREATMENT OF HUMAN COLON CANCER XENOGRAFTS

Subcutaneous Implants

Three xenograft lines were selected to test the hypothesis that topo I in human colon cancer presents a suitable target for chemotherapy. We review here the efficacy of 9-amino-20(*RS*), 10-amino-20(*RS*), 10,11-methylenedioxy-20(*RS*) and of its Na salt (29). Representative results of xenograft treatments are shown in Figures 24.2–24.5. A moderately-to-poorly differentiated human colon cancer, HT-29, and poorly differentiated colon cancer lines designated CASE and SW 48 (30,31) were implanted on day 0. The drugs were injected subcutaneously,

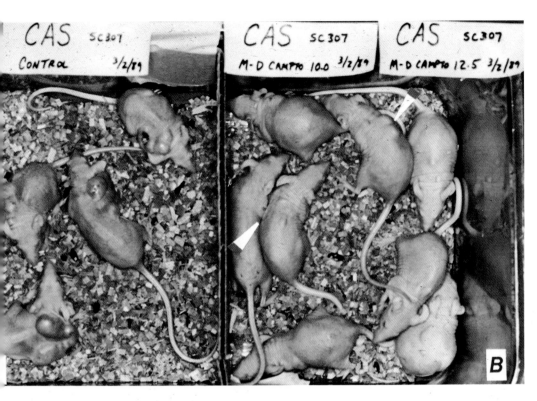

Figure 24.6. Human colon adenocarcinoma line CASE implanted subcutaneously (sc) into immunodeficient ("nude") NIH-1 mice. 10,11-methylenedioxy-20(RS)-camptothecin, formulated in Tween 80:0.15 NaCl, was injected sc into a site contralateral to tumor implants. The injections started on day 7 following tumor grafting. **A.** Control tumor-bearing mice injected sc with Tween-saline only. **B.** Mice bearing CASE xenografts were treated with 10.0 or 12.5 mg/kg/dose of the drug (total 50.0 or 62.5 mg/kg). No evidence of disease (NED) or minimal disease (tumors <0.1 cm³) was registered in 8/8 treated mice. Arrow, minimal disease in 2/8 mice; the rest, NED.

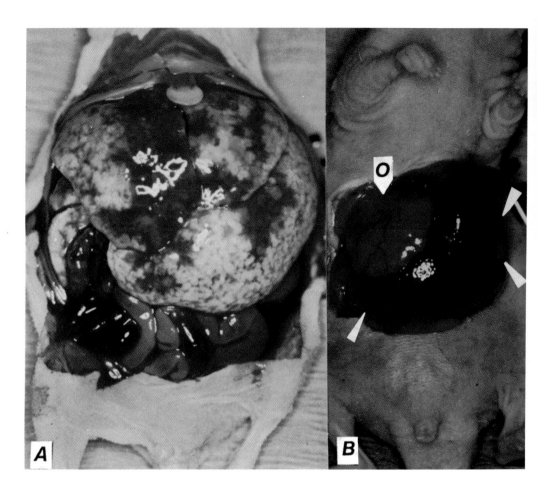

Figure 24.7. Human colon adenocarcinoma line McCN, 4 × 10⁶ cells injected into the spleen of immunodeficient NIH-1 mice on day 0. **A.** Day 28 autopsy of a mouse injected sc on day 7–14 with placebo; massive tumor infiltration of the liver confirmed by histology. **B.** Day 28 surgical inspection of a mouse injected sc on day 7–14 with 10,11-methylenedioxy-20(*RS*)-camptothecin, 6 mg/kg of body weight, total of 42 mg/kg; O, omentum; arrows, isolated tumor nodules.

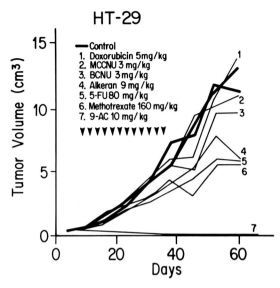

Figure 24.2. Treatment of human colon cancer xenografts carried by immunodeficient NIH-1 mice implanted with HT-29 human colon carcinoma. Each control of drug-treated group included 6 males; tumor fragments were implanted on day 0. For an implant, 50 mg of wet-weight finely minced tumor tissue in 0.5 ml EMEM (Gibco, Grand Island, NY) was injected under the skin over the right thigh. The treatments started on day 7, and continued twice a week for 3–6 weeks. The drugs were formulated in Tween 80:0.15 NaCl and injected subcutaneously, except doxorubicin, which was injected intravenously. MCCNU, methyl-1(2-chlorethyl)-3-cyclohexyl-1-nitrosourea; BCNU, 1,3-bis(2-chlorethyl)-1-nitrosourea, (median toxic doses for the schedule applied), and 9-AC, 9-amino-20(RS)-camptothecin. Controls were treated with the solvent only. The tumors were measured in three dimensions with a caliper, and tumor volume calculated. Means of tumor volumes in cm^3 were plotted against time; S.D. of the means was less than 15% of the value. All drug doses are per a single treatment, and arrows indicate individual injections. The care and treatment of experimental mice was in accordance with institutional guidelines.

with the exception of DXR, which was injected intravenously. The treatment started on day 7 and continued twice a week for 5–6 weeks. Drug doses were based on an established median toxic dose for the schedule applied. Among the 10 commonly used anticancer agents, only marginal growth–retardation of tumor implants was noticed in some cases (e.g., 5-FU, 80 mg/kg of body weight (b.w.)/dose or methotrexate, 160 mg/kg b.w./dose) (Figs. 24.2 and 24.3). This part of the experiment confirmed earlier results showing the ineffectiveness of tested drugs against 14 human colorectal xenograft lines (32). However, mice treated with camptothecin analogs showed marked inhibition of tumor growth. Five/6 mice with HT-29 tumors, injected subcutaneously twice a week with 9-amino-20(RS) 10 mg/kg b.w./dose, for a total of 6 weeks (Fig. 24.2), had no evidence of disease (NED) or minimal disease (tumor volume <0.1 cm^3). The appearance of a palpable nodule followed by continuous tumor regrowth signaled the end of a remission. As discussed later, no signs of drug toxicity were

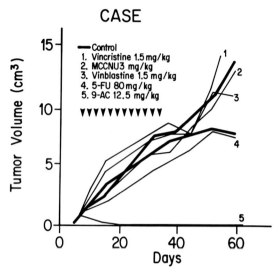

Figure 24.3. Treatment of human colon cancer xenografts carried by immunodeficient NIH-1 mice implanted with CASE human colon carcinoma. For details, see Figure 24.1.

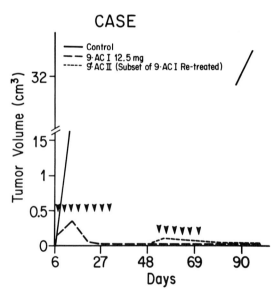

Figure 24.4. Treatment of human colon cancer xenografts carried by immunodeficient NIH-1 mice implanted with CASE human colon carcinoma. 9-AC I, first course of treatment with 9-amino-20(*RS*)-camptothecin; 9-AC II, second course of treatment. For the rest of details, see Figure 24.1.

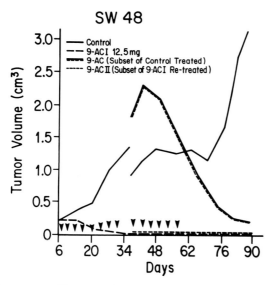

Figure 24.5. Treatment of human colon cancer xenografts carried by immunodeficient NIH-1 mice implanted with SW 48 human colon carcinoma. 9-AC I, first course of treatment with 9-amino-20(*RS*)-camptothecin; 9-AC II, second course of treatment. For the rest of details, see Figure 24.1.

detected. The first course of treatment was also well tolerated in mice with CASE or SW 48 human colon cancer. All mentioned tumor lines are extremely unresponsive to any kind of therapy (32). The first course of treatment of CASE (Figs. 24.3 and 24.4) or SW 48 tumors (Fig. 24.5) (12.5 mg/kg b.w., respectively) has resulted in NED or minimal disease in 6/6 mice of either group.

On day 51, mice with CASE tumors and minimal disease received a second course of therapy, consisting of a total of 6 injections, 12.5 mg/kg b.w./dose (Fig. 24.4). Following the first course of treatment, the second course (75 mg/ kg b.w. total dose) was also administered to mice with SW 48 tumors and minimal disease (Fig. 24.5). At the end of treatment, 5/6 mice had NED and the other had minimal disease.

A series of experiments comparing the efficacy of camptothecin, 9-amino-20(*RS*), and 10,11-methylenedioxy-20(*RS*) at the 10 mg/kg/dose level, is shown in Table 24.2. It appears that the two synthetic analogs are more potent anti-cancer drugs than their parent compound. Figure 24.6 (see color plate facing page 302) shows control mice with implanted CASE tumors, either untreated or treated with 10,11-methylenedioxy-20(*RS*).

Treatment of Advanced Tumors

The first course of treatments of the CASE and SW 48 lines always started with well-established tumors, averaging 0.2–0.25 cm³ in volume. In addition, day-35 SW 48 tumors (average size 2.5 cm³), were selected for the first treatment with 9-amino-20(*RS*). The disparity of tumor sizes between the control

Table 24.2. Treatment of Human Cancer Xenografts

Tumor (mouse strain)	Location	Treatment Schedule	Drug Efficacy[a]		
			CAM	9-AC	10,11-MDC
HT-29 colon cancer (NIH-1)	sc[b]	2x/week 10 mg/kg	PR[c]	CR[d]	CR
CASE colon cancer (NIH-1)	sc	2x/week 10 mg/kg		CR	CR
SW 48 colon cancer (NIH-1)	sc	2x/week 10 mg/kg		CR	

[a]CAM, camptothecin-20(S); 9-AC, 9-amino-20 (RS); 10,11-MDC, 10,11-methylenedioxy-20 (RS) camptothecins.
[b]sc, subcutaneous.
[c]PR, partial remission with toxic deaths.
[d]CR, complete remission.

and treated groups is intentional (Fig. 24.5). The largest tumors available were selected for treatment with 6 doses (12.5 mg/kg b.w./dose, delivered twice a week). There was a notable 91% reduction in the volume of the tumors in treated mice. In another experiment, 9-amino-20(RS) was also administered to mice with advanced HT-29 line tumors, average size of 8.0 cm³. A total dose of 60 mg/kg b.w. reduced the tumors by 46% (29).

Toxicity Data

The toxicity was evaluated in all experiments. The evaluation included the overall performance status, the body weight monitored twice a week, and animal survival. There was a considerable difference between the daily and the twice-a-week schedule. The daily "loading" was substantially the more toxic of the two. Consequently, the twice-a-week treatment schedule was used in most of the experiments.

Camptothecin, in escalating doses, caused animal deaths at most of the levels (Table 24.3). Only the lowest total dose, 28 mg/kg, did not cause deaths but reduced the tumor only partially. The first course of treatment with 10,11-methylenedioxy-20(RS) (100 mg/kg b.w. total dose) or with 9-amino-20(RS) (150 mg/kg b.w.) had no detectable toxic effects. It is noteworthy that the response of treated animals would have allowed either higher doses or a treatment course delivered over a longer time period. The treatments with 10-amino-20(RS) or 10,11-methylenedioxy-20(RS) Na salt led to toxic deaths or to substantial loss of body weight.

The second course of treatment with 50–75 mg/kg b.w. of 9-amino-20(RS) appeared to be more toxic than the first course. The body weight dropped by 19% on the average (CASE and SW 48 tumor lines) but recovered rapidly. The poorer performance of mice receiving the second course of treatment can be explained by a cumulative toxicity of the two treatments. There were, however, no signs of gastrointestinal toxicity or sterile hemorrhagic cystitis, which had been observed among patients treated with camptothecin Na salt (12,13).

Table 24.3. Toxicity—Twice a Week Treatment

Drug	Total Dose (mg/kg)	Overall Toxicity	Therapeutic Responses
20(*S*)-Camptothecin	70	Animal deaths	CR[a]
20(*S*)-Camptothecin	56	Animal deaths	PR[b]
20(*S*)-Camptothecin	50	Animal deaths	PR
20(*S*)-Camptothecin	42	Animal deaths	PR
20(*S*)-Camptothecin	28	Body weight loss >10%	PR
10,11-Methylenedioxy-20(*RS*)-camptothecin Na+	50	Body weight loss 20%	CR
10,11-Methylenedioxy-20(*RS*)-camptothecin Na+	62.5	Animal deaths	PR
10,11-Methylenedioxy-20(*RS*)-camptothecin	100	None	CR
10-Amino-20(*RS*)-camptothecin	100	Body weight loss <15%	PR
9-Amino-20(*RS*)-camptothecin	150	None	CR
9-Amino-20(*RS*)-camptothecin	175 (cumulative)	Body-weight loss ≤20%	CR

[a]CR, complete reduction of subcutaneous tumors.
[b]PR, partial reduction of subcutaneous tumors.

Long-Term Disease-Free Survival

Long-term survival was observed in mice implanted with SW 48 or CASE tumor lines and treated with 9-amino-20(*RS*) (Table 24.4). The treatments (one or two courses) are shown in Figures 24.4 and 24.5. At present, mice included in this experiment are approaching their natural life expectancy. Their overall performance status is unimpaired and there are no apparent signs of delayed or chronic toxicities.

Table 24.4. Long-Term Survival of Mice with Human Cancer Xenografts Treated with 9-Amino-20(*RS*)-Camptothecin

Line	Total Dose (mg/kg b.w.)	Number of Courses	Disease-Free Survival[a]	Performance Status[b]	Remission Duration[c]
SW 48	100	1	3/3 >11 m	1	
	175	2	3/3 >11 m	1	
CASE	100	1	2/3 >12 m	1	2 m[d]
	100	1	4/5 >6.5 m	1	2.5 m
	175	2	0/3	1	1,2,3.5 m

[a]Current number of mice alive with no evidence of disease/total number treated; duration of disease-free survival in months.
[b]Status during the disease-free survival without a detectable impairment.
[c]For relapsing tumors, the duration of disease-free survival in months.
[d]Expired without a tumor.

Table 24.5. Treatment of Liver Metastases

Drug	Treatment Schedule	Total Dose (mg/kg b.w.)	Body Weight	%ILS[a]
10,11-Methylenedioxy-20(RS)	Day 7–9[b]	30.0	Loss <20%	198
10,11-Methylenedioxy-20(RS) Na$^+$	Day 7–9	30.0	Loss <20%	200
5-Fluorouracil	Day 7–14	140.0	Loss >10%	106

[a]%ILS, increase in lifespan of treated mice over controls.
[b]Day 0, injection of McCN human colon cancer cells.

Treatment of Liver Metastases

The study used well-established methodology: a cell suspension of a human colon cancer xenograft line McCN was injected into the spleen, forcing the inoculum to retrograde through the vessels of the splenic peduncle. Resulting liver metastases of human colon cancer were treated subcutaneously with 10,11-methylenedioxy-20(RS) starting on day 7 following tumor cell injection. The treatment continued for 7 days at a daily dose of 6 mg/kg body weight. Control and drug–treated mice were inspected on day 28. Figure 24.7 (see color plate facing page 302) shows massive tumor infiltration of the liver in the controls, while the tumor involvement of the liver is substantially reduced in drug-treated animals.

In another experiment, shown in Table 24.5, mice with day-7 liver metastases were treated with three injections of 10,11-methylenedioxy or with its Na salt. The treatment improved the survival of experimental animals by ~100%. This should be compared with the treatment with 5-FU, 140 mg/kg b.w. total dose, which proved to be ineffective (33).

MULTIDRUG-RESISTANCE PHENOTYPE AND CAMPTOTHECINS

Resistance of human colon cancer lines to a variety of chemotherapeutic agents was demonstrated in xenograft experiments (29) and discussed earlier in this chapter. To determine whether the "classic" multidrug resistance phenotype, related to the MDR gene (35–37), is operational in our test lines, we have applied the standard immunoblotting technique. Monoclonal antibodies HYP.241 against P-glycoprotein react with membrane vesicles in resistant cells. Cells of the SW 48 line are positive, indicating the presence of the MDR gene product. The xenograft studies show that this line is resposive to the treatment with 9-amino-20(RS). It is also shown (Table 24.4) that the treatment of tumor-bearing mice resulted in long-term disease-free survival (37).

Table 24.6 compares drug effects on a wild KB-3-1 ovarian cancer-cell line and a mutant line KB-V1, resistant to colchicine (Col), DXR, and vinblastine (VBL). The MDR1 gene is expressed in the mutant line, while its mRNA is not detectable in the wild line. Relative resistance was determined by a clonogenic assay. It documents high resistance levels (Col, DXR, VBL) and no resistance to camptothecin and its analog 9-amino-20(RS). The results demonstrate that the two drugs clearly bypass the MDR1-related cell resistance (37).

Table 24.6. Drug Effects on Human Multidrug Resistant Cell Lines

Ovarian Cancer Lines	MDR1-mRNA Expression[a]	Relative Resistance[b]				
		Col	DXR	VBL	CAM	9-AC
KB-3-1	n.d.	1	1	1	1	1
KB-V1	320	170	420	859	1.2	2.6

[a]MDR1-mRNA expression, slot blots of total RNA were hybridized to the [^{32}P]labeled MDR1 probe. Levels of MDR1 expression were determined by densitometry of the 4.5-kb RNA in autoradiograms. The densitometric measurements were compared to the 4.5-kb peak of a reference KB-8 line, which has a mild resistance to colchicine. The band in this line has an arbitrarily assigned value of one; n.d., not detectable. The lines were developed in the laboratory of Dr. Ira Pastan, National Cancer Institute, NIH.
[b]Col, colchicine; DXR, doxorubicin; VBL, vinblastine; CAM, camptothecin-20(S); 9-AC, 9-amino-20(RS)-camptothecin.

DISCUSSION AND SUMMARY

Drug development is needed to improve chemotherapy of patients with locally advanced or metastatic colon cancer and unfavorable prognosis. Topo I, a nuclear enzyme important for solving topological problems arising during DNA replication and other cellular functions, has been identified as a principal target of a plant alkaloid, camptothecin, and its analogs prepared by total synthesis. Significantly increased levels of topo I were found, compared to normal tissues, in advanced stages of colon cancer and in several other human malignancies. Presumably, high topo I levels in colon cancer and low in normal colon mucosa contribute to therapeutic efficacy of camptothecins. There are also indications that the regulation of topo I levels may be qualitatively changed in tumor cells (38).

Two camptothecin analogs, 9-amino-20(RS) and 10,11-methylenedioxy-20(RS), were selected by tests with the purified topo I and tissue-culture screens. Unlike other anticancer drugs, or parent camptothecin, both analogs induced long-term disease-free remissions, which resulted from single-agent treatment of human colon cancer xenograft lines. Drug toxicity was low and allowed for repeated courses of therapy. The compounds effectively reduced the size of bulky tumors, and decreased the incidence of liver metastases. The experiments have also demonstrated that camptothecin and 9-amino-20(RS) bypass the MDR1-related cell resistance in colon cancer and overcome a less defined resistance to alkylating agents. Further studies of camptothecin analogs are necessary to evaluate their clinical usefulness. Recent improvements in the total synthesis procedure now permit the 20(RS) analogs to be prepared in the pure and more effective 20(S) form (M. E. Wall, unpublished data). The drugs can be a much needed addition to cancer chemotherapy and also a tool that allows detail studies of the molecular pathology of cancer.

REFERENCES

1. Sugarbaker, P. H., Gunderson, L. F., and Wittes, R. E. Colorectal cancer. In V. T. DeVita, S. Hellman, and S. A. Rosen-berg, eds. *Cancer.* Philadelphia: Lippincott, 1985, pp. 795–884.

2. Gastrointestinal Tumor Study Group.

Prolongation of the disease-free interval in surgically treated rectal carcinoma. N. Engl. J. Med. **312:** 1465–1472, 1985.

3. Astler, V. B. and Coller, F. A. The prognostic significance of direct extension of carcinoma of the colon and rectum. Ann. Surg. **139:** 846–852, 1954.

4. Moertel, C. G. Chemotherapy of gastrointestinal cancer. N. Engl. J. Med. **299:** 1049–1052, 1978.

5. Valone, F. H., Friedman, M. A., Wittlinger, P. S., Drakes, T., Eisenberg, P. D., Malec, M., Hannigan, J. F., and Brown, B. W., Jr. Treatment of patients with advanced colorectal carcinomas with fluorouracil alone, high-dose leucovorin plus fluorouracil, or sequential methotrexate, fluorouracil, and leucovorin: A randomized trial of the Northern California Oncology Group. J. Clin. Oncol. **7:** 1427–1436, 1989.

6. Poon, M. A., O'Connell, M. J., Moertel, C. G., Wieand, H. S., Cullinan, S. A., Everson, L. K., Krook, J. E., Mailliard, J. A., Laurie, J. A., Tschetter, L. K., and Wiesenfeld, M. Biochemical modulation of fluorouracil: Evidence of significant improvement of survival and quality of life in patients with advanced colorectal carcinoma. J. Clin. Oncol. **7:** 1407–1418, 1989.

7. The Nordic Gastrointestinal Tumor Adjuvant Therapy Group. Superiority of sequential methotrexate, fluorouracil, and leucovorin to fluorouracil alone in advanced symptomatic colorectal carcinoma: A randomized trial. J. Clin. Oncol. **7:** 1437–1446, 1989.

8. Laurie, J. A., Moertel, C. G., Fleming, T. R., Wieand, H. S., Leigh, J. E., Rubin, J., McCormack, G. W., Gerstner, J. B., Krook, J. E., Malliard, J., Twito, D. I., Morton, R. F., Tschetter, L. K., and Barlow, J. F., for the North Central Cancer Treatment Group and the Mayo Clinic. Surgical adjuvant therapy of large-bowel carcinoma: An evaluation of levamisole and the combination of levamisole and fluorouracil. J. Clin. Oncol. **7:** 1447–1456, 1989.

9. Chachoua, A., Green, M., and Muggia, F. Immune modulating therapy in gastrointestinal cancer. Am. J. Gastroenterol. **81:** 623, 1985

10. Arcamone, F. Clinically useful doxorubicin analogues. Cancer Treat. Rep. **14:** 159–161, 1987.

11. Wall, M. E., Wani, M. C., Cooke, C. E., Palmer, K. H., McPhail, A. T., and Slim, G. A. Plant antitumor agents. I. The isolation and structure of camptothecin, a novel alkaloidal and antitumor inhibitor from Camptotheca acuminate. J. Am. Chem. Soc. **88:** 3888–3890, 1966.

12. Gottlieb, J. A., Guarino, A. M., Call, J. B., Olivierio, V. T., and Block, J. B. Preliminary pharmacological and clinical evaluation of camptothecin sodium (NSC-100880). Cancer Chemother. Rep. **54:** 461–470, 1970.

13. Muggia, F. M., Creaven, P. J., Hansen, H. H., Cohen, M. N., and Selawry, D. S. Phase I clinical trials of weekly and daily treatment with camptothecin (NSC-100880): Correlation with clinical studies. Cancer Chemother. Rep. **56:** 515–521, 1972.

14. Hsiang, Y.-H., Liu, L. F., Wall, M. E., Wani, M. C., Kirschenbaum, S., Silber, R., and Potmesil, M. DNA topoisomerase I-mediated DNA cleavage and cytotoxicity of camptothecin analogs. Cancer Res. **49:** 4385–4389, 1989.

15. Jaxel, C., Kohn, K. W., Wani, M. C., Wall, M. E., and Pommier, Y. Structure-activity study of the actions of camptothecin derivatives on mammalian topoisomerase I. Evidence for a specific receptor site and for a relation to antitumor activity. Cancer Res. **49:** 1465–1469, 1989.

16. Hsiang, Y.-H., Hertzberg, R., Hecht, S., and Liu, L. F. Camptothecin induced protein-linked DNA breaks via mammalian DNA topoisomerase I. J. Biol. Chem. **260:** 14873–14878, 1985.

17. Hsiang, Y.-H. and Liu, L. F. Identification of mammalian topoisomerase I as an intracellular target of the anticancer drug camptothecin. Cancer Res. **48:** 1722–1726, 1988.

18. Hsiang, Y.-H., Lihou, M. G., and Liu, L. F. Arrest of replication forks by drug-stabilized topoisomerase I-DNA cleavable complexes as a mechanism of cell killing by camptothecin. Cancer Res. **49:** 5077–5082, 1989.

19. Wall, M. E., Wani, M. C., Natschke, S. M., and Nicholas, A. V. Plant antitumor agents. 22. Isolation of 11-hydroxycamptothecin from Camptotheca acuminata Decne: Total synthesis and biological activity. J. Med. Chem. **29:** 1553–1555, 1986.

20. Wani, M. C. and Wall, M. E. The structure of two new alkaloids from Camptotheca acuminata. J. Org. Chem. **34:** 1364, 1969.

21. Wall, M. E. and Wani, M. C. Camptothecin. In J. M. Cassady and J. D. Douros, eds. *Design and Synthesis of Potential Anticancer Agents Based on Natural Product Models.* New York: Academic Press, 1979, pp. 417–436.

22. Wani, M. C., Ronman, P. E., Lindley, J. T., and Wall, M. E. Plant antitumor agents. 18. Synthesis and biological activity of camptothecin analogues. J. Med. Chem. 23: 554, 1980.

23. Wani, M. C., Nicholas, A. W., and Wall, M. E. Plant antitumor agents. 23. Synthesis and antileukemic activity of camptothecin analogues. J. Med. Chem. 29: 2358, 1986.

24. Wani, M. C., Nicholas, A. W., Manikumar, G., and Wall, M. E. Plant antitumor agents. 25. Total synthesis and antileukemic activity of ring A-substituted camptothecin analogs, structure-activity correlation. J. Med. Chem. 30: 1774, 1987.

25. Wani, M. C., Nicholas, A. W., and Wall, M. E. Total synthesis and antitumor activity of 20(S) and 20(R) camptothecins. J. Med. Chem. 30: 2317, 1987.

26. Potmesil, M., Hsiang, Y.-H., Liu, L. F., Wu, H.-Y., Traganos, F., Bank, B., and Silber, R. DNA topoisomerase II as a potential factor in drug resistance of human malignancies. In M. Potmesil and W. E. Ross, eds. *Proceedings, The First Conference on DNA Topoisomerases in Cancer Chemotherapy. NCI Monogr.* 4: 105–109, 1987.

27. Potmesil, M., Hsiang, Y.-H., Liu, L. F., Bank, B., Grossberg, H., Kirschenbaum, S., Penzinger, A., Kanganis, D., Knowles, D., Traganos, F., and Silber, R. Resistance of human leukemic and normal lymphocytes to drug-induced DNA cleavage and low levels of DNA topoisomerase II. Cancer Res. 48: 3537–3543, 1988.

28. Hsiang, Y.-H., Liu, L. F., Hochster, H., and Potmesil, M. Levels of topoisomerase I and II in human colorectal carcinoma and normal mucosa. Proc. Ann. Meet. AACR 29: 172, 1988 (Abstract).

29. Giovanella, B. C., Wall, M. E., Wani, M. C., Nicholas, A. W., Liu, L. F., Silber, R., and Potmesil, M. Highly effective topoisomerase-I targeted chemotherapy of human colon cancer in xenografts. Science. 246: 1046–1048, 1989.

30. Leibovitz, A., Stinson, J. C., McCombs, W. B., McCoy, C. E., Mazur, K. C., Mabry, N. D. Classification of human colorectal adenocarcinoma cell lines. Cancer Res. 36: 4562–4569, 1976.

31. Fogh, J. and Trampe, G. In J. Fogh, ed. *New Human Tumor Cells In Vitro*, New York: Plenum Press, 1975, pp. 115–159.

32. Giovanella, B. C., Stehlin, J. S., Jr., Shepard, R. C., and Williams, L. J., Jr. Correlation between response to chemotherapy of human tumors in patients and in nude mice. Cancer. 52: 1146–1152, 1983.

33. Giovanella, B. C., Stehlin, J. S., Vardeman, D., Wall, M. E., Wani, M. C., Silber, R., and Potmesil, M. DNA topoisomerase-I targeted chemotherapy of human colon cancer metastases in xenografts. Proc. Am. Assoc. Cancer Res. 31: 448, 1990 (Abstract).

34. Shen, D.-W., Fojo, A., Chin, J. E., Roninson, I. B., Richert, N., Pastan, I., and Gottesman, M. M. Human multidrug-resistant cell lines: Increased mdrl expression can precede gene amplification. Science. 232: 643–645, 1986.

35. Moscow, J. A. and Cowan, K. H. Multidrug resistance. J. Natl. Cancer Inst. 80: 14–20, 1988.

36. Fline, R. L. Multidrug resistance. In H. M. Pinedo, D. L. Longo, and B. A. Chabner, eds. *Cancer Chemotherapy and Biological Response Modifiers Annual 10*. New York: Elsevier Amsterdam, 1988, pp. 73–84.

37. Potmesil, M., Wall, M. E., Wani, M. C., Silber, R., Cordon-Cardo, C., Stehlin, J. S., Kozielski, A., and Biovanella, B. C. DNA topoisomerase-I targeted chemotherapy of human colon cancer xenografts with mdr phenotype. Proc. Am. Assoc. Cancer Res. 31: 438, 1990 (Abstract).

38. Liu, L. F. DNA poisons as antitumor drugs. Annu. Rev. Biochem. 58: 351–375, 1989.

Chapter 25

Implications of Topoisomerase Mechanisms in the Therapy of Hematologic Neoplasms

FRANCO M. MUGGIA

AND PARKASH S. GILL

Topoisomerase I and II are key enzymes involved in the untwisting and duplication of DNA before the cell can undergo division (1–3). They are found in varying amounts in normal and tumor tissues, but there is incomplete information on how they are regulated individually or in concert. The levels of topoisomerase II vary significantly during various stages of cell cycle and are lowest during G_1-G_0 phases (4). Activities therefore are more readily identified in highly proliferative tumors than in low-grade neoplasms (5), and may bear a relationship to drug selectivity.

The majority of known DNA–topoisomerase II–inhibiting drugs are, in fact, most active against tumors with high growth fraction (Table 25.1), such as large cell lymphoma, ANLL, and CML blast crisis (6,7,8). These drugs have traditionally played a lesser role in neoplasms with low growth fraction. We review the regimens that have been studied and discuss subsequently how topoisomerase II action may be involved in drug activity or resistance. Finally, we shall indicate how these concepts can influence future strategies.

TREATMENT PROGRAMS

The hematologic neoplasms that have high growth fraction are treated mostly with the regimens containing combinations of one of more topoisomerase II inhibitors, with or without additional cytotoxic agents (Tables 25.2 and 25.3). These neoplasia include acute leukemias of both lymphoid and nonlymphoid type, high-grade non-Hodgkin's lymphomas, and Hodgkin's disease (6–10). Low-grade non-Hodgkin's lymphoma, multiple myeloma, and chronic leukemias may also be treated with topoisomerase inhibitors; however, the efficacy is limited and long-term disease-free survival is rare. Refractory myeloma has a higher growth fraction, however, and Barlogie therefore suggested refractory myeloma may begin to respond to S-phase specific agents (11). Such a concept

Table 25.1. Topoisomerase II Inhibitors in Hematologic Neoplasms

	Drug Classes
Anthracyclines	dauno-, doxo-, ida-, pirarubicin, aclacinomycin (aclarubicin), menogaril, AD-32
Synthetic intercalators	mitoxantrone, bisantrene, amsacrine (*m*-AMSA), anthrapyrazoles (oxantrazole)
Ellipticines	9-hydroxy ellipticinium
Podophyllotoxins	etoposide, teniposide

Table 25.2. Topoisomerase II Inhibitors in Acute Non-lymphoblastic (ANLL) and Lymphoblastic Leukemia (ALL)

Drug Regimen	Indication & Comments
araC + daunorubicin	ANLL first line (7 + 3)
araC + mitoxantrone	ANLL first line
araC + idarubicin	ANLL first line (ongoing)
hi araC + mitoxantrone	ANLL salvage
mitoxantrone + etoposide (VP-16)	ANLL salvage
aclacinomycin + etoposide (VP-16)	ANLL salvage
V Pred + L-asp + daunorubicin	ALL first line (high risk)
araC + teniposide (VM-26)	ALL salvage

Table 25.3. Topoisomerase II Inhibitors in Lymphoma (NHL) and Hodgkin's Disease (HD)

Drug Regimen	Indication & Comments
ABV dacarbazine	HD, first line and salvage
HOPE-bleo	HD, first line
OPEC	HD, salvage
EVA, EDAP	HD and NHL salvage
Mitoxantrone araC	NHL salvage
E ifos mitoxantrone	NHL salvage
CHOP, ProMACE, CHOPE, MACOP-B, M-BACOD	NHL high and intermediate grades, first line

V = vinblastine; araC = cytarabine; O = oncovin, vincristine; E = etoposide (VP-16); B,bleo = bleomycin; H,A = Adriamycin, doxorubicin hydroxyldaunorubicin; ifos = ifosfamide; C = cyclophosphamide; D = dexamethasone.

may be extended to expect sensitivity to topoisomerase II–acting drugs. More recently the VAD regimen given together with verapamil to reverse multidrug resistance has been shown to have considerable activity as a salvage regimen (12).

ISSUES WITH SPECIFIC DRUGS

Anthracyclines

Anthracycline analogs are very active in rapidly growing neoplasms, such as high-grade lymphoma and acute leukemias (6,8). Response rates are high when anthracyclines are used in combination with other topoisomerase inhibitors, such as epipodophyllotoxins (7). This could be related to preferential binding of these drugs to different sites of DNA–topoisomerase complexes, and more complete disruption of cellular function leading to cell death. The combination of topoisomerase inhibitors with other classes of active drugs in the treatment of acute leukemia, such as cell-cycle-specific antimetabolites, including cytosine arabinoside, have also been used clinically with significant activity (13,14). It is of interest to study if these classes of agents have synergy when used in combination, and if tumor response can be improved by variation of the schedule of these drugs. Work relevant to these issues include use of low-dose methotrexate followed by exposure to VP-16 in U937 cell lines (15). Methotrexate given for 16 h at low concentrations (0.02 μM) caused accumulation at the G1-S boundary. When methotrexate was removed, a wave of synchronization followed. The cytotoxic activity of VP-16 was potentiated for the first 4 h following withdrawal of methotrexate. This increased susceptibility coincided with an elevation of topoisomerase II levels. Thus, antimetabolites combined with topoisomerase inhibitors could result in further improvements in antitumor activity.

Interaction of alkylating agents and topoisomerase inhibitors may also be clinically significant. This may be illustrated by findings in Raji cell lines resistant to nitrogen mustard. Such cells are more sensitive to the cytotoxic activity of alkylating agents with the topoisomerase inhibitor and antimicrobial novobiocin. Thus, one may postulate that the topoisomerase inhibitor may prevent DNA repair associated with the recovery of tumor cells exposed to alkylating agents (15). Supportive data are available for platinum–DNA damage as well and have led to clinical trials of these drugs with novobocin. In other trials, the success of cis-platinum therapy followed by VP-16 and Ara-C, in relapsed or refractory non-Hodgkin's lymphomas (16), may represent other examples inadvertently or consciously exploiting such phenomena. Monitoring the topoisomerase levels in the tumor, during primary therapy and at the time of relapse, would be of interest.

It is interesting to note that anthracyclines also have activity in low-grade tumors (17) that have low topoisomerase activity. These clinical findings are consistent with *in vitro* studies, revealing perhaps that anthracyclines can act by alternate pathways to cause direct DNA binding and breaks. However, these agents are most active in rapidly dividing tumor types and parallel the activity of agents that predominantly act through topoisomerase inhibition (18). Future correlations are needed to determine whether anthracyclines predominantly mediate cytotoxicity through their interaction with topoisomerase II.

Separation of antitumor activity from cardiotoxicity may possibly relate to topoisomerase II actions in one but not the other; this remains to be established. However, such an aim is a noteworthy aspect for development of anthracyclines and related drugs. Thus, it is possible that one may specifically protect against cardiotoxicity, or that derivatives may be developed with no significant cardiac muscle effects while retaining cytotoxicity to tumor cells. Of numerous anthracyclines and related compounds that have been synthesized, some (such as nogalomycin derivatives, iminodaunorubicins, AD series, and anthrapyrazoles, for example) retain antitumor effects with minimal cardiotoxicity (19). In addition, mitoxantrone is also a very potent topoisomerase II inhibitor with significant activity in leukemia and lymphoma along with reduction in cardiac toxicity. The differences in the severity and frequency of cardiac toxicity among different anthracycline derivatives may be unrelated to their topoisomerase binding. The sparing of alopecia with mitoxantrone is another example of unexplained differences among topoisomerase II–acting drugs (20).

Podophyllotoxins

Various agents from the podophyllotoxin group of drugs have shown cytotoxic activity against neoplasia including hematologic malignancies. The agents studied most extensively are VP-16 and VM-26 (7,14). These agents do not directly intercalate with DNA, but mediate their activity through binding with topoisomerase II–DNA complex (21). In addition, these agents prevent annealing of DNA fragments following double-stranded DNA cleavage by topoisomerase II. Thus, the activity of these agents appears to depend on the amount of intracellular topoisomerase II at the time of drug delivery. As had previously been indicated for anthracyclines, topoisomerase II levels are elevated in cycling cells. Thus one can infer that podophyllotoxins have greater cytotoxic activity in cycling cells and, consequently, in tumors with high proliferative index. In fact, hematologic neoplasms including acute leukemias (myelogenous and lymphatic) and malignant lymphomas of high and intermediate grade respond well to VP-16 and VM-26. The response rates are higher with regimens that include other topoisomerase inhibitors such as daunorubicin and antimetabolites, such as methotrexate and cytosine arabinoside. A combination regimen (Pro-MACE), which includes prednisone, etoposide, cytarabine, bleomycin, vincristine, and methotrexate, produces response rates in nearly 80% of the patients with diffuse aggressive non-Hodgkin's lymphomas (7). It has previously been discussed that use of low-dose methotrexate at noncytotoxic levels synchronizes the cells and, when withdrawn, leads to enhanced VP-16 cytotoxicity for the first several hours. In addition, combination of VP-16 and cisplatin have synergistic activity, which may be explained through enhanced inhibition of DNA repair of cisplatin–DNA lesions of conversely through an increase in topoisomerase I–induced cleavage by cisplatin (22). Currently such regimens, utilizing VP-16 with the antimetabolite (cytosine-arabinoside) (cytarabine) and cisplatin, are in clinical trials in relapsed or refractory Hodgkin's and non-Hodgkin's lymphoma (16). Furthermore, a combination of VP-16 and cytarabine, and VP-16 and daunorubicin have shown 40–50% response rates in acute myelogenous leukemia. More recently VP-16 has been incorporated in various preparatory regimens for bone marrow transplantation, for the treatment of leukemias, lymphomas, and Hodgkin's disease. VP-16 has been combined with either total nodal irradiation, or cytoxan and cisplatin, or carmustine, cytarabine, and melphalan (BEAM regimen). The response rates following such regimens and bone marrow transplantation are over 50% (23,24). Finally, drug scheduling remains to be explained in terms of topoisomerase action, and must be further studied. The availability of oral VP-16 has stimulated trials of continuous exposure to this drug.

IMPLICATIONS IN DRUG RESISTANCE MECHANISMS

Topoisomerase-Mediated Resistance

It is apparent that the cytotoxic activity of topoisomerase inhibitors correlates with topoisomerase levels, and that there is cross-sensitivity among various topoisomerase inhibitors. Furthermore, low topoisomerase II levels are associated with low response rates, and short disease-free survival when topoisomerase inhibitors are used. Thus one mechanism of drug resistance may be related to topoisomerase levels. Additionally, drug resistance may be generated through the alterations in binding of DNA–topoisomerase and drug complex, and mutations in the topoisomerase enzymes (25,26,27). These data are beginning to appear, and they will be useful in future human clinical trials to guide in the design of treatment regimens that maximize chances for synergy and to avoid regimens with low predicted antitumor activity.

Multidrug Resistance (MDR)

Patients relapsing after initial therapy are rarely cured with second line therapy. This is in part related to the emergence of drug resistance to multiple classes of drugs. One mechanism of drug resistance is related to enhanced expression or amplification of MDR1 gene, which is associated with phenotypic changes in the cells and expression of p170 on the cell membrane (27,28). It is important to consider whether there is any correlation between MDR and resistance to topoisomerase inhibitors. In some instances, resistance to DNA cleavage in naked nuclei suggests this is mediated solely by topoisomerases. *In vivo,* however, multiple mechanisms may be operative. One such study reveals that when a cell line (K562) is made to become resistant to anthracyclines, a lower degree of resistance is limited to topoisomerase inhibitors only. However, when the sublines are made to become highly resistant, the lines express MDR while also maintaining resistance to topoisomerase inhibitors (29).

Clinical Implications

In vitro studies of drug resistance mechanisms have served to point the way for questions to be posed in clinical settings. These problems include devising optimal sequencing and combinations, seeking optimal drug scheduling, identifying cross-resistance patterns, and correlating drug failure with tumor biology and/or prior therapeutic exposure. Some of these aspects were reviewed in the prior topoisomerase symposium (30). Studies with clinical specimens and various topoisomerase findings are proceeding in coordination with some laboratories, but the methodology does not yet allow simple characterization of enzyme content, activity, and type from clinical material. The progress made in the last few years devising simplified new techniques provides hope that much will soon be learned about resistance mechanisms in relation to topoisomerase in hematologic malignancies.

REFERENCES

1. Gellert, M. DNA topoisomerases. Annu. Rev. Biochem. **50:** 879, 1981.
2. Liu, L. F. DNA topoisomerases: Enzymes that catalyze the breaking and rejoining of DNA. Crit. Rev. Biochem. **15:** 1, 1983.
3. Vosberg, H. P. DNA topoisomerases: Enzymes that control DNA conformation. Curr. Top. Microbiol. Immunol. **114:** 19, 1985.
4. Markovits, J., Pommier, Y., Kerrigan, D., et al. Topoisomerase II. Mediated DNA breaks and cytotoxicity in relation to cell cycle. Cancer Res. **47:** 2050, 1987.
5. Potmesil, M., Hsiang, Y. H., Bank, B., et al. Resistance of human leukemic and normal lymphocytes to drug induced DNA cleavage and low levels of DNA topoisomerase II. Cancer Res. **48:** 3537, 1988.
6. Shipp, M. A., Harrington, D. P., Klatt, M. M., et al. Identification of major prognostic subgroups of patients with large cell lymphoma treated with m-BACOD or M-BACOD. Ann. Intern. Med. **104:** 751, 1986.
7. Fisher, R. I., DeVita, V. T., Jr., Hubbard, S. M., Longo, D. L., et al. Diffuse aggressive lymphoma. Increased survival after alternating flexible sequences of proMACE and MOPP chemotherapy. Ann. Intern. Med. **98:** 304, 1983.
8. Rees, J. K. H., Sandler, R. M., Challener, J., Hayhoe, F. G. J. Treatment of acute myeloid leukemia with a triple cytotoxic regimen: DAT. Br. J. Cancer. **36:** 770, 1977.
9. Bonadonna, G. and Santoro, A. ABVD chemotherapy in the treatment of Hodgkin's disease. Cancer Treat. Rep. **9:** 21, 1982.
10. Bonadonna, G., Valagussa, P., and Santoro, A. Alternating non-cross-resistant combination chemotherapy or MOPP in Stage IV Hodgkin's disease. Ann. Intern. Med. **104:** 739, 1986.
11. Barlogie, B., Smith, L., and Alexanian, R. Effective treatment of advanced multiple myeloma refractory to alkylating agents. N. Engl. J. Med. **310:** 1353, 1984.
12. Dalton, W. S., Grogan, T. M., Meltzer, P. S., et al. Drug resistance in multiple myeloma and non-Hodgkin's lymphoma: Detection of p-glycoprotein and potential circumvention by addition of verapamil to chemotherapy. J. Clin. Oncol. **7:** 415, 1989.
13. Preisler, H. D., Epstein, J., Barcos, M., et al. Prediction of response of non-lymphocytic leukemia to therapy with high dose cytosine arabinoside. Br. J. Hematol. **58:** 19, 1984.
14. Tschopp, L., VonFliedner, V. E., Sauter, C., et al. Efficacy and clinical cross-resistance of a new combination therapy (AMSA/VP16) in previously treated patients with acute nonlymphocytic leukemia. J. Clin. Oncol. **4:** 318, 1986.
15. Lorico, A., Boicchi, M., Rappa, G., et al. Synchronization of human U937 lymphoma cells by low doses of methotrexate increases topoisomerase II-mediated DNA breakage and cytotoxic activity of VP16. The Second Conference on DNA Topo-

isomerases in Cancer Chemotherapy, Program and Abstracts, New York, 1988.

16. O'Donnell, M. R., Foreman, S. J., Levine, A. M., et al. Cytarabine, cisplatinum and etoposide chemotherapy for refractory non-Hodgkin's lymphoma. Cancer Treat. Rep. **71:** 187, 1987.

17. Ezdinli, E. Z., Anderson, J. R., Melvin, F., et al. Moderate versus aggressive chemotherapy of nodular lymphocytic poorly differentiated lymphoma. J. Clin. Oncol. **3:** 769, 1985.

18. Gewirtz, D., Ellis, A., Woods, K., Munger, C. Factors conferring intrinsic resistance to the anthracycline antibiotics in rat hepatoma. The Second Conference on DNA Topoisomerases in Cancer Chemotherapy, Program and Abstracts, New York, 1988.

19. Muggia, F. M., Green, M. D., Blum, R. Anthracyclines and anthracenediones: A perspective from recent clinical trials. In J. W. Lown, ed. *Anthracycline and Anthracenedione-Based Anticancer Agents.* Elsevier, 1988, pp. 667–714.

20. Prentice, H. G., Robbins, G., Ma, D.D.F., et al. Mitoxantrone in relapsed and refractory acute leukemia. Semin. Oncol. **11:** (Suppl I): 32, 1984.

21. Long, B. H., Musial, S. T., Brattain, M. G. Single and double strand DNA breakage and repair in human lung adenocarcinoma cells exposed to etoposide and teniposide. Cancer Res. **45:** 3506, 1985.

22. Durand, R. E., and Goldie, J. H. Interaction of etoposide and cisplatinum in an in vitro tumor model. Cancer Treat. Rep. **71:** 673, 1987.

23. Carella, A. M., Congio, A. M., Goazza, E., et al. High-dose chemotherapy with autologous bone marrow transplantation in 50 advanced resistant Hodgkin's disease patients: An Italian study group report. J. Clin. Oncol. **6:** 1411, 1988.

24. Philip, T., Boiron, P., Philip, I., et al. Massive therapy and autologous bone marrow transplantation in pediatric and young adults Burkitt's lymphoma (30 courses of 28 patients: a 5-year experience). Eur. J. Cancer Clin. Oncol. **22:** 1015, 1986.

25. deJong, S., Ziglstra, J. G., DeVries, E.G.E., and Mulder, N. H. Reduced DNA topoisomerase II activity and drug induced DNA cleavage activity in extracts from an Adriamycin resistant human small cell lung carcinoma cell line. The Second Conference on DNA Topoisomerases in Cancer Chemotherapy, Program and Abstracts, New York, 1988.

26. Woynarowski, J. M., Sigmund, R. D., and Beerman, T. J. Modulation of topoisomerase II and enzyme-mediated effects of topoisomerase II targeted drugs by agents binding to the minor groove in DNA. The Second Conference on DNA Topoisomerases in Cancer Chemotherapy, Program and Abstracts, New York, 1988.

27. Drake, F. H., Hofmann, G. A., Bartus, H. F., et al. Comparison of the 170 kDa and 180 kDa forms of topoisomerase II. Proceedings from Second Conference on DNA Topoisomerases in Cancer Chemotherapy, Program and Abstracts, New York, 1988.

28. Shen, D-W., Fojo, A., Chin, J. E., et al. Human multidrug resistant cell lines. Increased mdrl expression can precede gene amplification. Science. **232:** 643, 1985.

29. Vasanthakumar, G., Ahmed, N. K. Topoisomerase I and II activity in k562 resistant sublines. The Second Conference on DNA Topoisomerases in Cancer Chemotherapy, Program and Abstracts, New York, 1988.

30. Muggia, F. M., McVie, G. Treatment strategies in relation to drug action. NCI Monogr. **4:** 129, 1987.

INDEX